The International Library of Bioethics

Founding Editors

David N. Weisstub
Thomasine Kimbrough Kushner

Volume 93

Series Editor

Dennis R. Cooley, North Dakota State University, History, Philosophy, & Religious Studies, Fargo, ND, USA

Advisory Editor

David N. Weisstub, Faculty of Medicine, University of Montreal, Montréal, QC, Canada

Editorial Board

Terry Carney, Faculty of Law Building, University of Sydney, Sydney, Australia

Marcus Düwell, Philosophy Faculty of Humanities, Universiteit Utrecht, Utrecht, Utrecht, The Netherlands

Søren Holm, Centre for Social Ethics and Policy, The University of Manchester, Manchester, UK

Gerrit Kimsma, Radboud UMC, Nijmegen, Gelderland, The Netherlands

Daniel P. Sulmasy, Edmund D. Pellegrino Center for Clinical, Washington, DC, USA

David Augustin Hodge, National Center for Bioethics, Tuskegee University, Tuskegee Institute, AL, USA

Nora L. Jones, Center for Urban Bioethics, Temple University, Philadelphia, USA

The *International Library of Bioethics* – formerly known as the International Library of Ethics, Law and the New Medicine comprises volumes with an international and interdisciplinary focus on foundational and applied issues in bioethics. With this renewal of a successful series we aim to meet the challenge of our time: how to direct biotechnology to human and other living things' ends, how to deal with changed values in the areas of religion, society, and culture, and how to formulate a new way of thinking, a new bioethics.

The *International Library of Bioethics* focuses on the role of bioethics against the background of increasing globalization and interdependency of the world's cultures and governments, with mutual influencing occurring throughout the world in all fields. The series will continue to focus on perennial issues of aging, mental health, preventive medicine, medical research issues, end of life, biolaw, and other areas of bioethics, whilst expanding into other current and future topics.

We welcome book proposals representing the broad interest of this series' interdisciplinary and international focus. We especially encourage proposals addressing aspects of changes in biological and medical research and clinical health care, health policy, medical and biotechnology, and other applied ethical areas involving living things, with an emphasis on those interventions and alterations that force us to re-examine foundational issues.

More information about this series at https://link.springer.com/bookseries/16538

Pamela Grace · Aimee Milliken
Editors

Clinical Ethics Handbook for Nurses

Emphasizing Context, Communication and Collaboration

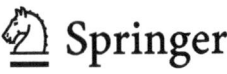

Editors
Pamela Grace
William F. Connell School of Nursing
Boston College
Chestnut Hill, MA, USA

Aimee Milliken
William F. Connell School of Nursing
Boston College
Chestnut Hill, MA, USA

ISSN 2662-9186   ISSN 2662-9194 (electronic)
The International Library of Bioethics
ISBN 978-94-024-2153-8   ISBN 978-94-024-2155-2 (eBook)
https://doi.org/10.1007/978-94-024-2155-2

© Springer Nature B.V. 2022
This work is subject to copyright. All rights are solely and exclusively licensed by the Publisher, whether the whole or part of the material is concerned, specifically the rights of translation, reprinting, reuse of illustrations, recitation, broadcasting, reproduction on microfilms or in any other physical way, and transmission or information storage and retrieval, electronic adaptation, computer software, or by similar or dissimilar methodology now known or hereafter developed.
The use of general descriptive names, registered names, trademarks, service marks, etc. in this publication does not imply, even in the absence of a specific statement, that such names are exempt from the relevant protective laws and regulations and therefore free for general use.
The publisher, the authors and the editors are safe to assume that the advice and information in this book are believed to be true and accurate at the date of publication. Neither the publisher nor the authors or the editors give a warranty, expressed or implied, with respect to the material contained herein or for any errors or omissions that may have been made. The publisher remains neutral with regard to jurisdictional claims in published maps and institutional affiliations.

This Springer imprint is published by the registered company Springer Nature B.V.
The registered company address is: Van Godewijckstraat 30, 3311 GX Dordrecht, The Netherlands

Preface

A few years ago, one of us, Pam, was contacted by Springer Science and Technology to consider developing a book that would help point-of-care nurses to develop their confidence in ethical decision making in practice. This resource was to be broadly applicable to nursing practice across countries. An additional aim was to assist nurse educators and leaders in their roles related to developing nurses who could and would exercise moral agency on behalf of good patient care. The dearth of this sort of critically needed practical resource for nurses, that could also be useful for other healthcare clinicians, is notable. Emerging literature has exposed and continues to highlight the problem for nurses and other clinicians of the experience of moral distress and its effects upon them personally and professionally which have only been exacerbated by the current global pandemic. The impact of moral distress on clinicians, also and ultimately, plays out in patient care. Moral distress is the disequilibrating feeling experienced in trying to do the right thing for patients under conditions of ambiguity or when obstructions occur. While we both practice and teach in the USA, we are aware from the literature and discussions with non-US-based colleagues that most if not all of the problems faced by nurses in their daily practice in the USA are shared by clinicians internationally. Thus, the content and strategies provided in this book are aimed specifically at preparing nurses regardless of country, region, or practice specialty to identify, analyze, and act to resolve ethical issues in practice.

Our combined experiences as practicing nurses, educators, and clinical ethicists provided both the impetus for the book and the wherewithal to develop it as a resource for others both in the USA and internationally. Grace has been involved in developing nurse moral agency for the past 20 years, both as a clinician and an educator. Most saliently, for several years she was involved, with colleagues in the Boston area, in presenting annual daylong clinical ethics education programs which were enthusiastically received each year. The end-of-program evaluations highlighted the desire for many more such opportunities where participants could develop skills in ethical decision making and clinical ethics. She also served as an ethics resource for a local hospice, the clinical research unit of a major academic medical center, and as faculty for other clinical education programs both funded and unfunded (Grace,

Robinson, Jurchak, Zollfrank, A., & Lee, S., 2014) and authored several editions of an advanced practice ethics book (Grace, 2009, 2014, 2018), that is used internationally. She has also been involved in clinical ethics education initiatives internationally. As an academic, she has been responsible, over the past 20+ years, for developing the ethical decision-making skills of both pre-licensure and graduate (postgraduate) students. What is most evident from all of these experiences is that developing and maintaining nurse ethical decision-making skills and moral agency should be seen as an ongoing endeavor that is nurtured beyond formal nursing studies and continues into the clinical setting.

Milliken is an experienced critical care nurse, an educator, and serves as the director of clinical ethics in a major academic medical center. She has been responsible for developing multi-disciplinary as well as nursing specific ethics rounds on multiple inpatient units. In this role, she is witness to the many problems encountered by nurses as they strive to provide good patient care and advocate for patient needs to be met. Her most recent project had been to analyze the reasons that ethics consults have been sought over a 15-year period which provided additional insights into the complexity of problems present in contemporary healthcare settings. She is concerned to develop nurse ethical awareness of their responsibilities in everyday practice as well as in situations where there is conflict.

Both of us from our various and extensive nursing and teaching experiences as well as our ethics work have been concerned with two main issues related to nurses' ability to practice in accord with professional goals and perspectives. The first, and perhaps most serious, is that nurses are not always aware of the inherently ethical nature of all healthcare practice. Thus, they do not always intentionally practice with the 'good' of the patient or patients as their foremost priority. Instead, they may be influenced by the non-patient care concerns of the institution or of powerful others. For such reasons, they may not always recognize when patients are receiving suboptimal care, and they may not recognize their responsibilities to act to address such situations. This problem of not understanding their primary obligation to provide for the patient's good is multifactorial in origin, but in large part has to do with the lack of attention given to developing the ethical awareness of nursing students during nursing education. The second is that nurses who are aware of the ethical nature of their work, nevertheless, may not be adequately prepared, or may not perceive themselves to have an obligation or capacity to articulate the essential aspects of a patient care problem. Additionally, they may not know how to discover and access appropriate supports and resources to help them resolve problems.

Thus, we developed this work as a practical handbook the content of which we believe is accessible to, and comprehendible by, practicing nurses and allied health professionals working at the bedside. Additionally, we provide strategies for educators and leaders to use in supporting the development of nurse moral agency. While it is first and foremost a 'nursing ethics' handbook, it will be a helpful accessory for all healthcare personnel who face ethical issues in the course of their work and who work with nurses to resolve these issues. It provides the tools for developing confidence and skill in ethical decision making in interdisciplinary settings such as acute and chronic care hospitals and ambulatory clinics. Both authors are experienced nurses and nurse educators with strong ethics education backgrounds. We believe from our experiences and prior research that nurses have the knowledge and capacity to recognize developing ethical issues in their practice settings and act to address them and can benefit from the opportunity to practice and develop these skills. Nurses are often the first line of defense related to patient safety and quality care. Thus, their ability to appropriately and accurately transmit patient values, preferences, and desires to the healthcare team as well as evaluate how a proposed course of action is liable to reflect these elements is often critical in ensuring that the 'real' needs of patients are understood and met. Some of the obstacles to optimal patient care are institutional, some due to hospital hierarchies and dynamics, and others the result of inadequate communication. As such, a variety of strategies aimed at addressing these challenges are required and are provided in the book.

The book is separated into three parts. The first part provides foundational information related to nursing ethics, the ethics of other healthcare professions, clinical ethics including the development of bioethics and explores areas of differentiation as well as overlap. The language and tools of healthcare ethical decision making are introduced and illustrated with case examples and strategies for nursing and other healthcare providers to use in analyzing problems and conceptualizing resolutions. The second part provides for the further development and refinement of ethical decision-making skills facilitative of moral agency on behalf of good patient care. It includes a chapter on improving intra- and interdisciplinary communication and provides practice exercises. The ability to communicate clearly is critical to ethics discussions, and in a prior project, to develop nurse confidence in their advocacy skills, practice using a validated communication method was highly valued. This is followed by an exploration of the types of resources available in institutions and countries related to resolving conflictual situations and includes the idea of preventive ethics with an emphasis on nurses roles in identifying and resolving emerging problems. A section on advance care planning is provided and exemplified in a synthesized encounter demonstrating how nurses can initiate such conversations. Included in the part is a chapter exploring cultural and religious perspectives and their influences on ethical decision making. Finally in the third part, with the assistance of contributing authors, we explore different aspects pertaining to ethical issues in particular settings and populations. Specifically, we address issues related to genetics, mental health, organizations, and injustice.

Throughout the chapters, cases and exercises are introduced to help nurses with practical strategies to improve their confidence in ethical decision making both as individuals and in collaboration with others. These exercises and cases can be used in a variety of settings to structure discussion and practice skills, particularly in areas where robust ethics resources may not be readily available to coordinate such efforts. For example, nurses could use the case studies to facilitate ethics rounds on their units even in the absence of a trained nurse ethicist. Exercises that promote self-reflection and reflection on practice are infused throughout the book. A major strength of the book is the rich variety of well-developed cases we have synthesized from actual situations. These are drawn from the public domain, the authors' experiences as ethics consultants, nurse educators, and are based on the extensive practice experiences of the editors and guest authors.

Chestnut Hill, USA   Pamela Grace
                                                                                  Aimee Milliken

Acknowledgements

This book developed as a result of our combined experiences as nurses, ethicists, and scholars and a recognition of the dire need for an accessible handbook that nurses working in healthcare environments could access and that nurse educators and leaders could refer to for supportive strategies. The problems nurses face in their daily practice are multifaceted and complex and are often difficult to describe to those not in the profession. Several decades ago, Daniel Chambliss (1996) undertook an in-depth ethnographic study of the social organization of ethics using nurses and hospitals as representative subjects. His report opens with the words 'Nursing is a noble profession but too often a terrible job' (p. 1). With this book, we hope to mitigate the experience of nursing as a terrible job by empowering the moral agency of nurses.

We used the insights from countless numbers of our nursing and ethics colleagues and students to augment the content of the book. Special thanks are owed to the guest authors and contributors whose topical expertise undoubtedly provided knowledge that raised the quality of the book and its likely helpfulness as a practical tool to facilitate ethical decision making both in daily practice and in conflictual situations. In many cases, we worked with our guest experts to develop the ethical analyses of cases. We learned so much from these collaborations.

We are grateful for our many and varied experiences, both formative and challenging, and for the support and encouragement of a host of others in our lives and careers. Those influences include family, friends, teachers, colleagues, mentors, students, each other, and above all the patients and families we have been privileged to serve. The echoes of these countless prior influences are redound in the book. We both feel fortunate to have found our home in a profession that serves a critical human need and is replete with meaningful interactions.

Many thanks to Aimee, who despite her extraordinarily busy life agreed to co-edit this book with me ... a gifted nurse, scholar, and clinical ethicist. Her collaboration on this project was invaluable.

Finally, I am so thankful for my husband Chris Hayford whose patience and humor continue to bring joy into my life—Pam.

Thank you to my husband Travis, and to our son Finn, who are my anchors and constant source of inspiration. To my parents and sister, for your unwavering support. Thank you to Pam, for your years of mentoring and colleagueship, and for bringing me on to this project. I am grateful for the privilege of working with you—Aimee.

Contents

Part I Foundations of Professional and Clinical Ethics

1 Introduction 3
Pamela J. Grace and Aimee Milliken

2 Developing Ethical Awareness and Ethical Sensitivity 21
Aimee Milliken and Pamela J. Grace

3 The History, Language and Tools of Ethics: Application
in Healthcare Settings 35
Pamela J. Grace and Aimee Milliken

Part II Essential Knowledge and Skills for Ethical Deliberations

4 Effective Communication—Improving Communication Skills 59
Ben Benjamin, Aimee Milliken, and Pamela Grace

5 Models of Ethics Deliberation and Consultation 85
Aimee Milliken, Settimio Monteverde, and Pamela Grace

6 Cultural, Religious, Language and Personal Experiences:
Influences in Ethical Deliberations 115
Annette Mendola, Pamela J. Grace, and Aimee Milliken

Part III Ethical Issues Associated with Practice and Research

7 Neonatal and Pediatric Acute and Palliative Care 135
Pamela J. Grace, Aimee Milliken, and Melissa Uveges

8 Genetics: Nurses Roles and Responsibilities 153
Melissa K. Uveges and Andrew A. Dwyer

9 Ethical Issues in Psychiatric and Mental Health Care 175
Julie P. Dunne, Emma K. Blackwell, Emily Ursini,
and Aimee Milliken

10 **Research on Human Subjects: Nurses Roles and Responsibilities** 205
Pamela J. Grace and Aimee Milliken

11 **Organizational Influences on Ethical Action** 227
Aimee Milliken and Pamela Grace

12 **Social Justice, Structural Disparities and Nursing Responsibilities** 237
Pamela Grace, Aimee Milliken, and John Welch

Index 255

Part I
Foundations of Professional and Clinical Ethics

Chapter 1
Introduction

Pamela J. Grace and Aimee Milliken

Abstract This Chapter provides an outline of reasons for developing a clinical ethics handbook for nurses that is both practical in orientation and relevant internationally. Foundational to the rest of the book, are definitions of various concepts we rely upon to make our points. Defining 'health' in the context of clinical settings is a priority for mutual understanding among the different professions. A 'clinical setting' is any organized inpatient or outpatient location providing healthcare services. Differences and similarities in branches of healthcare and professional ethics and their mutual goals along with distinct perspectives on how to meet those goals are clarified. Both mutual goals and the distinct perspectives of the different healthcare professions are ethical in nature. They aim to provide for the individual and social good of healthcare. We delineate aspects of the struggle to practice well within the increasing complexity of contemporary healthcare environments, noting that nurses often bear the largest burden in the struggle because of their proximity to patients and their families. The knowledge, skills, and attributes needed for nurse moral agency—ability to practice ethically—in interdisciplinary settings are outlined. Highlighted is the importance of preventive ethics and of understanding context, engaging in effective communication, and collaborative efforts to provide good care. We describe how our prior mutual and individual work to inform the structure of the book.

1.1 The Challenges of Contemporary Healthcare Environments

Contemporary healthcare environments are increasingly complex and challenge all of us who work within them as we strive to achieve our professional goals (Austin, 2012; Institute of Medicine, 2010; Jurchak et al., 2017; World Health Organization, 2015).

P. J. Grace (✉) · A. Milliken
William F. Connell School of Nursing, Boston College, Chestnut Hill, MA, USA
e-mail: Gracepa@bc.edu; pamela.grace.2@bc.edu

A. Milliken
e-mail: aimee.milliken@bc.edu

© The Author(s), under exclusive license to Springer Nature B.V. 2022
P. Grace and A. Milliken (eds.), *Clinical Ethics Handbook for Nurses*, The International Library of Bioethics 93,
https://doi.org/10.1007/978-94-024-2155-2_1

Each conscientious and ethically aware healthcare professional faces obstacles to providing the care that their clinical judgment identifies as needed for an individual, group, or for public health. Yet the reason that healthcare systems exist, and within them healthcare professionals, is that individuals cannot meet all of their own health needs for various reasons (Grace, 1998). We discuss in more detail later the reasons why certain professions, namely those that provide human services facilitative of effective human functioning within a society, are at their core ethical rather than commercial in nature. Additionally, and infused throughout the book, are some of the ways managerial and market values complicate the work of nurses and other healthcare professionals as they strive to provide humane, ethical patient-centered healthcare.

1.2 A Practical Strategic Resource for Point of Care Nurses, Nurse Educators and Leaders

The reasons for a book like this, that is practical in focus and international in scope, are various. Primarily, there is both hard and anecdotal evidence of a dire need for just such a resource for bedside nurses who face innumerable challenges to good practice on a day-to-day basis and bioethics textbooks tend not to speak to the contextual issues faced by nurses. Our recognition of the need stemmed from our practice experiences, work with students both undergraduate and graduate, interactions with point-of-care nurses, memberships in ethics committees and involvement in ethics consultations. Additionally, both the international literature and interactions with international educators and ethics colleagues corroborate that similar problems arise in other countries. What is certain is that having ethics education in a nurse's preparatory or even ongoing education is necessary but not sufficient to maintain confidence in the ability to advocate for good care when obstacles to good practice are ever-present (Lee et al., 2019).

This finding resulted from research into the effectiveness of the Clinical Ethics Residency for Nurses program (CERN) (Lee et al., 2019) for which Grace was a co-PI. An analysis of end of program essays (N = 65) revealed several themes including the perception that the 96-h program (taking place over 9 months) gave a good basis for increasing confidence in ethical decision making and action but that learning needed to be fortified in ongoing opportunities. Opportunities for continuing education, rounding, and debriefing on wards and units, access to ethics resources, and supportive environments are all critical to the development and maintenance of nurse moral agency.

Preparatory to the ensuing discussions some definitional clarity is provided. Definitions are important so that the reader understands what is meant by various terms and concepts. In a sense term and concept are similar but we take 'term' to be the broader label encompassing both a more abstract concept that requires a definition for its contextual meaning to be understood—such as 'moral distress', and 'advocacy'—and a circumscribed, concrete label for an entity the meaning of which is generally obvious. As an example of a more concrete term, a bus stop is a place where a bus stops to pick up passengers.

1.3 Clarifying Concepts and Terms

1.3.1 *The Meaning of Health*

A generally acceptable definition of health is foundationally important for discussions in the remainder of this book. It is critical for purposes of communication and collaboration with colleagues, patients, and families. Regardless of the different perspectives of each discipline on the reasons why their services are needed, and the associated responsibilities of their members, understanding that they share mutual goals related to patient health, patient interests and patient well-being provides an anchor for collaborations on behalf of good care.

One thing is indisputable: health, as experienced by individuals, is not merely the absence of physical problems. Furthering health and well-being necessarily includes accounting for contextual features of a person's life, as well as their subjective understanding of health. Yet what constitutes health remains the subject of both philosophical and political debate (Bambra et al., 2005; Boorse, 1997; Nordenfelt, 2006; Schramme, 2007) and definitions are numerous. So, what is needed is a definition that can accommodate the foci of disparate healthcare disciplines.

We know that what is perceived as health to a person with chronic physical illness or mental health issues may well differ from what is perceived as health for an elite athlete. Additionally, what people take to be health at one period in life may not be the same idea that person has of health at a different life-phase. So even within a person's life trajectory, what constitutes health is a fluid concept. If a person does not *feel* healthy then they are *not* healthy from their perspective and this deviation from their norm or perspective on what is optimal health for them is an important consideration for the various healthcare professions. But additionally, healthcare professionals are also responsible for anticipating, where possible, the future health concerns and needs of individuals, communities, and society and this includes engaging in *preventive ethics*. Preventive ethics is the term used for recognizing emerging ethical problems and addressing them before they progress to crisis point. Nurses, because they are often the ones in closest and more sustained contact with patients and their families, and thus understand their ideas, values, and preferences related to health and wellbeing, are ideally positioned to engage in preventive ethics actions.

Here we review some existing definitions of health and settle on one that we think most healthcare professionals will find acceptable as an anchor for interdisciplinary communication about patient care situations. The World Health Organization (WHO) in 1948 defined health as "a state of complete physical, mental and social well-being and not merely an absence of disease or infirmity", and their definition has not changed. There were good reasons for the WHO's definition, emphasizing as it does the responsibilities of societies for their constituents, and noting that social conditions can interfere with people being able to live, what Powers and Faden (2006) call a 'minimally decent life'. However, while at the time the definition represented a new way of looking at health, it has been criticized as too ambitious, nonspecific, and impractical for contemporary purposes (Huber et al., 2011). One compelling reason is that many people live with chronic diseases and cannot obtain complete physical health. A broadly acceptable definition for all healthcare professionals is needed.

We live in an era when due to biotechnological and other advances people, at least in more developed countries, are living longer and experiencing chronic illness in larger numbers than ever before and a definition that can accommodate 'health' within or despite disease is necessary (Willis et al., 2008). For such reasons, Huber et al. (2011), subsequent to a two-day invitational conference in the Netherlands on defining health, propose that a better conception of health is the "ability to adapt and self-manage in the face of social, physical, and emotional challenges" (p. 235). We do not think that this definition quite captures the experience of health from either a nursing or other health disciplines' perspective as it neglects populations who cannot self-manage, such as small children and those with severe cognitive impairments. More recently, a nursing-focused definition considered health as a multifaceted-concept that is signified by sense of integrity or wholeness regardless of physical limitations or disease processes, or trajectory towards death (Willis et al., 2008). As Nordenfelt (2006) points out "etymologically health is connected with the idea of wholeness" (p. 3). For the purposes of this book, we accept Willis et al. (2008) definition, while recognizing that the various healthcare professions may emphasize different facets that contribute to wholeness, but all must account for the patient's perspective where this is possible either as reported by the person or his or her 'proxy' or substitute decision maker. Since this is a clinical ethics handbook, dealing with issues in the hospital or clinic, we believe this definition captures the range of healthcare disciplines who work collaboratively in the interests of patients. Those working in public health would necessarily have an expanded definition of health.

1.3.2 Connecting and Distinguishing Bioethics, Professional Ethics, Medical Ethics and Nursing Ethics

Another point of clarity that provides a foundation for the rest of the book is how the different fields of study related to ethics and human service professions are both distinct in focus and overlapping in substance. First, it is important to note that we use the terms *Ethical* and *Moral* throughout the book as synonymous concepts, even though outside of a healthcare setting the two terms can be used to evaluate different aspects of human action. In everyday life, 'ethics' tends to be used to describe cultural guidelines about acceptable actions—where culture can be micro (institutional) or macro (societal) in nature. Whereas 'moral' tends to be used appraise more personal (Weston, 2011) characteristics and predispositions. The historical root meanings of both terms are similar but derived from different languages. Health care professions exist to provide a 'good', and there are ways of determining what that good is, based on the given profession's goals or reason for existence. Thus, it is reasonable to assume that when an individual becomes a professional, actions taken within that role are subject to ethical appraisal and that is the equivalent of moral appraisal. The parent field of study underlying professional ethics is moral philosophy (Grace, 2018). Moral philosophy also is the parent field of study for any other discipline that is concerned with determining what constitutes a good human action toward other people, animals, and the environment as well as for determining why and under what circumstances. When ideas from moral philosophy are applied to actions this is called *applied ethics*.

Since World War II, with its accompanying unprecedented development of biotechnology and subsequent applications for human disease and incapacity, moral philosophers became more involved in analyses of, and decision-making about, the use of such technologies (Jonsen, 1998) as they were posing dilemmas for society outside of the usual medical ethics type problems. For example, in 1960 a patient in kidney failure received the first arteriovenous shunt permitting him to receive hemodialysis from a specially designed machine, however there were more people in need of these machines than available machines presenting a moral dilemma (Jonsen, 1998). A *moral dilemma* is a particular type of ethical problem where a person is forced to choose between two equally undesirable alternatives. It comes from the Greek *di* meaning two and *lemma* meaning premise or assumption (Brown, 1993). As this issue of allocating a scarce resource—dialysis machines—was not purely a medical issue but rather a social one, it required broader ethical analyses and different tools than clinical decision-making. Thus, the knowledge, skills and input of other humanities and social sciences disciplines were sought. Hence, the discipline of Bioethics was born in the 1960s. Bioethics, according to *The Encyclopedia of Bioethics* (Reich, 1995) is "the study of the moral dimensions- including moral vision, decisions, conduct and policies – of the life sciences and health care, employing a variety of ethical methodologies in an interdisciplinary setting" (p. xxi).

Historically, *medical ethics* as a field of study explored medical practice, the characteristics of medical practitioners and the responsibilities they owe to patient and themselves and as a set of normative principles medical ethics describes how physicians ought to act in providing care to patients. *Normative principles* are those that provide a reason for one to act and have moral force. For example, Professional Codes of Ethics tell professionals how they are expected to act and that they can be held accountable for not acting in ways prescribed by its intent and tenets. For instance, among the World Medical Association (WMA) International Code of Medical Ethics statements are the following: that a physician should "always exercise his/her independent professional judgment and maintain the highest standards of professional conduct...not allow his/her judgment to be influenced by personal profit or unfair discrimination… (and) be dedicated to providing competent medical service in full professional and moral independence, with compassion and respect for human dignity" (WMA, 2018).

While the field of study about physicians and their conduct is medical ethics, *Nursing Ethics* is a field of study concerned with understanding "why nursing exists, (what needs and) purposes it serves, its relationship to other professions and disciplines, and what characteristics are needed for nurses to practice well" (Grace, 2018, p. 36). Additionally, nursing ethics inquiries are about what knowledge development and educational endeavors are necessary for supporting good nursing practice in dynamic environments. The tentative answers to such questions structure the profession and its responsibilities to both individuals and society. They are tentative answers because as societies and conditions change, codes of ethics are revised to align with the changes.

There is good evidence that nursing ethics as a field of study, has been developing since Florence Nightingale's reformation of nursing. Her work was anchored in the ethical principles of providing a good and improving healthcare (Hoyt, 2010). Nursing has been self-reflective about its need for guidelines to good nursing conduct over the decades and this has resulted in the development of Codes of Ethics that are specific for professional practice in individual countries. A given country's code of ethics often has legal standing and tenets can be invoked to hold nurses accountable. For example, a 1994 ANA position statement remains valid states that American Nurses Association Code of Ethics for Nurses with Interpretive Statements (regardless of iteration) is not:

> open to negotiation in employment settings, nor is it permissible for individuals, groups of nurses or interested parties to adapt of change the language of this code. The *Code for Nurses* encompasses all nursing activities and may supersede specific policies of institutions, of employers, or of practices. Therefore the content of the Code of Ethics for Nurses with Interpretive Statements is nonnegotiable. (ANA, 1994)

It has been used to defend US nurses when they followed the Code of Ethics guidelines but were sanctioned by their institutions for so doing. In the US a Navy nurse who refused to force feed a detainee on hunger strike at Guantanamo Bay Naval Base for ethical reasons was threatened with court martial and decommissioning for this refusal, He was accused of dereliction of duty for disobeying orders. Various forces, including the ANA Code of Ethics, were brought to bear in arguing that nurses must be free to follow their conscience and, after a variety of hearings, and a letter of support from the Navy Surgeon General the officer was reinstated (Rosenberg, *Miami Herald*, May 6, 2016).

The International Council of Nurses (ICN), which is a federation of 130 plus national nursing organizations, based in Geneva, Switzerland, constructed a Code of Ethics from the input of its member nursing organizations and is more Global in pertinence. However, the essential intent of the tenets is similar and both the ICN and the Codes of Ethics from other countries rely for their foundation on the goals of the profession as these have been developed and articulated over time.

Various healthcare professions have been more or less reflective about their work and reason for being. Many also have Codes of Ethics delineating expectations of members. Each of these professions can also be said to have an 'ethics' associated with their professional practice. Thus, nursing ethics, medical ethics, physiotherapy ethics, pharmacy ethics, human subject research ethics and so on, are all branches of professional ethics which in turn are 'applied ethics' or the tools and insights from moral philosophy applied to practices. As might be expected, because each of these is concerned with providing or optimizing the human good of 'health' there will necessarily be areas of overlap. All of the different healthcare professions encounter Bioethical problems in the course of their work. For this and associated reasons, some have argued that Bioethics should be the umbrella term covering the ethics of healthcare professions others disagree (DeVries et al., 2009; Kopelman, 2006), and we are among the dissenters. We believe that each profession has its own historically developed perspective on how to achieve its purposes and that bioethics cannot adequately capture the distinctions, unique purposes, and ongoing discussions within each profession about how to continue to meet its responsibilities despite increasing complexity within the healthcare environment.

Clinical ethics is the term used to describe the process of resolving ethical issues that arise in the course of patient care and involves the input of different practice professions as well as non-clinicians who have expertise and education in philosophy, bioethics or related humanities disciplines. Nurses are involved in both clinical ethics conflicts and obstacles to everyday practice.

1.4 Problems Faced by Nurses: Major Themes in the Literature

1.4.1 Moral Distress

Moral distress has been recognized as a ubiquitous problem for all healthcare providers (Borhani et al., 2014; Browning, 2013; Carse, 2013; Corley et al., 2005), but is perhaps experienced especially frequently by nurses because of their proximity to the patient, patient suffering, and family concerns. Essentially moral distress is not the same as emotional distress although moral distress does have emotional aspects. *Moral distress* was originally described as the feeling of unease that arises when one has a good idea of what is required for a patient's wellbeing but one cannot supply that need for various reasons (Jameton, 1984). Others have expanded the definition to include the idea of moral stress (Fourie, 2015, 2017; Lützen et al., 2010) caused by the environment or by uncertainty about the situation or what to do. What is known about moral distress is that it can cause nurses to distance themselves from patients or to leave the profession, neither of which is good for patients (Catlin et al., 2008; Epstein & Hamric, 2009).

1.4.2 Complexity in Contemporary Practice Environments

The growing complexity of healthcare environments is beyond dispute and recent studies continue to highlight the problems posed for nurses and other providers by workplace complexity (Dauwerse et al., 2011; Jurchak et al., 2017; Lee et al., 2019; Lysdahl & Hofmann, 2016). In the Jurchak et al (2017) study documenting reasons why prospective participants in a clinical ethics residency for nurses (CERN) desired to enter the program, the increasing complexity of their environments and its accompanying 'grey zone' practice issues were prominent themes. "Grey zones are complex situations where the right action is not clearly evident, it is difficult to judge benefits over harms, or there are conflicts among the healthcare team or the team and others" (Jurchak et al., 2017, p. 448). Besides the complexity caused by biotechnological innovations are difficulties associated with cultural diversity, associated communication difficulties and value conflicts as well as unrealistic patient and family expectations.

Thus, complexity in the contemporary healthcare environment is multifactorial and besides factors such as unprecedented advances in biotechnology, the increasingly multi-cultural makeup of many societies, and communication difficulties, there are issues of hierarchy and power. Additionally, there are pressures to contain costs (and in the U.S. to make profits), exclusion or disempowerment of healthcare professionals from institutional administrations in some countries, institutional hierarchies and medical specialization which can lead to fractured care, among other problems. All of these factors contribute to the difficulties nurses face in trying to practice well on a day-to-day basis. While the predominance of any of one of these factors may vary among countries, evidence points to the shared experience of complexity across countries.

1.4.2.1 Biotechnological Advances: Contributions to Complexity

The emergence of bioethics as a discipline, as discussed earlier, is attributable to the exponential advances in biotechnology available since World War II (1939–1945) (Jonsen, 1998). Such advances include biological, surgical, prosthetic, mechanical, informational, genetic, pharmacological, and other innovations, including the advent of specialized intensive care units within hospitals. These innovations, while increasing the overall life span of populations in developed countries that have some form of organized healthcare system, have also led to an increase in the number of people who are living longer with chronic illnesses and co-morbid conditions. This is not intrinsically problematic, as many people are assisted to enjoy a good quality of life by these advances and other social supports despite chronic illness, but these advances have also led to what has been termed the 'technological imperative' in healthcare (Baily, 2011; Hofmann, 2002). This is the idea that, perhaps insidiously, physicians and others have come to feel that because technological advances exist they should be used. Thus "pharmacologic and technological advances (are sometimes used) to extend life without appropriate evaluation of how these fit with patients' goals" (Grace, 2018, p. 385). Sometimes such interventions are continued even after it becomes clear that the physiologic goals for the person cannot be met.

Adding to the complexity problem is that biotechnological advances can be profitable for the entities that develop and market them. This in turn causes rhetoric to be developed that is persuasive to both clinicians and the public, leading to some unrealistic expectations of modern medicine and associated demands for treatments that cannot always meet a person's goals. Complexity surrounding healthcare contexts is also augmented when one considers the recent availability of unprecedented, albeit unfiltered, access to information facilitated by the advent social media and informational technologies (ITs). Informational technologies are those innovations that provide instant access to information, help us build knowledge, stimulate thinking and imagination, and articulate ideas to others (Carr, 2011; Cuchetti & Grace, 2020). However, the information gained is not always validated, sound or contextualized. Additionally, social media and ITs can expose people to inadvertent erosion of their privacy.

1.4.2.2 Culturally Diverse Societies: Contributions to Complexity

In the U.S., especially in large cities, coastal, and border areas, healthcare professionals provide care to diverse communities. Nurse frequently encounter patients and sometimes physicians with whom they have difficulty interacting due both to differences in cultural values and language difficulties. We know from the literature that issues related to providing healthcare in increasingly multicultural societies are factors not just in the US healthcare environment but in many countries (Brunton & Cook, 2018; McCarthy et al., 2013). There is a need to how to better relate to others who might not share one's values, and how to communicate effectively when culture and language difficulties exist (Jurchak et al., 2017). Chapter 7 provides an in-depth look at cultural, religious and other contextual influences on ethical decision making, along with strategies to help nurses resolve difficulties.

Also needed are strategies for healthcare providers to deal with political forces (institutional and social) that pressure nurses to prioritize acting as agents of their governments policies over the good of persons. For example, in some regions nurses may be asked to report patients they suspect lack legal documentation of their presence in the country. At the time this book was in process, overt political antagonism toward undocumented persons existed in parts of the US and we believe it will continue. Among the sequelae of such pressures, is that undocumented immigrants may not seek healthcare for fear of reprisals. They may also refrain from seeking healthcare for their children who do have citizenship as a result of similar fears. For example, as reported in 2019 by New York Times the administration headed by Donald Trump discontinued a program that allowed immigrants with serious health conditions—including children and people with disabilities—and their families to remain in the United States while receiving life-saving medical treatment. This meant that such children would be sent back to their home countries and to almost certain death. Luckily, the public outcry resulting from activism on behalf of and by these children caused the Trump administration to reverse its decision. Thus, both communication problems and social or political mandates that conflict with the humanitarian goals of healthcare are faced by healthcare professionals, in many countries. Such problems are fairly widely documented in the nursing and health literature internationally. For example, a special issue of *Eurohealth* (vol 22[3], 2016) is devoted to the topic.

1.4.2.3 Cost Controls, Economics, and Managerialism: Contributions to Complexity

Other factors contributing to complexity in the healthcare system include profit-motive and cost-containment measures that shift proper focus of healthcare institutions from being primarily about human good, to primarily the economic concern of controlling costs and even maximizing profits (Relman, 2007). In the UK, Europe, Asia, Scandinavia and elsewhere those at the point of care have felt the influence of managerialism on their practices (Bamford & Porter O'Grady, 2000; Hau, 2004; Komesaroff et al., 2015). Managerialism is the term used to describe how business principles are used to direct care management (Frith, 2013; Gilbert, 2005). Among the problems associated with managerialism are that the professional practice autonomy can be undermined by those who are not healthcare professionals but rather have a business focus. According to Komesaroff et al. (2015), "The particular system of beliefs and practices defining the roles and powers of managers ... is referred to as managerialism. This is defined by two basic tenets: (i) that all social organisations must conform to a single structure; and (ii) that the sole regulatory principle is the market" (p. 519). They worry that when market principles dominate then other principles important to human good are diminished. "(O)ther criteria such as loyalty, trust, care and a commitment to critical reflection, ... become displaced and devalued" (p. 519). Among the implications of this for healthcare professionals is that they cannot act alone in refocusing actions. Molina-Mula et al. (2018), noted of the Canadian context that,

> a health system based on market ethics, which standardises and institutionalises patients, loses the sense of patient-centred healthcare. Quality goals are promoted that are not aimed at meeting the needs of patients and their self-determination but are rather aimed at a health institution's performance indicators. For this reason, nurses who are pressured by the healthcare organisation are compelled to prioritise activities that ensure these indicators are met rather than patient care. (p. 7)

To effectively advocate for patients, nurses need specific ethics-related knowledge and skills as well as motivation and experience. When nurses gain or refine these attributes they can support and influence others in doing the right thing even when there are impediments (Lee et al., 2019). They can also help develop supportive environments.

1.5 Knowledge, Skills and Attributes Needed for Nurse Moral Agency

Earlier we noted that moral agency is the ability and motivation to practice ethically even in difficult circumstances. On those occasions when it is impossible for various reasons to influence a problematic situation, for example, there is inadequate staffing for the acuity level of the patients, then nurses still have responsibilities to try and influence unit, clinic, or institutional policies (formal or informal) after the fact (Grace, 2001). There are many reasons that nurses do not speak up about issues that face, or that they see patients struggling with, including trying to get their preferences for treatment heard.

1.5.1 Disempowered Nurses

As Manojlovich (2007) noted, "powerless nurses are ineffective nurses" (para 1). Among the reasons nurses do not exercise moral agency as noted in the literature, and anecdotally from our extensive experiences, is that nurses may be influenced by the ongoing hierarchical system in many institutions that situate nursing and nursing activities at the lower end of the power structure. Various countries accord nurses more or less power over their practice. Some nurses do not think that it is their role to speak up for patients or are afraid to do so. In a study of new nurses Kelly (1998) found, "They sacrificed their standards of care and ideals by assuming the norms and values of the hospital system in order to be respected by the team" (p. 1141). In other cases, nurses are afraid they will lose their position, will anger their co-workers, and perhaps cause conflict with physicians interfering with collaborative practice. Nurses may feel too overworked to take the time to advocate for a particular patient, may be uncertain how to articulate the issue, may have become numbed to the sorts of problems that have occurred in the past and that they were unable to positively influence. They may offer resistance of various sorts (Peter et al., 2004) that can result in ethical actions but in a less straightforward or economical way. Many nurses have talked about lack of unit support and 'toxic' work environments that deter them from disturbing the status quo when this obstructs optimal patient care.

1.5.2 Status of Nurse Perception of Power Internationally

Nurses' perception of their power to advocate for patients varies with both education level and supportive environments but also from country to country. In those countries that have been particularly male-dominated, or dominated by the need to respect elders, power differentials may be especially strong. For example, in South Korea, Yi (2018) notes that while things are improving for Korean nurses (and thus for patients) "In a very paternalistic hospital and healthcare environment, nursing, as a women-dominated discipline, is still regarded as inferior to male-dominated jobs or professions, such as medicine. Even when nurses themselves recognize their contributions, they cannot be assertive and show their impact on patient outcomes to others" (p. 58). In reviewing the literature from a wide variety of countries, we developed a synthesized list of nurses' shared experiences of feeling powerless. These feelings of powerlessness, as synthesized from the literature and anecdotally from nurses' stories as told in an ethics class over the past 20 years, are associated with:

- Ability "to provide competent quality care" related to severe injuries such as burns (Kornhaber & Wilson, 2011, p. 172)
- Inability to influence ethical decisions
- Inability to change institutional or unit culture
- Ability to act in situations of dual loyalties (e.g. Rules of prison work versus professional responsibilities to the prisoner patient)
- Inability to implement professional values
- Bias and prejudice toward patients and colleagues
- Ability to effectively articulate the nuances of a problem

Building one's knowledge, skill, and experience base are all important factors in developing confidence in one's moral agency and in overcoming feelings of powerlessness. Additionally, developing supportive environments and having ongoing ethics discussion opportunities all strengthen nurse moral agency. As reported by Lee et al. (2019) who analyzed the final essays from 3 cohorts of point of care and advanced practice nurses (N = 65) participating in a year-long clinical ethics residency (CERN) (2010–2013) the majority of participants upon completing the program recognized that they had developed important knowledge and skills to enable them to recognize, analyze and address practice issues, develop decision-making confidence, and build supportive environments.

> Six major themes corresponding to questions posed to the participants included the ability to advocate for good patient care; to support and empower colleagues, patients, and families; they experienced personal and professional transformation; they valued the multimodal nature of the program; and were using their new knowledge and skills in practice. However, they also recognized that their development as moral agents needed to be viewed as an ongoing developmental process. (Lee et al., 2019, abstract)

1.5.3 Attributes Needed for Nurse Moral Agency

1.5.3.1 Personal Attributes

From the nursing and healthcare literature, insights from the behavioral sciences, and the first author's work exploring characteristics of a 'good' nurse (unpublished data) and philosophical insights we have derived a (non-exhaustive) list of personal attributes that facilitate nurse moral agency by predisposing the nurse to attunement

1 Introduction

with patient, family, colleagues, and the ethical aspects of both everyday and dilemmatic situations. These characteristics lead to a predisposition to act. Additionally, an unpublished dissertation by Dr. Suellen Breakey (2006) focused on the characteristics of ICU nurses who actively engaged in end-of-life decision-making. This resulted in a grounded theory of "Optimizing Stewardship". A question remains, however, to what extent can these characteristics be developed and honed if they are weak or nonexistent. We have some evidence about which characteristics can be developed (De Cremer, 2016; Lee et al., 2019) but more work is needed in this area. Each of these characteristics could be described in great detail which we have not done here. However, in various chapters these characteristics along with they can be developed are discussed in more detail. For now we just provide a brief description of each. Important characteristics include:

• Self-reflective and reflective about practice, admits when things have not gone well and learns from these situations, understands the nature and role of biases and prejudice • Ethical awareness and sensitivity—see Chapter 2. Understands the ethical nature of all nursing practice • Conscientiousness—sense of moral responsibility for one's actions—acts with care and honesty • Proactive—notices likely problems before, or as they arise • Capacity to separate reason from emotion • Empathy and ability to relate to patients. To try to grasp another person's concerns from their perspective not yours. Requires deep listening	• Articulate and communicative, separates emotions from reasoning when discussion a situation. Chapter 4 provides more detail • Assertiveness—willing to speak up on behalf of a patient, colleague or self for needed change • Motivation—emotional engagement that results in action • Persistence • Mettle (Breakey, 2006) described as a strong sense of character and warranted confidence in what one knows and can follow through even when others do not agree • Trustworthiness- honest, transparent, and reliable

Possessing such personal attributes, as described above and in more detail in Chapter 2, or being able to develop them, while necessary, is not sufficient for clinical wisdom (Haggerty & Grace, 2008), ethical decision-making and moral agency. Certain types of knowledge are also required.

1.5.3.2 Knowledge

The types of knowledge facilitative of nurse moral agency include:

- Role-Related or professional responsibilities associated with the development of nursing as a profession (albeit in various stages of maturity in different countries), its goals and perspectives on the human being and its role in human wellbeing.
- Knowledge from the different sciences, physiologic, psychologic, social, cultural as delivered in nursing curricula and necessary for a given practice setting but applied using nursing's perspective of the human as a contextually situated being.

- Knowledge of the language and tools of ethics, such as principles and their role in problem analysis.
- Knowledge of the goals and perspectives of other members of the healthcare team and how this both coheres with nursing's and in what ways they might differ.

1.5.3.3 Skills and Experiences

However, while possessing personal characteristics and the types of knowledge described above are critical for moral agency, the development of certain skills are also important. Skill development often requires experience, practice, and mentorship. The types of skills nurses need to advocate for their patients, support and educate colleagues and collaborate with other members of the health care team include effective communication skills—which in turn involves careful listening and the ability to elicit the perspectives of all involved. The ability to defuse and mediate heightened tensions, and to articulate accurately the facts of a given situation using the tools of ethics, such as professional goals and ethical principles are important additional skills. Chapter 4 provides exercises and techniques designed to improve intra and interdisciplinary communication.

1.6 Summary

This chapter provided some foundational ideas that will be elaborated upon and exemplified throughout the book. We highlighted and defined some important basic concepts that should help with future discussions. While the list of characteristics, knowledge and skills needed for moral agency may seem overwhelming, we suspect that many nurses already possess these to a degree and the role of the book will be to show how these can be enhanced on behalf of good patient care and ethical practice. In future chapters we provide exercises and other strategies to help nurses develop the capacities they desire.

References

American Nurses Associtation. (1994). *The nonnegotiable nature of the Code of ethics for nurses.* Author. http://ojin.nursingworld.org/MainMenuCategories/Policy-Advocacy/Positions-and-Resolutions/ANAPositionStatements/Position-Statements-Alphabetically/prtetcode14446.html

American Nurses Association. (2015). *Code of ethics for nurses with interpretive statements.* Author. https://www.nursingworld.org/practice-policy/nursing-excellence/ethics/code-of-ethics-for-nurses/

Austin, W. (2012). Moral distress and the contemporary plight of health professionals. *HEC Forum, 4*(1), 7–38. https://doi.org/10.1007/s10730-012-9179-8

Baily, M. A. (2011). Futility, autonomy and cost in end-of-life care. *Journal of Law, Medicine, and Ethics, 39*(2), 172–182.

Bambra, C., Fox, D., & Scott-Samuel, A. (2005). Towards a politics of health. *Health Promotion International, 20*(2), 187–193. https://doi.org/10.1093/heapro/dah608

Bamford, A., & Porter-O'Grady, T. (2000). Shared governance within the market orientated health care system of New Zealand. *International Nursing Review, 47*(2), 83–88.

Beardwood, B., Walters, V., Eyles, J., & French, S. (1999) Complaints against nurses: A reflection of 'the new managerialism' and consumerism in health care? *Social Science and Medicine, 48*(3), 363–374.

Boorse, C. (1997). A rebuttal on health. In J. M. Humber & R. F. Almeder (Eds.), *What is disease?* Humana Press.

Borhani, F., Abbaszadeh, A., Nakhaee, N., & Roshanzadeh, M. (2014). The relationship between moral distress, professional stress, and intent to stay in the nursing profession. *Journal of Medical Ethics and History of Medicine, 7*, 3.

Breakey, S. (2006). *Optimizing stewardship: A grounded theory of nurses as moral leaders in the intensive care unit* (Order No. 3221256). Available From ProQuest Dissertations & Theses Global (304913628). Retrieved from https://proxy.bc.edu/login?

Brown, L. (Ed.). (1993). *The new shorter Oxford English dictionary*. Oxford Clarendon Press.

Browning, A. M. (2013). CNE article: Moral distress and psychological empowerment in critical care nurses caring for adults at end of life. *American Journal of Critical Care, 22*(2), 143–151. https://doi.org/10.4037/ajcc2013437

Brunton, M., & Cook, C. (2018). Dis/Integrating cultural difference in practice and communication: A qualitative study of host and migrant Registered Nurse perspectives from New Zealand. *International Journal of Nursing Studies, 83*, 18–24.

Carr, N. (2011). *The shallows: What the Internet is doing to our brains*. W. W. Norton.

Carse, A. (2013). Moral distress and moral disempowerment. *Narrative Inquiry in Bioethics, 3*(2), 147–151. https://doi.org/10.1353/nib.2013.0028

Catlin, A., Armigo, C., Volat, D., Vale, E., Hadley, M. A., Gong, W., Bassir, R., & Anderson, K. (2008). Conscientious objection: A potential neonatal nursing response to care orders that cause suffering at the end of life? Study of a concept. *Neonatal Network, 27*(2), 101–108.

Corley, M. C., Minick, P., Elswick, R. K., & Jacobs, M. (2005). Nurse moral distress and ethical work environment [Research Support, Non-U.S. Gov't]. *Nursing Ethics, 12*(4), 381–390.

Cuchetti, C., & Grace, P. J. (2020). Authentic intention: Tempering the dehumanizing aspects of technology on behalf of good nursing care. *Nursing Philosophy, 21*(1), e12255.

Dahlqvist, V., Soderberg, A., & Norberg, A. (2009). Facing inadequacy and being good enough: Psychiatric care providers' narratives about experiencing and coping with troubled conscience. *Journal of Psychiatric and Mental Health Nursing, 16*(3), 242–247.

Dauwerse, L., Abma, T., Molewijk, B., & Widdershoven, G. (2011). Need for ethics support in healthcare institutions: views of Dutch board members and ethics support staff. *Journal of medical ethics, 37*(8), 456–460.

De Cremer, D. (2016, December 22). 6 traits that predict ethical behavior at work. *Harvard Business Review*. Accessed July 27, 2019 from https://hbr.org/2016/12/6-traits-that-predict-ethical-behavior-at-work

De Vries, R., Dingwall, R., & Orfali, K. (2009). The moral organization of the professions: Bioethics in the United States and France. *Current Sociology, 57*(4), 555–579.

Epstein, E. G., & Delgado, S. (2010, September 30). Understanding and addressing moral distress. *OJIN: The Online Journal of Issues in Nursing, 15*(3), Manuscript 1.

Epstein, E. G., & Hamric, A. B. (2009). Moral distress, moral residue, and the crescendo effect. *Journal of Clinical Ethics, 20*(4), 330–342.

Eurohealth (2016). Demographics and diversity in Europe: New solutions for health. *Eurohealth, 22*(3). Accessed August 5, 2019. http://www.euro.who.int/en/about-us/partners/observatory/publications/eurohealth

Fourie, C. (2015). Moral distress and moral conflict in clinical ethics. *Bioethics, 29*(2), 91–97.

Fourie, C. (2017). Who is experiencing what kind of moral distress? Distinctions for moving from a narrow to a broad definition of moral distress. *AMA Journal of Ethics, 19*(6), 578–584.

Frith, L. (2013). The NHS and market forces in healthcare: The need for organisational ethics. *Journal of Medical Ethics, 39*(1), 17–21.

Gilbert, T. P. (2005). Trust and managerialism: Exploring discourses of care. *Journal of Advanced Nursing, 52*(4), 454–463.

Grace, P., & Milliken, A. (2016). Educating nurses for ethical practice in contemporary health care environments. *Hastings Center Report*, Special Supplement. Nurses at the table: Nursing, ethics, and health policy. Hastings Center, 46(5), S13–17. https://doi.org/10.1002/hast.625

Grace, P. J. (1998). *A philosophical analysis of the concept 'advocacy': Implications for professional-patient relationships* (Order No. 9923287). Available from ProQuest Dissertations & Theses Global (304456718). https://search.proquest.com/dissertations-theses/philosophical-analysis-concept-advocacy/docview/304456718/se-2?accountid=9673

Grace, P. J. (2001). Professional advocacy: Widening the scope of accountability. *Nursing Philosophy, 2*(2), 151–162.

Grace, P. J. (2018). *Nursing ethics and professional responsibility in advanced practice* (3rd ed.). Jones and Bartlett.

Grace, P. J., Robinson, E., Jurchak, M., Zollfrank, A., & Lee, S. (2014). The Clinical ethics residency for nurses (CERN): An educational model for ethics leadership at the bedside. *Journal of Nursing Administration, 44*(12), 640–646.

Haggerty, L. A., & Grace, P. J. (2008). Clinical wisdom: The essential component of 'good' nursing care. *Journal of Professional Nursing, 24*(4), 235–240.

Hau, W. W. (2004). Caring holistically within new managerialism. *Nursing Inquiry, 11*(1), 2–13.

Hofmann, B. (2002). Is there a technological imperative in health care? *International Journal of Technology Assessment in Health Care, 18*(3), 675–689.

Hoyt, S. (2010). Florence Nightingale's contribution to contemporary nursing ethics. *Journal of Holistic Nursing, 28*(4), 331–332.

Huber, M., Knottnerus, J. A., Green, L., van der Horst, H., Jadad, A. R., Kromhout, D., Leonard, B., Lorig, K., Loureiro, M. I., van der Meer, J. W. M., Schnabel, P., Smith, R., van Weel, C., & Smid, H. (2011). How should we define health? *British Medical Journal, 343*(7817), 235–237.

Hsieh, H. F., & Shannon, S. E. (2005). Three approaches to qualitative content analysis. *Qualitative Health Research, 15*(9), 1277–1288.

Institute of Medicine. (2010). *The future of nursing: Leading change, advancing health*. National Academies Press. Retrieved from http://www.nap.edu/catalog.php?record_id=12956

International Council of Nurses (ICN). (2012). *Code of ethics for nurses*. Author. https://www.icn.ch/sites/default/files/inline-files/2012_ICN_Codeofethicsfornurses_%20eng.pdf

Jameton, A. (1984). *Nursing practice: The ethical issues*. Prentice Hall.

Jonsen, A. (1998). *The birth of bioethics*. Oxford University Press.

Jordan, M., & Dickerson, C. (2019, August 29). Sick migrants undergoing lifesaving care can now be deported. *New York Times*. https://www.nytimes.com/2019/08/29/us/immigrant-medical-treatment-deferred-action.html

Jurchak, M., Grace, P. J., Lee, S., Zollfrank, A., & Robinson, E. (2017, June 12). Developing abilities to navigate through the grey zones in complex environments: Nurses reasons for applying to a clinical ethics residency for nurses. *Journal of Nursing Scholarship, 49*(4), 445–455. https://doi.org/10.1111/jnu.12297

Kelly, B. (1998). Preserving moral integrity: A follow-up study with new graduate nurses. *Journal of advanced nursing, 28*(5), 1134–1145.

Komesaroff, P. A., Kerridge, I. H., Isaacs, D., & Brooks, P. M. (2015). The scourge of managerialism and the Royal Australasian College of Physicians. *Medical Journal of Australia, 202*(10), 519–521.

Kopelman, L. M. (2006). Bioethics as a second-order discipline: Who is not a bioethicist? *The Journal of Medicine and Philosophy, 31*(6), 601–628.

Kornhaber, R. A., & Wilson, A. (2011). Building resilience in burns nurses: A descriptive phenomenological inquiry. *Journal of Burn Care & Research, 32*(4), 481–488.

Lee, S., Robinson, E. M., Grace, P. J., Zollfrank, A., & Jurchak, M. (2019). Developing a moral compass: Themes from the Clinical Ethics Residency for Nurses' final essays. *Nursing Ethics.* https://doi.org/10.1177/0969733019833125

Lützen, K., Blom, T., Ewalds-Kvist, B., & Winch, S. (2010). Moral stress, moral climate and moral sensitivity among psychiatric professionals. *Nursing Ethics, 17*(2), 213–224.

Lysdahl, K. B., & Hofmann, B. (2016). Complex health care interventions: Characteristics relevant for ethical analysis in health technology assessment. *GMS Health Technology Assessment, 12.*

Machteld, H., Knottnerus, J. A., Green L., van der Horst, H., Jadad, A. R., Kromhout, D., Leonard, B., Lorig, K., Loureiro, M. I., Van der Meer, J. W., & Schnabel, P. (2011). How should we define health? *BMJ, 343,* d4163. https://doi.org/10.1136/bmj.d4163

Manojlovich, M. (2007, January 31). Power and empowerment in nursing: Looking backward to inform the future. *OJIN: The Online Journal of Issues in Nursing, 12*(1), Manuscript 1.

McCarthy, J., Cassidy, I., Graham, M. M., & Tuohy, D. (2013). Conversations through barriers of language and interpretation. *British Journal of Nursing, 22*(6), 335–339.

Molina-Mula, J., Peter, E., Gallo-Estrada, J., & Perelló-Campaner, C. (2018). Instrumentalisation of the health system: An examination of the impact on nursing practice and patient autonomy. *Nursing Inquiry, 25*(1), e12201.

Nordenfelt, L. (2006). *Animal and human health and welfare: A comparative philosophical analysis.* CABI publishing.

Peter, E., Lunardi, V. L., & McFarlane, A. (2004). Nursing resistance as ethical action: Literature review. *Journal of Advanced Nursing, 46*(4), 403–416.

Powers, M., & Faden, R. (2006). *Social Justice: The moral foundations of public health and health policy.* Oxford University.

Reich, R. T. (1995). Introduction. In R. T. Reich (Ed.), *Encyclopedia of bioethics* (Rev. ed.). Simon Schuster Macmillan.

Relman, A. S. (2007). Medical professionalism in a commercialized health care market. *JAMA, 298*(22), 2668–2670.

Robinson, E., Jurchak, M., Zollfrank, A., Lee, S., Frost, D., & Grace, P. J. (2014). Enhancing moral agency: Clinical ethics residency for nurses. *Hastings Center Report, 44*(5), 12–20. https://doi.org/10.1002/hast.353

Rosenberg, C. (2016, May 6). Navy reinstates nurse who refused to force-feed at Guantánamo. *Miami Herald.* https://www.miamiherald.com/news/nation-world/world/americas/guantanamo/article75398072.html

Schramme, T. (2007). A qualified defence of a naturalist theory of health. *Medicine, Health Care and Philosophy.* https://doi.org/10.1007/s11019-006-9020-8.

Starr, P. (2013). *Remedy and reaction: The peculiar American struggle over health care reform.* Yale University Press.

Weston, A. (2011). *A practical companion to ethics* (4th ed.). Oxford University Press.

Willis, D. G., Grace, P. J., & Roy, C. (2008). A central unifying focus for the discipline: Facilitating humanization, meaning, choice, quality of life, and healing in living and dying. *Advances in Nursing Science, 31*(1), E28–E40.

World Health Organization. (1948). Preamble to the Constitution of WHO as adopted by the International Health Conference, New York, 19 June–22 July 1946; signed on 22 July 1946 by the representatives of 61 States (Official Records of WHO, no. 2, p. 100) and entered into force on 7 April 1948.

World Health Organization. (2015). *Global health ethics-key issues.* WHO. https://www.who.int/ethics/publications/global-health-ethics/en/

World Medical Association. (2018, July). *International code of medical ethics.* Author. https://www.wma.net/policies-post/wma-international-code-of-medical-ethics/

Yi, M. (2018). Leadership in nursing in Korea. *Asian/pacific Island Nursing Journal, 3*(2), 56.

Chapter 2
Developing Ethical Awareness and Ethical Sensitivity

Aimee Milliken and Pamela J. Grace

Abstract The goals of nursing and other healthcare professions fundamentally involve providing a good to individuals and society, regardless of country or setting. These goals have been established by the healthcare professions over time and codified in codes of ethics, as described in Chapter 1. In this chapter, we build upon this foundation by describing the role of the nurse in fulfilling these goals, first by recognizing ethical issues as they arise in practice, and then by addressing them. We turn to nursing and healthcare ethics literature to provide a framework for ethical action and highlight the importance of nurses and other clinicians building these skill sets, both individually and as interdisciplinary teams. The nurse, in particular, is optimally positioned to identify ethical concerns, but must be prepared with the language, skills, confidence, and motivation to communicate these concerns to the interdisciplinary team in a productive way in order to achieve the patient's goals to the extent that they are achievable. Finally, we discuss methods for cultivating the practice of self-reflection in order to identify one's own values and biases and recognizing how they may impact care and provide several exemplar cases with questions for discussion.

2.1 Foundations for Ethical Nursing Practice

As described in Chapter 1, the goals of nursing and other healthcare professions fundamentally involve providing good to individuals and society (Grace, 2001). These goals have been established by the healthcare professions over time and codified in codes of ethics (American Medical Association, 2016; American Nurses Association, 2015; International Council of Nurses, 2012). Though nursing and other healthcare professions share intersecting goals, including the promotion of health and

---

A. Milliken (✉) · P. J. Grace
William F. Connell School of Nursing, Boston College, Chestnut Hill, MA, USA
e-mail: aimee.milliken@bc.edu

P. J. Grace
e-mail: pamela.grace.2@bc.edu; Gracepa@bc.edu

prevention of illness, what makes nursing's goals distinct is the particular perspective on these goals that the profession has developed (Grace & Milliken, 2016). To that end, nursing scholars have synthesized the profession's specific goals into a central unifying focus to guide practice, education, and research: "facilitating humanization, meaning, choice, quality of life, and healing in living and dying" (Willis et al., 2008, p. E28).

In Chapter 1 we noted that because nursing is one of the healthcare professions that provides an important human service and came into being to meet healthcare needs that were not otherwise met, nursing actions are aimed at providing a benefit (a 'good' in ethical terms). Thus, we can assert that the profession is intrinsically ethical in nature. In other words, we can be ethically criticized when we do not have patient or societal good as the primary focus for our actions. In this chapter, we build upon the assertion that nursing is an ethics-laden profession by describing the role of the nurse in fulfilling professional goals, first by recognizing ethical issues as they arise in practice, and then by developing the skills to address them. We provide a framework for ethical decision making and action that is synthesized from prior work in moral philosophy, ethics, and nursing literature. The Four Component Model of moral agency as developed by James Rest (1982) is particularly helpful for understanding the processes of decision-making. Additionally we draw upon the work of other scholars, and our own research on nurses' professional responsibilities and ethical awareness (Grace, 2001, Grace, 2018; Milliken, 2018; Milliken & Grace, 2015). We highlight the importance of nurses and other clinicians building these skill sets, both individually and as interdisciplinary teams, by identifying the deleterious effects that unresolved ethical issues can have on patient care and the caring professions. Particular attention is paid to the role of the nurse, as nurses are optimally positioned to identify ethical concerns, but must be prepared with the language to communicate these concerns to the interdisciplinary team in a productive way in order to achieve the patient's goals. Finally, we discuss methods for cultivating the practice of self-reflection in order to identify one's own values and biases and recognizing how they may impact care. We conclude with several exemplar cases and questions for discussion.

2.2 Challenges in the Ethical Preparation of Nurses

Literature on nursing ethics, and healthcare ethics more broadly, consistently demonstrates the importance of providing nurses and other clinicians with the education and training to recognize and address ethical issues as they arise in practice (Robichaux, 2012; Rushton, 2016). Ethics is considered a fundamental component of nursing practice (Holt & Convey, 2012; Lechasseur et al., 2016). Recognition of the ethical import of all nursing practice actions, including routine, day-to-day actions, has been described as foundational to safe and effective nursing care (Austin, 2007; Milliken et al., 2018; Ulrich et al., 2010).

A major challenge with nursing ethics education involves the fact that nursing ethics often is subsumed under the umbrella of bioethics or medical ethics in nursing education (Woods, 2005). Ethics curricula, when it is incorporated into nursing education, often focuses on ethical dilemmas, where principals are in conflict (Truog et al., 2015), and other landmark, precedent-setting cases. Everyday ethical issues tend to receive little attention in ethics education yet are significant sources of stress for practicing nurses (Maiden et al., 2011; Oh & Gastmans, 2013; Ulrich et al., 2007, 2010).

Furthermore, there is growing evidence to suggest that nurses do not consistently feel prepared to face ethical issues that arise. Some authors have argued that nurses are in fact ill-equipped to meet the ethical demands they encounter in practice, despite advances in nursing's technical education (Woods, 2005). Others have argued that nurses do successfully recognize intractable ethical issues but fail to notice burgeoning issues or issues that arise in the course of routine care (Krautscheid, 2015; Truog et al., 2015). In either case, ethical problems may go unnoticed, and nurses may not feel equipped to address issues even when they are aware of them (Robinson et al., 2014). Under-preparation for the ethical demands of practice can lead to suboptimal patient care, moral distress, burnout, and attrition (Hamric, 2012; Meltzer & Huckabay, 2004; Parker et al., 2013).

In order to fulfill nursing's ethical obligations, nurses must first develop an awareness of their ethical responsibilities, and then reason through the processes of moral action in order to act as moral agents. In the following section, we describe these processes, beginning with ethical awareness, proceeding to the iterative Four Component model of moral action as described by James Rest, and concluding with moral agency, or the nurse's willingness and ability to provide "good" (meaning ethical) patient care.

2.3 Developing Ethical Awareness

Ethical awareness involves the nurse's recognition that all nursing actions are ethical in nature (Milliken et al., 2018; Milliken & Grace, 2015). We know from the literature, and anecdotally from our work, many nurses do not understand that even the most routine of nursing actions have some ethical aspects. For example, we can fail to practice well when we do not focus on a patient's particular needs related to some aspect of care, such as the insertion of an intravenous (IV) cannula or turning a patient in bed. There is some risk in every nursing action that either the individual patient's best interests are not served, or that we did not reduce necessary harms. Lack of ethical awareness may also result in nurses not noticing more serious ethical issues or burgeoning issues. Chambliss (1996), in his study of intensive care nurses (ICU) realized that nurses could become immune to noticing ethical issues especially when they happened frequently. Ethical awareness should prompt nurses to notice the ethical aspects of both everyday practice, and more complex problems, and should ideally result in nurses taking action to resolve those problems.

Ethical nursing actions, then, are those that are in-line with the profession's goals, which necessarily also means that they accord with a patient's values and preferences. In other words, every action a nurse takes on behalf of a patient has potential ethical implications for that patient. Though routine actions have a low likelihood of violating an ethical principle such as beneficence (to provide a good) or non-maleficence (avoid or reduce harm), there is still potential risk that the action may not be in line with nursing goals or with the patient's preferences. In contemporary healthcare settings, especially, there are many factors that work against an intentional focus on the good of the patient including an emphasis on economic or expediency concerns.

Exemplifying further the ways in which we can violate an ethical principle in routine practice, is the practice of administering medications. In giving a routine medication there is a risk of giving the wrong dose (risk for harm), the patient having an adverse reaction (risk for harm), or the patient not being fully informed about the purpose of the medication (risk for violating autonomy). Recent studies, conducted by the first author, have suggested that nurses reliably recognize the ethical implications of ethically high-risk nursing actions, such as disconnecting the ventilator for a patient near the end of life, but less reliably recognize the implications of more routine actions, such as starting an intravenous line, performing a dressing change, or giving daily medications (Milliken et al, 2018, 2020). The implications of the research also, are that a substantial number of nurses fail to notice emerging or repeating ethically problematic situations.

Among the implications then of nurses having ethical awareness is that they will recognize burgeoning ethical problems early and institute appropriate actions thereby reducing harms and optimizing benefits. Preventive ethics is the term used to describe early interventions that prevent or forestall emerging ethical problems from worsening (Epstein, 2012; Foglia et al., 2012; Splaine et al., 2012).

As the first step in the process of ethical action, ethical awareness prompts nurses to recognize ethical issues. However, an awareness of ethical responsibility is not sufficient to ensure patients get the care they need. Nurses must also be sensitive to the range of possible options, have the reasoning processes to choose an optimal path, and possess the skills needed to take action. These processes are described in Rest's model of moral action.

2.4 Ethical Sensitivity and Rest's Four Component Model of Moral Action

Rest's Four Component model was derived from reflections on teaching ethics to students, and how ethics education could be improved from insights from research in moral psychology. Rest did not assume that the actual consequences of these cognitive processes would result in 'good' actions. That is, he did not have in mind some ultimate principle from which one could ethically appraise the action. Rather, he deduced that these are the processes that the human mind engages when trying to determine what the right thing to do is in a given situation and ways to accomplish the action. It is described as an iterative framework, meaning the components are not linear in nature and all are necessary for moral action. Simply put, Rest (1982) describes the components in the following way: How does the person interpret the situation and how do they view possible actions as impacting others' welfare? How does the person figure out what the morally ideal course is? How do they decide what to do? Do they implement what they intend to do? In other chapters we discuss various aspects of the framework in more detail using examples from a variety of settings. Here we start with a brief explanation of the components.

2.4.1 The First Component is Ethical (Moral) Sensitivity

This concept has been defined by scholars as "interpreting the situation" and involves an awareness of how our actions affect other people (Bebeau et al., 1999). Ethical sensitivity also involves sensing the range of possible actions, and the impact of these actions on others: namely, the patient.

2.4.2 The Second Component is Moral Judgment

Moral judgment is about the process of determining what action is right or wrong in a given situation (Bebeau et al., 1999). It involves developing a justification for choosing a particular line of action. Once a nurse is aware of an ethical issue and has a sense of the possible options, moral judgment would involve choosing an option and being able to describe the rationale for that choice.

2.4.3 The Third Component is Moral Motivation

Moral motivation is defined as "prioritizing moral values over other values", including one's own values (Bebeau et al., 1999). This can be particularly challenging, especially in situations where one's personal values conflict with one's professional responsibilities. For example, a nurse may be faced with caring for a patient who values "life at any cost" and is undergoing intensive interventions that the nurse may not choose for themselves or for a loved one. The nurse may then experience distress arising from the situation. However, reflecting on this distress, the nurse may be able to recognize that the personal values underlying their distress differ from the patient's values, and that judgments of quality of life are inherently value-laden and influenced by many personal and contextual factors.

2.4.4 The Final Component of the Four Component Model Involves Moral Character

Rest and colleagues define moral character as involving strength of convictions, having courage, persisting, and having the skills to implement a moral judgment (Bebeau et al., 1999). This would involve the ability to do the "right" thing, or act as a moral agent, even in the face of conflict or challenge.

2.5 Moral Agency, Advocacy, and Moral Distress: Implications for Good Patient Care

In this section, we discuss some concepts related to the processes of ethical action described above as well as the ability to take action when it is needed.

2.5.1 Moral Agency

Moral agency is defined as the nurse's willingness and ability to take ethical action (Jurchak et al., 2017). This requires that nurses are not only aware of the ethical import of their practice actions, but that they embody this perspective as well (Nelson, 2007) by acting in accord with their clinical judgment and assessment of which actions are required to promote a patient's good or to minimize harm.

Possessing moral agency means that one has appropriate knowledge, skills, and experience. Enacting moral agency additionally requires certain characteristics such as motivation. The ability to communicate concerns in a way that is thoughtful, non-confrontational, articulate and persuasive is especially important, particularly in interdisciplinary contexts. Though strong emotions such as anger, frustration, or worry are often the first sign that something is amiss, effective communication about ethics issues requires that one uncovers the reasons for discomfort and identifies the intellectual or fact-based aspects of the challenging situation (Reilly & Jurchak, 2017). In order to accomplish this, nurses have to be prepared with the language to communicate these concerns to the interdisciplinary team in a constructive way in order to achieve the patient's goals. Chapter 4 outlines common communication challenges, and best practices for avoiding these, including the SAVI system.

2.5.2 Advocacy

Moral agency is an essential component of nurse advocacy, which involves an attention to the immediate needs of the patient, and also to the broader societal issues that impact patient care (Grace, 2001). Often, disparate and dysfunctional societal social structures give rise to challenges seen at the point of care. Nurses, in their role as advocates, must also be attuned to these matters.

For example, as discussed in Chapter 1, healthcare structures and insurance coverage systems may detrimentally impact both the ability of people to access care, including primary care, and the quality of care patients receive. Clinical nurses are responsible for understanding how broader policy decisions and societal institutions have impacted, and do impact, the patients within their practice environments. They may need to collaborate with other nurses and allied healthcare providers to influence change at institutional and social policy levels. These structures and systems vary internationally. For example, in Chapter 12, we provide strategies and resources for nurses in a variety of countries and settings to advocate for policy or environmental changes. However, the main focus of this book is on enabling moral agency in clinical settings. In this setting, when the nurse does not or feels that they do not have moral agency, then, moral distress may be experienced. The concept of moral distress was discussed briefly in Chapter 1, here the relationships among moral agency, advocacy and moral distress are elaborated.

2.5.3 Moral Distress

Evidence is mounting that moral agency, through its relationship to advocacy and action, can serve as an antidote to moral distress (Grace et al., 2014; Jurchak et al., 2017). Moral distress was originally conceptualized by philosopher Andrew Jameton (1984) and has been defined as a "disjuncture between moral choice and moral action as a consequence of external constraints, with the moral agent experiencing anger, frustration, guilt and powerlessness as a result" (Musto & Rodney, 2016, p. 76). Others have extended the meaning of moral distress as occurring also under conditions of uncertainty, where one is not sure of the best or right action (Fourie, 2015). While originally identified in nurses, the concept has since been examined in other types of healthcare professionals as well (Musto & Rodney, 2016; Peter & Liaschenko, 2013). Evidence has shown that moral distress significantly contributes to burnout, attrition, and disengagement (Rodney, 2017). These factors inevitably are detrimental to patient care.

While the experience of some moral distress is inevitable in healthcare, because of the nature of services rendered, having the ability to analyze difficult situations and act to resolve them can alleviate or ameliorate the experience and lessen the detrimental psychological and physical sequelae. Many interventions have focused on alleviating moral distress, including those targeted at increasing resilience (Guo et al., 2018; Rushton et al., 2015, 2017), and those focused on fostering interdisciplinary communication about ethical issues (Liaschenko & Peter, 2016; Rushton, 2016). A commonality in many of these interventions is the development of the nurse's agency. Increased confidence in identifying, communicating about, and acting on ethical issues can help decrease feelings of powerlessness (Robinson et al., 2014) thereby decreasing moral distress.

2.6 The Nurse's Role in Interdisciplinary Contexts and Moral Communities

As described, an important component of the nurse's role as a moral agent is communication in interdisciplinary contexts. Recent studies have highlighted distinctions in the way different types of healthcare professionals view their respective scopes of moral responsibility (Pavlish et al., 2019). These different professional lenses can naturally give rise to situations of conflict or disagreement about what is best for a patient, and reasonable people may arrive at different ethically defensible conclusions about the plan of care. Because the nurse brings an important perspective to the care team, and often spends the most one on one time with the patient and family, it is imperative that the nurse is able to use the language of ethics to communicate concerns in a respectful and coherent way.

One way of promoting this type of dialogue is to create "moral communities" within healthcare institutions. Originally conceptualized by Margaret Urban Walker (Walker, 1993), moral communities are "places, both literally and figuratively, that 'keep moral space open'" (Liaschenko & Peter, 2016, p. S20). Authors have argued that these types of spaces should include actual physical locations where there is time carved out for discussion and ethical discourse in an interdisciplinary environment.

Liaschenko and Peter (2016) suggest engaging around the following set of questions: "What is your understanding of the situation? What counts as a good outcome? What is at stake for you? How do you view your responsibilities in the situation? What is most important to you? What will your view of yourself or others be if option A is taken or option B?" (p. S20). Other methods may include interdisciplinary case conferences, role play, and simulation (Brock et al., 2013; Robinson et al., 2014; Vanlaere et al., 2010). These discussions can help foster an understanding of different perspectives, build respect, promote teamwork, and promote individual nurse agency (Jurchak & Pennington, 2009).

2.7 Self-Reflection and Reflective Practice

An important component of ethical practice is developing habits for self-reflection and reflective practice. This includes the identification of personal, cultural, religious, and professional biases and values which may impact the care nurses provide and the ethical issues they are sensitive to. For example, writing and reviewing narratives may help nurses develop and reflect upon their professional identities, learn from challenging cases, and aid in decreasing moral distress (Ramos et al., 2014; Wald,

2015). Using narratives as a component of reflective practice may be especially useful in reviewing prior clinical experiences, creating spaces for dialogue such as those already mentioned, and in bridging the theory–practice gap (Choperena et al., 2019). Lim and Shi (2013) recommend journaling, diary or letter writing, and private blogging as some mechanisms for narrative reflection. They also suggest reading the reflections of others as a starting point, and describe Florence Nightingale as a pioneer of reflective practice in her work "Notes on Nursing" (Nightingale, 1989). Reflection is an important component of developing a robust moral character, an essential component of the Rest model of moral action (Bebeau et al., 1999; Rest, 1982). An exercise to facilitate self-reflection is provided at the end of the chapter.

2.8 Summary

The nurse plays a pivotal role in ensuring safe and ethical patient care. This chapter describes the role ethical awareness and sensitivity play in ethical nursing practice. In order to fulfill this responsibility, and lessen the effects of moral distress, nurses must find ways to equip themselves with the skills to recognize and address ethical issues as they arise and the language to communicate about these concerns in interdisciplinary contexts. By practicing these skills, which are founded in nursing's professional aims, and taking the opportunity for reflection as outlined in this chapter, nurses can develop a robust sense of moral agency, can create moral communities where discussion about challenging ethical issues can occur, and can more effectively advocate on behalf of their patients.

2.9 Exercise: Practicing Self-Reflection

The practice of self-reflection comes easily to some and not so easily to others. When a class of nurses or nursing students is asked to signal if they consider themselves self-reflective, all hands are generally raised. However, genuine self-reflection requires that we admit we have biases, prejudices, and distorted judgments that can cause us to fail to do right by our patients, sometimes by being judgmental or making unwarranted assumptions. Admitting one could have done things differently is difficult and unsettling, yet without this recognition we cannot grow as nurses and as ethical professionals. Consider a patient care situation that did not go well for some reason (the patient's attitude toward you, your attitude toward the patient, patient's family, co-workers etc.). Write down or consider:

- What was your role in the situation?
- Were you uncomfortable, annoyed, frustrated, or surprised?
- Have you encountered similar issues before?

- Were your feelings visible to those involved and did that contribute to or escalate the problem?
- What assumptions did you make?
- What values did you hold about the situation?
- Did your values conflict with those involved?
- How did you learn those values?
- How might you reframe the problem to try and understand why the person is acting that way.
- What is the perspective or what are the values of the perceived antagonist?
- How might one's psychosocial or physiologic knowledge base help one understand the reason the other person is actig the way they do.
- What could you do to prepare yourself to be more effective in the future?

References

American Medical Association. (2016). *AMA code of medical ethics*. Retrieved from https://www.ama-assn.org/delivering-care/ama-code-medical-ethics

American Nurses Association. (2015). *Code of ethics for nurses*. Retrieved from http://www.nursingworld.org/DocumentVault/Ethics_1/Code-of-Ethics-for-Nurses.html

Austin, W. (2007). The ethics of everyday practice: Healthcare environments as moral communities. *ANS. Advances in Nursing Science, 30*(1), 81–88. https://doi.org/10.097/00012272-200701000-00009

Bebeau, M. J., Rest, J. R., & Narvaez, D. (1999). Beyond the promise: A perspective on research in moral education. *Educational Researcher, 28*(4), 18–26. https://doi.org/10.3102/0013189X028004018

Brock, D., Abu-Rish, E., Chiu, C.-R., Hammer, D., Wilson, S., Vorvick, L., Blondon, K., Schaad, D., Liner, D., & Zierler, B. (2013, November). Interprofessional education in team communication: working together to improve patient safety. *BMJ Qual Saf, 22*, 414–423. https://doi.org/10.1136/bmjqs-2012-000952

Choperena, A., Orovigoicoechea, C., Salcedo, A. Z., Moreno, I. O., & Jones, D. (2019). Nursing narratives and reflective practice: A theoretical review. *Journal of Advanced Nursing, 00*, 1–11. https://doi.org/10.1111/jan.13955

Epstein, E. G. (2012). Preventive ethics in the intensive care unit. *AACN Advanced Critical Care, 23*(2), 217–224. https://doi.org/10.1097/NCI.0b013e31824b3b9b

Foglia, M. B., Fox, E., Chanko, B., & Bottrell, M. M. (2012). Preventive ethics: Addressing ethics quality gaps on a systems level. *Joint Commission Journal on Quality and Patient Safety, 38*(3).

Fourie, C. (2015). Moral distress and moral conflict in clinical ethics. *Bioethics, 29*(2), 91–97.

Grace, P. J. (2001). Professional advocacy: Widening the scope of accountability. *Nursing Philosophy, 2*, 151–162. https://doi.org/10.1046/j.1466-769X.2001.00048.x

Grace, P. J. (2018). *Nursing ethics and professional responsibility in advanced practice* (3rd Ed.). Burlington, MA: Jones and Bartlett.

Grace, P. J., Robinson, E. M., Jurchak, M., Zollfrank, A. A., & Lee, S. M. (2014). Clinical ethics residency for nurses. *JONA: The Journal of Nursing Administration, 44*(12), 640–646. https://doi.org/10.1097/NNA.0000000000000141

Grace, P., & Milliken, A. (2016). Educating nurses for ethical practice in contemporary health care environments. *Hastings Center Report, 46*. https://doi.org/10.1002/hast.625

Guo, Y. F., Luo, Y. H., Lam, L., Cross, W., Plummer, V., & Zhang, J. P. (2018). Burnout and its association with resilience in nurses: A cross-sectional study. *Journal of Clinical Nursing*, *27*(1–2), 441–449. https://doi.org/10.1111/jocn.13952

Hamric, A. B. (2012). Empirical research on moral distress: Issues, challenges, and opportunities. *HEC Forum*, *24*, 39–49. https://doi.org/10.1007/s10730-012-9177-x

Holt, J., & Convey, H. (2012). Ethical practice in nursing care. *Nursing Standard*, *27*, 51–56. Retrieved from http://ezproxy.umsl.edu/login?, http://search.ebscohost.com/login.aspx?direct=true&db=afh&AN=83809034&site=ehost-live&scope=site

International Council of Nurses. (2012). *The ICN code of ethics for nurses*. Retrieved from http://www.icn.ch/images/stories/documents/about/icncode_english.pdf

Jameton, A. (1984). *Nursing practice: The ethical issues*. Retrieved from https://repository.library.georgetown.edu/handle/10822/800986

Jurchak, M., & Pennington, M. (2009). Fostering moral agency in new intensive care unit nurses. *Critical Care Nurse*, *29*(6), 80–80. https://doi.org/10.4037/ccn2009519

Jurchak, M., Grace, P. J., Lee, S. M., Willis, D. G., Zollfrank, A. A., & Robinson, E. M. (2017). Developing abilities to navigate through the grey zones in complex environments: Nurses? Reasons for applying to a clinical ethics residency for nurses. *Journal of Nursing Scholarship*, 1–11. https://doi.org/10.1111/jnu.12297

Krautscheid, L. (2015). Microethical decision making among baccalaureate nursing students: A qualitative investigation. *Journal of Nursing Education*, *53*(3), S19–S25. https://doi.org/10.3928/01484834

Lechasseur, K., Legault, A., & Caux, C. (2016). Ethical competence: An integrative review. *Nursing Ethics*, *1*(13), 1–13. https://doi.org/10.1177/0969733016667773

Liaschenko, J., & Peter, E. (2016, October). Fostering nurses' moral agency and moral identity: The importance of moral community. *Hastings Center Report*, *46*. https://doi.org/10.1002/hast.626

Lim, F., & Shi, T. (2013). Florence Nightingale: A pioneer of self-reflection. *Nursing 2013*, *43*(5), 1–3. https://doi.org/10.1097/01.NURSE.0000428713.27120.d2

Maiden, J., Georges, J. M., & Connelly, C. D. (2011). Moral distress, compassion fatigue, and perceptions about medication errors in certified critical care nurses. *Dimensions of Critical Care Nursing: DCCN*, *30*(6), 339–345. https://doi.org/10.1097/DCC.0b013e31822fab2a

Meltzer, L. S., & Huckabay, L. M. (2004). Critical care nurses' perceptions of futility and its effect on burnout. *American Journal of Critical Care*, *13*(3), 202–208. Retrieved from http://www.ncbi.nlm.nih.gov/pubmed/15149054

Milliken, A., Courtwright, A., Grace, P. J., Fagan-Bengston, E., Visser, M., & Jurchak, M. (2020). Ethics consultations at a major academic medical center: A retrospective. *Longitudinal Analysis, AJOB Empirical Bioethics*, *11*(4), 275–286. https://doi.org/10.1080/23294515.2020.1818879

Milliken, A. (2018). Nurse ethical sensitivity: An integrative review. *Nursing Ethics*, *25*(3). https://doi.org/10.1177/0969733016646155

Milliken, A., Ludlow, L., Desanto-Madeya, S., & Grace, P. (2018). The development and psychometric validation of the ethical awareness scale. *Journal of Advanced Nursing*. https://doi.org/10.1111/jan.13688

Milliken, A., & Grace, P. (2015). Nurse ethical awareness: Understanding the nature of everyday practice. *Nursing Ethics*, 0969733015615172-. https://doi.org/10.1177/0969733015615172

Musto, L. C., & Rodney, P. A. (2016). Moving from conceptual ambiguity to knowledgeable action: Using a critical realist approach to studying moral distress. *Nursing Philosophy*, *17*(2), 75–87. https://doi.org/10.1111/nup.12104

Nelson, S. (2007). Embodied knowing? The constitution of expertise as moral practice in nursing. *Texto & Contexto - Enfermagem*, *16*(1), 136–141. https://doi.org/10.1590/S0104-07072007000100017

Nightingale, F. (1989). *Notes on nursing*. Retrieved from http://uploads.worldlibrary.net/uploads/pdf/20131204225351nightingale.pdf

Oh, Y., & Gastmans, C. (2013). Moral distress experienced by nurses: A quantitative literature review. *Nursing Ethics*, *22*(1), 15–31. https://doi.org/10.1177/0969733013502803

Parker, F. M., Lazenby, R. B., & Brown, J. L. (2013). The relationship of moral distress, ethical environment and nurse job satisfaction. *Online Journal of Health Ethics, 10*(1). https://doi.org/10.18785/ojhe.1001.02

Pavlish, B. C. L., Brown-Saltzman, K., Raho, J. A., & Chen, B. (2019). A national survey on moral obligations in critical care. *American Journal of Critical Care, 28*(3), 183–192. https://doi.org/10.4037/ajcc2019512

Peter, E., & Liaschenko, J. (2013). Moral distress reexamined: A feminist interpretation of nurses' identities, relationships, and responsibilites. *Journal of Bioethical Inquiry, 10*(3), 337–345. https://doi.org/10.1007/s11673-013-9456-5

Ramos, F. R. S., de Farias Brehmer, L. C., Varcas, M. A., Trombetta, A. P., Silveira, L. R., & Drago, L. (2014). Ethical conflicts and the process of reflection in undergraduate nursing students in Brazil. *Nursing Ethics, 22*(4), 428–439. https://doi.org/10.1177/0969733014538890

Reilly, K. M., & Jurchak, M. (2017). Developing professional practice and ethics engagement: A leadership model. *Nursing Administration Quarterly, 41*(4), 376–383. https://doi.org/10.1097/NAQ.0000000000000251

Rest, J. R. (1982). A psychologist looks at the teaching of ethics. *The Hastings Center Report, 12*(1), 29–36. Retrieved from http://links.jstor.org/sici?sici=0093-0334(198202)12:1%3C29:APLATT%3E2.0.CO;2-Q

Robichaux, C. (2012). Developing ethical skills: From sensitivity to action. *Critical Care Nurse, 32*(2), 65–72. https://doi.org/10.4037/ccn2012929

Robinson, E. M., Lee, S. M., Zollfrank, A., Jurchak, M., Frost, D., & Grace, P. (2014). Enhancing moral agency: Clinical ethics residency for nurses. *The Hastings Center Report, 44*(5), 12–20. https://doi.org/10.1002/hast.353

Rodney, P. A. (2017). What we know about moral distress. *American Journal of Nursing, 117*(2), S7–S10. https://doi.org/10.1016/j.amepre.2009.01.018

Rushton, C. H. (2016, October). Creating a culture of ethical practice in health care delivery systems. *The Hastings Center Report, 46*(Suppl. 1), S28–31. https://doi.org/10.1002/hast.628

Rushton, C. H., Batcheller, J., Schroeder, K., & Donohue, P. (2015). Burnout and resilience among nurses practicing in high-intensity settings. *American Journal of Critical Care, 24*(5), 412–421. http://dx.doi.org/10.4037/ajcc2015291

Rushton, C. H., Schoonover-Shoffner, K., & Kennedy, S. M. (2017). Executive summary: Transforming moral distress into moral resilience. *American Journal of Nursing, 117*(2), 52–56. https://doi.org/10.1097/01.NAJ.0000512298.18641.31.Executive

Splaine, M., Nelson, W., & Gardent, P. (2012). Editorial: Broadening implementation of a preventive ethics approach. *The Joint Commission Journal on Quality and Patient Safety, 38*(3), 99–102. https://doi.org/10.1016/S1553-7250(12)38013-6

Truog, R. D., Brown, S. D., Browning, D., Hundert, E. M., Rider, E. A., Bell, S. K., & Meyer, E. C. (2015). Microethics: The ethics of everyday clinical practice. *Hastings Center Report, 45*(1), 11–17. https://doi.org/10.1002/hast.413

Ulrich, C. M., O'Donnell, P., Taylor, C., Farrar, A., Danis, M., & Grady, C. (2007). Ethical climate, ethics stress, and the job satisfaction of nurses and social workers in the United States. *Social Science and Medicine, 65*(8), 1708–1719. Retrieved from http://www.ncbi.nlm.nih.gov/pubmed/17619068

Ulrich, C. M., Taylor, C., Soeken, K., O'Donnell, P., Farrar, A., Danis, M., & Grady, C. (2010). Everyday ethics: Ethical issues and stress in nursing practice. *Journal of Advanced Nursing, 66*(11), 2510–2519. https://doi.org/10.1111/j.1365-2648.2010.05425.x

Vanlaere, L., Coucke, T., & Gastmans, C. (2010). Experiential learning of empathy in a care-ethics lab. *Nursing Ethics, 17*(3), 325–336. https://doi.org/10.1177/0969733010361440

Wald, H. (2015). Professional identity (trans)formation in medical education: Reflection, relationship, resilience. *Academic Medicine, 90*(6), 701–706. https://doi.org/10.1097/ACM.0000000000000731

Walker, M. U. (1993). Keeping moral space open: New images of ethics consulting. *The Hastings Center Report, 23*(2), 33–40. https://doi.org/10.2307/3562818

Willis, D. G., Grace, P. J., & Roy, C. (2008). A central unifying focus for the discipline. *Advances in Nursing Science, 31*(1), E28–E40. https://doi.org/10.1097/01.ANS.0000311534.04059.d9

Woods, M. (2005). Nursing ethics education: Are we really delivering the good(s)? *Nursing Ethics, 12*(1), 5–18. https://doi.org/10.1191/0969733005ne754oa

Chapter 3
The History, Language and Tools of Ethics: Application in Healthcare Settings

Pamela J. Grace and Aimee Milliken

Abstract In this Chapter we provide some history behind the contemporary use of ethics language and tools in healthcare settings. We discuss the relationships among philosophical inquiry, moral theory, applied ethics, professional ethics, and ethical decision making frameworks and associated tools. This background context provides a foundation for understanding in which cases, for which purposes, and under which conditions philosophical inquiry, moral theories and principles help us promote individual and/or societal good. Discussed in turn are the historical development of medicine and healthcare professions, the nascent discipline of Bioethics, and? the relationships of philosophical inquiry and 'language of ethics' to healthcare goals. A nuanced discussion of moral principles and their application is provided. Finally, some practical decision-making frameworks and strategies are introduced. These are meant to be helpful to the point-of-care clinicians, nurse educators and leaders, and to others who provide services supportive of healthy work environments and good patient care.

3.1 History of Bioethics: Role of Philosophy and the Humanities

3.1.1 History of Medicine: Goods and Harms

Although the existence of 'physicians', or healers of human maladies of various sorts, is traceable back to the ancient Greeks in the Western World and to a similar time frame in the Eastern World, the extent of these healers' powers to cure was somewhat limited. They used drugs to manage pain and assorted signs and symptoms along with other strategies such as acupuncture in the East and trepanning (making

---

P. J. Grace (✉) · A. Milliken
William F. Connell School of Nursing, Boston College, Chestnut Hill, MA, USA
e-mail: Gracepa@bc.edu

A. Milliken
e-mail: aimee.milliken@bc.edu

© The Author(s), under exclusive license to Springer Nature B.V. 2022
P. Grace and A. Milliken (eds.), *Clinical Ethics Handbook for Nurses*, The International Library of Bioethics 93,
https://doi.org/10.1007/978-94-024-2155-2_3

a hole in the cranium) in the West. Trepanning in early times was used to relieve 'evil spirits' but sometimes provided relief from cerebral pressure (Faria, 2015). Herbs and physical interventions such as these could work to the benefit of persons when based on consistent observations, for example, the use of Willow bark for pain which has aspirin-like properties. However, they could also be harmful when used indiscriminately or when based on unproven beliefs, custom or folklore rather than consistent observations. For example, bloodletting was based on the belief that the four humors of the body (blood, phlegm, yellow bile and black bile) were out of balance and releasing blood could restore the balance. Hippocrates (often cited as the father of medicine) and later Galen (129–200 AD) (Greenstone, 2010) promoted this theory based on their findings from anatomical dissections. However, Hippocrates also proposed that the practice of medicine was moral in nature involving attention to the good (wellbeing) of others and included a concern for humanity. He wrote that one must also anticipate and safeguard against possible harms to the person being treated (Askitopoulou & Vgontzas, 2018). This idea has been since captured in the Latin saying "Primum Non Nocere" meaning first do no harm and which is incorporated into modern day Oaths taken by physicians. It signifies a general acknowledgement that in the course of trying to provide the good of medical care to someone, harms of various sorts can be caused. Beauchamp and Childress (2019) identify this as the principle of nonmaleficence as discussed in more detail shortly.

In contemporary times we are aware that treatments meant to cure physical or psychological ills can, in some situations, actually cause more harm than benefit and their effective use depends upon a variety of factors including the considered desires and preferences of individual persons. At the writing of this chapter the world is being overmastered by COVID-19 as named by the World Health Organization (2020). The acronym stands for corona virus disease of 2019. While some experiencing the virus have mild symptoms, a significant proportion experience acute and in some cases refractory respiratory distress requiring prolonged use of mechanical ventilation which is sometimes successful and sometimes, especially in the presence of multiple organ failure, just prolongs suffering. Thus, it has become more important than ever to inform persons of the possible trajectory of their illness given other factors such as age and co-morbid conditions and to solicit their wishes in anticipation of a rapid deterioration. Of course, a confounding reason for increased interest in eliciting preferences for treatment in the context of this catastrophic pandemic is the shortage of ventilators and a scarcity of other resources such as hospital beds, protective equipment, healthcare providers and so on. More on this problem and the issue of individual versus social good and of the critical importance of remaining transparent in our decision-making is in later chapters. Truog et al. (2020) article, *The toughest triage: Allocating ventilators in a pandemic,* provides a good discussion of the issue.

3.1.2 Scientific Advances and the Beginnings of Modern Medicine

The advancement of medical knowledge from Ancient to Medieval times proceeded slowly and often relied on unproven theories. In the Western world scientific development, in general, was hampered by the strong belief, reinforced by religious leaders, that the earth upon which human beings live is the center of the universe around which everything else including the sun revolves. Having this perspective worked for centuries against theorizing about alternate explanations that could then be explored and tested empirically—to challenge this view was considered heresy and could lead to punishment, banishment or even death. To gain a broader view about the natural world and its physical laws, science "had to break through the constraints of an outdated worldview that had permeated even the most basic observational description" (Godfrey-Smith, 2003, p. 114) distorting it.

The astrological observations of Copernicus, supported several decades later by Galileo's observation of the sky using a telescope he invented, toppled the prior paradigm and opened the way to a new view of the world and how it worked. Copernicus died before his work was published and thus avoided punishment, Galileo, however, was sentenced to life imprisonment. It took some time for his ideas to be accepted. However, gradually it became acknowledged there are immutable laws governing the natural world that could allow prediction (Lange, 1999). Understanding these laws permits human beings to envisage future events and, in some cases, control them. In turn, progress in the natural sciences led to ideas about the possibility of improvement in the human condition. Thus medical science also progressed, although not all medical practices were based on rigorous scientific research, perhaps because of the recognition that physical explanations could not predict individual differences in a person's physical response because of the confounding influences of concurrent physical, psychological, and contextual factors. Throughout the 19th Century and into the 20th Century the idea that both doctors and nurses had responsibilities to patients began to be discussed in more detail as these occupations developed into modern professions, at least in many developed countries.

3.1.3 Professional Ethics

The responsibilities of both physicians and nurses are ethical in nature because they are about providing a service or 'good' to patients and depend on having a knowledge and skill base and an intention to provide the services that are the reason professions exist. In general, physicians and nurses were and are trusted to know and provide what is needed for an individual's health and wellbeing, or to relieve suffering. Medicine, along with ministry and law, developed from religious orders in the Middle Ages. These bodies have been considered professions longer than other providers of healthcare services. The term 'profession' derives from Middle

English and denotes the vows taken while entering religious orders (Windt, 1989). The meaning of the term 'profession' has evolved over time and is often used loosely to describe various skilled as well as academically based vocations. While there is no single agreed upon definition of modern human service professions, they are generally supposed to be self-organized bodies that have some control over their practices. Flexner (2015), an educator, was worried about the lack of rigor and consistency in medical education and saw the need to improve medical curricula. His rigorous study of medical education in the US and Canada led to the Flexner Report (2015). In it he proposed "that professions have an extensive and specialized knowledge base, take responsibility for developing and using their knowledge, (and) have a practice or action orientation" (Grace, 2018, p. 43). Professions set their own standards for practice giving them some autonomy over the scope, boundaries, and nature of their services. Additionally, they have a lengthy education process that results in the provision of services rather than goods (Kepler, 1981). In a sense professions 'promise' that they can meet unmet needs in a society, and what has been termed a 'social contract' exists between the profession and the society served (Grace, 2018). These promises are implicitly attached to healthcare professional practice and are also often explicitly articulated in codes of ethics. Most importantly, there is an accountability assumed by members of a profession about how services should be provided, and they are answerable to the society they serve. In Chapter 1, we delineated the meaning of ethics for the professions of nursing and medicine. Here we focus on tracing the development of Bioethics as a relatively new discipline that could aid in resolving ethical dilemmas given birth by the rapid development of biotechnological advances that occurred during the mid-20th Century.

3.1.3.1 Medical Ethics

As described in more detail in Chapter 1, Medical ethics was historically the field of inquiry about good medical practice and the desired characteristics of physicians. Among the first to talk specifically about 'medical ethics', according to McCullough (1998) were Scottish physicians John Gregory (1724–1173) and Thomas Percival (1740–1804). Percival authored a book titled *Medical Ethics* in 1803. In this he discussed physician responsibilities to patients and each other as well as the need to uphold public trust (Jonsen, 1998). So Medical Ethics was about delineating and refining guiding standards for the practice of medicine. Standards were determined largely by physicians themselves a small proportion of whom also had backgrounds in philosophy or the humanities. Physicians in many countries have developed their own codes of ethics. These tend to be based in ideals common across medical practice, as well as having culturally or societally specific provisions. Additionally the World Medical Association (WMA) adopted a code of ethics in 1949—partly influenced by atrocities of WWII in which some German Physicians were complicit in unethical and even torturous practices. The WMA code of ethics has been amended several times the latest being 2006 (WMA, 2020). How then did Medical Ethics as a field of inquiry come to include the input of scholars from the humanities and how did it undergo a metamorphosis into Biomedical ethics and later Bioethics? Albert Jonsen (1998), in his book *The Birth of Bioethics* provides a meticulous account of this move. He was among the philosophers whose input was sought to resolve the dilemmas and complex issues incurred by the rapid advance of biotechnology.

3.1.4 The Beginnings of Bioethics

The term Bioethics, as noted by Reich (1995) was coined by Van Rensselaer-Potter, a research oncologist. His idea was for a field of study in ethics that accounted for the health of both humans and the "biosphere as a whole" (Kuhse & Singer, 2006, p. 1); he was interested in human survival (Whitehouse, 2003). However, as Reich (1994) notes, others such as Hellegers a Dutch Obstetrician and one of the founders of the Kennedy Institute of Ethics at Georgetown University began to use "the term more narrowly to apply to the ethics of medicine and biomedical research… I was also aware, at the outset, that Potter's use of the term "bioethics" was marginalized, whereas the Hellegers/Georgetown biomedical connotation of the word came to dominate the emerging field of bioethics in academic circles and in the mind of the public" (p. 334). For Hellegers, bioethics would be a unique discipline drawing on scientific advances, medical science and moral philosophy (Reich, 1994) to explore contemporary problems especially as these related to medical research and practice.

For clarity, a *discipline* is generally understood to be a field of inquiry as opposed to a *profession* which is action or practice oriented and has a set of implicit or explicit goals to which actions are directed. A discipline when associated with professional practice, is generally understood as the knowledge development arm for the practice of a science or a profession (Donaldson & Crowley, 1978; Keiner, 2002). For professions, ideally, the discipline's scholars work to 'fill-in' knowledge for those areas of practice about which not much is known. Inevitably the discipline and the practice inform each other. Scholars in a practice discipline cannot provide knowledge for the profession in the absence of the insights of the practitioners about what is needed to practice well.

Bioethics, then, is not itself, generally considered a practice or profession so much as a field of inquiry, however the practice of clinical ethics and ethics consultation has developed as an offspring of the larger project of Bioethics. This movement is discussed in more detail in Chapter 6. Kopelman (2009) brought attention to this idea that Bioethics is a discipline that does not have a directly related practice arm. Rather Bioethics comprises scholars from a multitude of disciplines and bioethics is a secondary discipline for many. What she means is that physicians, nurses, chaplains etc. have as primary their originating profession and secondarily an interest in bioethics most often as a result of problems encountered in practice.

The impetus for the development of Bioethics as a discipline was the result of various events. Albert Jonsen (1998), a philosopher and theologian, as noted earlier, was among the early non-medical scholars co-opted into assisting physicians to resolve emerging healthcare dilemmas. A *true dilemma* is a problem that has no discernable right or best answer. In healthcare, true dilemmas exist, but explorations of a dilemmatic problem may reveal one option to be more ethically sound than another. Regardless, it is important to explore what appear to be dilemmas in order to find the fairest or most just answer either for the individuals involved or for the society. Jonsen (1998) describes how the rapid progress of biotechnological innovations since the turn of the century, and particularly since WWII, led to ethical problems in healthcare that could not be effectively explored or answered by medical clinicians alone.

One reason for this was that such advances had societal implications going beyond the individual physician–patient relationship. Physicians for the most part simply did not have the type of educational background or skills to address such questions as how to best allocate scarce resources. Jonsen's (1998) book is recommended for those wishing a more detailed account of the development of bioethics up to 1998. Bioethics has become a generally accepted term internationally, for the study of ethical problems arising in healthcare, including research settings, although universal agreement about the nature and essential aspects of the discipline is not discernable across countries in part because of local differences (Holm & Williams-Jones, 2006).

The new discipline of Bioethics, sometimes referred to, at least in the early years, as biomedical ethics, emerged after WWII. The advent of WWII (1939–1945) brought about exponential increases in biological and technological innovations. These increases occurred for variety of reasons: to remedy the physical damage caused by modern weapons, as a result of experiments conducted by many countries ostensibly to safeguard combatants, and in the interests of national security (Moreno, 2015). Applications of biotechnological advances in the context of healthcare gave rise to new sorts of quandaries that were beyond the ability of the medical community to resolve on its own. Medical education and expertise is clinical in nature, and medical practice is largely focused on the care of individual patients. However, medical ethics, as discussed previously and in earlier chapters had historically been concerned with the proper education and conduct of physicians in relation to their patients or practice area. As Pellegrino and Thomasma (2004), note it stems from "a philosophy of medicine in which the good of the patient determines the obligations and virtues of the health professional" (p. 17). That is, it is about how physicians should address patient needs and what physicians' responsibilities to patients are related to helping them get what is needed for their cure or comfort. It was understood that physicians were not, in general skilled in evaluating philosophical, social, or moral questions that attend contemporary biotechnological innovations, as these were not a focus of medical education at the time. Yet, the rapid development of biotechnology and its applications to human disease and incapacity, were posing just these sorts of questions. The complexity of such problems, as "who should receive dialysis in the context of scarce availability of dialysis machines"? warranted the analyses of those skilled in unpacking complex problems and exploring aspects of social justice. These were life and death issues that went beyond medical expertise to resolve. Deeper explorations were needed to understand how to account for both the ethical care of individual patients and the interests of society. The question of justice in allocating scarce resources required critical analyses from those trained in philosophical inquiry and its associated techniques.

Some of the initial foci of bioethical inquiry, such as how to fairly allocate scarce dialysis machines, have more or less reached resolution as more machines became available and in-depth analyses resulted in helpful decision-making frameworks. However, exponential advances in biotechnology, genetics and other contemporary innovations continue to raise new dilemmas that have both clinical and social implications. The current (as of this writing) Global COVID-19 pandemic exemplifies the need for an 'all hands-on deck' approach to resolution. In the US at least, but almost certainly elsewhere also, it is often the least well off and most disadvantaged who are at the highest risk of serious illness and death. All of the following are needed to curb the spread and preserve the most lives: healthcare and public health professionals, sociopolitical critique, philosophic inquiry, political will, and public understanding.

3.2 Relationship of Moral Philosophy and Moral Theory to Healthcare and Nursing Goals

Central to the discipline of Bioethics is an understanding of moral theory. Moral theories develop from centuries of philosophical inquiry into what is the meaning of 'good' in human life and in human interactions with the world. This branch of philosophy is called moral philosophy. Philosophy is the encompassing discipline that seeks to understand the nature of the world, its origins, and the place or human beings within it. Philosophical inquiry has several branches including moral philosophy, epistemology which is about knowledge, logic which is about reasoning, metaphysics which is about questions that cannot be resolved by empirical observations such as the nature and causes of existence and others.

For Centuries philosophers and theologians have been engaged in the project of theorizing about the beginnings and nature of the world, its underlying structure and humankind's place within it and more recently the nature and meaning that 'existence' holds for persons. In the words of Nagel (1987) another concern of philosophy "is to question and understand very common ideas that all of us use every day" (p. 5) but without giving a thought to their deeper meanings. As noted, our concern here is with the relationships among moral philosophy, moral theorizing and professional ethical responsibility. Moral philosophy is the field of inquiry that explores the meaning of 'good' and its relationship to human action. Since Ancient Greek times in the West and a similar time frame in the East philosophers have theorized about whether there is or could be an absolute good towards which all human beings should strive in order to live well (given or designed by a power that is outside of or 'above' the human world). This has been termed the "summum bonum" or the ultimate good. They have questioned whether, if such a good exists, can we discern what it is and if not what sort of framework would help people live together and flourish (a social construction).

Theories developed from these philosophical inquiries about the good are called moral theories. "It is, however, important to remember that these insights are always necessarily influenced" by the political and social contexts of the times within which these philosophers lived and their "conscious or unconscious motivations for trying to make sense of the world" (Grace, 2018, p. 10). One thing that is broadly recognized is that moral theories necessarily differ from one another in significant ways and can give conflicting direction in particular cases or situations because they are based in different belief systems. For such reasons, ethical decision-making in healthcare settings almost never relies exclusively on one moral theory to direct actions. Rather, determining what is in the best interest of a given patient serves as the focus or anchor and principles derived from moral theories can help us gain clarity related to we might consider in our deliberations. However, in cases where scarce resources are the issue the best interests of groups of patients may change the focus of ethical analysis.

Nevertheless, moral theories provide insights related to ethical decision-making in healthcare settings. When their limits and flaws are understood, they and the principles derived from them can help us think carefully about what is at stake, what are important considerations and why.

3.3 Moral Theory and Ethical Principles: Purpose, Scope and Limits in Healthcare

Two normative moral theories that are considered especially important in shedding light on problems occurring within contemporary health care settings are deontology and consequentialism. A normative theory is one that essentially says if this theory is correct then we are committed to act as the theory directs in order to promote a good. The proponents of these normative theories were influenced by the times in which they lived. Thus they should not be straightforwardly applied in contemporary times without understanding sociopolitical and value differences. A brief discussion of two (among many) of these theories highlights how they can give different directions for action.

3.3.1 Deontology

Duty-based theories are those based in the idea that there are certain rules which if followed by everyone will result in good or 'right' actions. Duty-based theories may either use religious precepts as foundational, for example, the Ten Commandments or, as in Immanuel Kant's (1724–1804) writings, the idea that man is a rational animal and can make moral rules that if applied universally lead to good actions. The Deontological theoretical stance focuses on something other than consequences as the main consideration in decision-making. It argues for the critical importance of treating individual human beings with equal moral respect. They are either worthy of moral respect because of a religious precept, or because they are rational animals who can use reason determine what morally appropriate actions are in a given situation. But because everyone is to be treated as of equal moral worth, they should never be treated merely as a means for someone else's ends (Kant 1967/1785). It is beyond this chapter's scope to explain in detail Kant's very precise and meticulous exploration of man's capacity for reasoned decision-making and why this ability makes each individual human being worthy of moral respect. Suffice it to say, Kant argued that a human being by virtue of possessing the capacity to reason has a duty to use reason to determine the correct action(s) for a particular circumstance (Kant (1967/1785). Likely as a result of beliefs during that historical period, Kant did not include women and children in the class of persons who have the absolute ability to reason—this is partly attributable to the era he lived in. Nevertheless the potential for reason permits women at least to be included in the idea of freedom to choose and moral worth (Varden, 2017). The rule that allows good/right (accords with duty) decision-making is the *Categorical Imperative*. The Categorical Imperative is in essence a formula or structure that can be used to determine right actions. Roughly stated, a person can ask themselves would I be okay with anyone else taking the action that I am about to take in my current context and circumstances. If the answer is 'no' then I am not justified in taking the action. In fact, I am morally obligated not to take the action. As an example, "would I be justified in lying to someone"? The answer is that it would not be reasonable to do so because if everyone lied we would not be able to rely on what anyone says, and this is irrational. As an example of how this might be used in practice, Ms. J with stage 4 breast cancer asks me "is this serious?" it would be wrong on a Kantian view for me to say no as lying: a) does not treat her with respect and b) we would not be able to use as a universal rule that it is okay to lie to cancer patients when they ask us about their prognosis. One critique of deontologic theories is that they may work well in abstract circumstances but when it comes to an individual, harm may be caused (this consequence is not as important to a deontologist as following a generally reasonable rule). For example, if I tell the truth in a way that does not account for the negative effect it will have on the person in question, I might cause harm to the person and in healthcare settings we are ethically responsible for trying to minimize harms. Another critique is that the rules can be quite abstract and not provide guidance in a complex situation for which multiple aspects are in play. Finally, we might agree that every person should be treated with dignity and equal moral worth as everyone else, but not agree that any of us makes totally objective decisions. We are all influenced by a host of other factors conscious and subconscious.

3.3.2 Consequentialism

With consequentialist moral theories the important aspects have to do both with the results of actions and the extent to which good consequences are spread across both persons and groups of persons. Good actions are defined as those that have good consequences. Perhaps the best-known consequentialist theories are those of the Utilitarians, Jeremy Bentham (1748–1832) and John Stuart Mill (1806–1873). Bentham and later Mill were heavily influenced by the ideas of Scottish philosopher David Hume (1711–1776). Hume is thought to have introduced the idea of a utility principle. This principle represents the idea that "human responses are fortified in relation to the usefulness of their actions to others and the pleasure gained from this" (Grace, 2018.p. 14.). Bentham and Mill were social reformers, as well as philosophers. They were concerned with social problems caused by the industrial revolution in England. A few people had a lot of power (factory owners and the like) and masses of people were living in poverty. Conditions for the majority of people were dire.

As noted in the Stanford Encyclopedia of Philosophy (2014),

> Utilitarianism is also distinguished by impartiality and agent-neutrality. Everyone's happiness counts the same. When one maximizes the good, it is the good impartially considered. My good counts for no more than anyone else's good. Further, the reason I have to promote the overall good is the same reason anyone else has to so promote the good. It is not peculiar to me. (The History of Utilitarianism, para 4)

Two important points about utilitarianism from Mill's point of view is that happiness or pleasure, two forms of "good," are not surface level but involves qualitative components, such as the ability to live a good life including the pursuit of intellectual pleasures. The second point is that pleasure is cumulative across society. Hence the popularized saying that "the greatest good for the greatest number". Criticisms of utilitarian ideas include that it might be permissible to ignore one person's good if several other people would benefit (Grace, 2018). Again, in healthcare settings our goals are to provide for individual good and minimize the impact of necessary harms on individuals.

The tension between these moral theories is visible during our current pandemic. Healthcare providers are, for the most part, involved in and concerned with the wellbeing of individuals. The Codes of Ethics of the various professions stress this as an obligation of professional practice. However, when there are not enough healthcare providers to attend to each person, or not enough resources to be distributed as in a pandemic, Utilitarian ideas tend to underlie public health ethics which prevail in crisis triage situations.

Both deontologic and consequentialist theories "provide important insights about human values and characteristics: Utilitarianism for its ability to critique social justice and deontology for its implications that there are general rules that all (cognitively able) people can agree upon" (Grace, 2018, p. 16) as well as its emphasis on the moral worth of each individual human being.

Moral theories of social justice — which are discussed in more depth in *: Social Justice, disparities, and nursing responsibilities*—call attention to the idea that in a pandemic situation it is often the least well off who suffer the most as a result of structural inequities and racism. It is well documented that the poor and otherwise disadvantaged, are disproportionately likely to experience chronic illnesses and thus be most vulnerable to viruses such as COVID-19.

3.3.3 Moral or Ethical Principles in Healthcare Decision-Making

The use of moral theories, perspectives and the principles derived from them in the process of healthcare decision-making whether on the individual or societal level is called applied ethics. We have proposed that while moral theories can provide some insights into what is important in human lives, they cannot be uncritically applied to decision-making in healthcare settings because of their respective flaws. What then about the roles of ethical or moral principles (we treat ethical and moral as equivalent concepts related to healthcare practice)? How can ethical principles be useful in resolving the thorny problems that arise in contemporary healthcare? Ethical principles are derived from a variety of places but mostly from different moral theories. Some of the principles include autonomy, beneficence, non-maleficence, and justice. They tend to have stood the test of time in helping humans live well together. Depending on culture, certain principles may be prioritized over others. For example, in the Western World the value of the principle of autonomy tends to be prioritized, however, in the Eastern World different principles are prioritized. For example, Tai (2013) writes,

> Confucian scholars believe that any principle without compassion as a base cannot endure. The eastern teachings regard internal virtues as the foundation of morality that spontaneously motivate a person to act in an ethical way. Without having this inner drive, any regulations, principles or law are but superficial. Eastern society also regards family as a basic unity therefore, familial autonomy is more important than individual autonomy. (p. 64)

This Eastern perspective is especially congruent for nurses who work closely with patients and see them in all of their individuality and context. Compassion and empathy are highly valued by the profession as characteristics that help to 'humanize' the often cold and sterile environments in which healthcare is provided.

Additionally, ethical principles can provide conflicting directions as discussed shortly. The role of ethical principles in healthcare settings, then, is to draw our attention to important considerations in a particular case or situation. They help us examine in more depth than we otherwise might, the implication of certain actions. However related to individuals, it is the particular goals of the profession—the reason the profession exists—in concert with knowledge of the patient's preferences and goals that serve as the anchor for further clarity and analysis. Ethical principles allow us to probe in some depth the nuances of a case. They stimulate us to gather more facts or clarify the values and biases of those involved. Professional goals provide motivation for action. We provide some decision-making heuristics shortly that can help with unpacking difficult situations in order to understand them better.

3.3.4 The Georgetown Principles

Four ethical principles that are useful in healthcare settings have been described in-depth by philosophers Beauchamp and Childress who taught at Georgetown University in Washington DC and were affiliated with the Kennedy Institute of Ethics. The first edition of their book *Principles of Biomedical Ethics* was published in 1977 (Beauchamp & Childress, 2019) and at the writing of this handbook is in its 8th Edition. Described below briefly are these four principles that have become widely relied upon in the settings of clinical and professional ethics. Additionally, we add two principles that are important for nurses and those who work closely with patients, these are veracity and fidelity. Later we also discuss how other philosophical perspectives such as feminism and critical social theory can broaden our view of the nature and origins of ethical issues that emerge in the healthcare environment. The principles of autonomy, beneficence, nonmaleficence and justice as fairness are the focus of Beauchamp and Childress' book. For good communication among clinicians and other members of the healthcare team, it is important that all persons involved understand in what sense the term is being used. When unsure, a good rule of thumb is to ask.

3.3.4.1 Autonomy

The principle of autonomy is more complex than is generally understood. Its origins are in the Greek language and, straightforwardly, 'autonomy' means self-rule. Originally the term referred to the self-governance of towns but gradually came to denote individual self-governance. This change in meaning became strengthened as a result of Immanuel Kant's theory. The concept can be viewed in two ways depending on context. The first sense of autonomy is about according a person respect simply because they are a human being, "regardless of who they are, where they come from or what they have done" (Grace, 2018, p. 18). In essence, the idea that human beings all have moral worth as individuals has been argued from religious, philosophical, and secular perspectives and underlies conceptions of human rights. At its most basic this means that persons should not be treated as less than fully human as has happened in the past. For example, slavery treats persons as means to another's ends, not as individually important. Indeed, for Kant punishing a criminal by restricting their freedom still upholds the principle because it ensures that they are accountable for their autonomously chosen actions (Fleischacker, 2009), however this logic cannot be applied to the enslavement of groups of people. Treating people or groups of people as if they are not worth as much as others has led to past atrocities. We are all at risk of becoming among the members of a group considered not morally worthy.

Indeed, most of our arguments about human rights rely on this sense of the principle of autonomy. For nurses, this first sense of autonomy tells us essentially not to judge the worth of patients based upon our assessment of their past or present behavior or presentation. While this can be hard to do, nevertheless, it frees us to treat everyone with respect and means we do not have to evaluate who is worthy of our good care and who is not.

The second sense of autonomy is also informed by Kant's moral theory. It is the right to make personal decisions because as human beings we have the ability to reason and make rational (good) decisions as a result of that facility. Additionally, we might be supposed to know ourselves better than anyone else does. Finally, this right respects our autonomy in the first sense as described above. It respects us as individuals with individual goals and values. This second sense of autonomy underlies such actions as informed consent to treatment, privacy, and confidentiality. "However, autonomy is often interpreted by nurses and others as the right to make bad healthcare decisions. This is a distorted view (Grace, 2018, p. 19). Patients, for the most part do not have our knowledge base and/or they may have trouble processing information because of physical or psychological impairments, as examples: lack of oxygen, delirium, dementia. Thus, they cannot necessarily be expected to make the best decisions for themselves without our help. In the US, the *President's Commission for the study of Ethical Problems in Medicine* (1982) formulated a minimum set of capacities needed for patient decision-making capacity. The person should evidence:

- Possession of a set of values and goals.
- The ability to communicate and understand information.
- The ability to reason and deliberate about one's choice (p. 57).

For those who do not meet the criteria for autonomous decision-making, their autonomy is supported either by a surrogate who knows the person's wishes and desires, written instructions prepared in advance of loss of capacity, seeking to understand how the patient has lived his or her life and so on. In some instances, this information can be difficult to ascertain, particularly in the absence of a surrogate. Later Chapters take up the issue of decision-making capacity and surrogate decision-making.

3.3.4.2 Non-Maleficence and Beneficence

These principles are often described together, or in the case of *The Belmont Report* (1979) in the US that details the ethical treatment of research subjects, the principle of beneficence includes the injunction to do no harm (nonmaleficence). Nonmaleficence is "closely associated with the maxim primum non nocere: Above all (or first) do no harm" (Beauchamp & Childress, 2009, p. 149). In the world outside of healthcare nonmaleficence means not doing intentional harm to others. However, in healthcare settings it is recognized that some harms are necessary in order to do good. On balance, however, the potential harms should be considered proportional to the likely benefits. For example, surgery involves invasive procedures which by definition cause harm to bodily integrity. Hydrating a patient, requires the placement of a gastric tube or an intravenous (IV) cannula. Getting someone out of bed for the first time after surgery can be very painful. So nonmaleficence cannot be merely about not intentionally harming someone. Nonmaleficence can be considered a negative principle, meaning it sometimes requires withholding actions that may, on balance, be more harmful than helpful for the patient. Nonmaleficence for healthcare providers, then means all of the following:

- Accurately assessing for unmet needs or failing to protect from harm (for example, assessing a patient for risk of falls).
- Balancing benefits of treatments over potential harms caused (getting a post-surgery patient out of bed to prevent complications that might lead to death outweighs the pain caused).
- Protecting the patient from the incompetent or careless actions of others.
- Helping a patient resist pressure from others to accept treatment that is not in alignment with their values and preferences.
- Anticipating and minimizing the potential for harm (for example, providing pain medications before getting a post-surgery patient out of bed, addressing a patient's fear of injections).
- Addressing a patient's decision that is not in-line with their own best interests due to inadequate information or cognitive impairment.

The principle of beneficence is in a sense, a more positive principle. This principle supports the idea that we have obligations to benefit others; in other words we must take action to accomplish a "good." As Beauchamp and Childress (2009) note, it "connotes acts of mercy, kindness, and charity" (p. 23) towards others. As discussed earlier, the principle of utility described by David Hume and then taken up by Bentham and Mill, stresses the important for human beings of the pursuit of happiness and avoidance of pain (Mill, 1965/1861). However, while utilitarianism is about maximizing overall benefits to groups or societies, beneficence in healthcare is about providing a good for an individual in terms of their health or wellbeing. Thus beneficence, in a sense, is about upholding the goals of the healthcare profession to provide the 'good' promised by way of the profession's self-determined goals, codes of ethics, and practice standards. This means that members of the healthcare profession have stronger duties to patients when acting within their roles than they would normally have towards others in everyday life.

Beneficence is the duty in healthcare to maximize benefits and minimize harms for patients. This necessarily means that we treat people as individuals whose contexts, influences, values, and preferences are mostly unique to them. The principle of beneficence is also sometimes called the 'best interest' principle because when a person has lost decision-making capacity (the ability to make autonomous decisions as described above), and we have no evidence of their prior wishes (either stated or written) we must try to ascertain what action would achieve the most benefit. "Under the best interest standard. A surrogate decision maker must determine the highest net benefit among available actions, assigning different weights to interests the patient has in each option and discounting or subtracting inherent risks or costs" (Beauchamp & Childress, 2009, p. 102). When healthcare providers are evaluating what is being proposed as good for, or the most beneficent action, for someone who cannot speak for themself, or has temporarily or permanently lost capacity this is called *Paternalism*. Beauchamp and Childress (2009) argue that paternalistic actions in health care are only warranted if:

1. The patient is at risk of a significant preventable harm.
2. The paternalistic action will probably prevent the harm.
3. The projected benefits … outweigh its risk to the patient.
4. There is no reasonable alternative.
5. (It is) the least autonomy-restrictive alternative… (p. 216).

Paternalism in healthcare is meant to protect the vulnerable from harm but can also be misused as it can in general life. Someone a physician, nurse or family member may decide that they know better than the person what will benefit that person. Such decisions need careful consideration about a person's capacity for making a task-related decision as described in the section above on autonomy.

3.3.4.3 Justice as Fairness

This is the fourth principle in Beauchamp and Childress' (2009) lexicon. We discuss the ethical responsibilities associated with different perspectives on justice in more detail in Chapter 12. "There are two broadly socially oriented ideas regarding justice" (Grace, 2018, p. 25). The first is that meritorious people should be rewarded for their talents, diligence, and efforts. However, some persons have had all the opportunities needed to contribute to society, whereas others have been disadvantaged in a variety of way such as impoverished childhoods, lack of support, victims of violence and this has undermined their ability to be moral agents (Blacksher, 2002). Relying on merit then as a way to distribute the benefits and burdens of societal living further disadvantages the already least well off. A different view proposed by John Rawls (1971) in his theory of justice. Rawls' theory takes into account that people may be disadvantaged by society in various ways. Rawls relies on Kant's concept that human beings are in essence rational beings. He constructs a hypothetical account of what justice would look like in a society if members of that society did not know what talents, impediments, access to material goods and standing they would have. He postulated that from this group would emerge two rules that would protect them should they be among the least well off. "First: each person is to have an equal right to the most extensive liberty compatible with a similar liberty for others. Second: social and economic inequalities are to be arranged such that they are both (a) reasonably expected to be to everyone's advantage, and (b) attached to positions and offices open to all" (Rawls, 1971, p. 60). A newer conception of social justice is that of Powers and Faden (2006). They argue that a comprehensive theory of social justice is not possible. What we should be doing as healthcare providers is using ideas of injustice to try and discover what sorts of things get in the way of a person being able to live a minimally decent life. These perspectives on justice are taken up in more detail in Chapter (xxx) and exemplified with cases.

3.3.4.4 Veracity and Fidelity

Veracity or the need to be truthful is important for all healthcare professionals. It is perhaps especially important for nurses. As a rule, we spend more time at the bedside than others. We are privy to the stories of patients and their families. They often turn to us for clearer more comprehendible accounts of what they have been told. They entrust us with their stories, and they rely on us to be truthful. Not being truthful or even the perception of a lack of truthfulness undermines their trust in the profession. When trust is undermined a patient may not reveal to us information that will help us to help them. However, being truthful is often not as easy as it sounds. Beauchamp and Childress (2009) note, "veracity in the health care setting refers to comprehensive, accurate, and objective transmission of information, as well as to the way the professional fosters the patient's or subject's understanding" (p. 289). But as we know stark truthfulness can sometimes be harmful to patients. Additionally, sometimes nurses do, and sometimes do not have the complete pathophysiological picture, nor a good understanding of possible courses of action. What we do have is our clinical judgment, ability to collaborate, access to evidence, knowledge of the patient (including cultural needs), and ethical decision-making frameworks (Grace, 2018). Transparency about what we know and what we do not is critically important as is the ability to reassure a patient that we will try to get them what they need to make a decision or understand what is going on with them. We need to be able to self-reflect on our biases and prejudices and the boundaries of our knowledge as well as reflecting on why the patient is asking of us what they are asking. We have to be careful not to make promises to patients that cannot be kept. For example, if a patient says something like "if I tell you something I have been worrying about will you promise not to tell"? our impetus might be to say yes. However, what if the patient tells you they are having suicidal thoughts? A better response would be, "I will keep your confidence but if there is a risk of harm to you, or others, I may need to tell someone who can help you."

So veracity is crucial to help patients trust us. Trust is needed for patients to reveal things that would allow us accurate assessments of their needs. Trust is the concept behind Fidelity. Fidelity means that we adhere to the tenets of our profession (the reason the profession exists) and can be trusted to do so. Persons in need of healthcare services are made more-than-usually vulnerable. They need our help because they are unable to meet their own healthcare needs. They are expecting that we will put their best interests first and foremost. Yet so many things can interfere with our ability to keep the good of the patient at the center of our activities. These can include pressures from administration, our colleagues, physicians, patients' family members among other distractions as discussed in Chapter 2.

3.4 Other Ethical Perspectives: Care, Feminist, Narrative, Virtue

Several other perspectives on ethical decision-making in health care allow for us to incorporate aspects that are not so clearly visible within historical moral theories or even the four principles. Especially important in nursing is the perspective of 'care'. The care perspective has been proposed as important for nurses coming as it does from a feminist understanding of the work of women and from Carol Gilligan's (2014) rebuttal to her mentor's Lawrence Kohlberg's work. Kohlberg (1981) derived a hierarchy of moral development from research with young men that postulates the highest level of moral reasoning to be one of impartialist justice. In impartialist theories of justice everyone is treated as the same as everyone else. Individual characteristics are not considerations. Kohlberg's work takes as a starting point the idea that, as in Immanuel Kant's theory, human beings are capable of objective reasoning and that allows them to determine the ethically correct action undistracted by other influences. Interestingly, women did not generally score as 'highly' on Kohlberg's scale as did men and this led to Gilligan's work on care. Gilligan (2014), proposed that women were more concerned with relationships and that, an.

> ethic of care, (is) grounded in voice and relationship, as an ethic of resistance both to injustice and to self-silencing. It is a human ethic, integral to the practice of democracy and to the functioning of a global society. More controversially, it is a feminist ethic, an ethic that guides the historic struggle to free democracy from patriarchy (Gilligan, 2011, p. 175).

Authors have defined 'care' variously. However, a simple definition that captures the meaning for nurses is a "focused attention on, and when possible engagement with, a patient to determine that person's particular needs and the use of clinical judgement to meet those needs" (Grace, 2018, p. 423).

An ethic of care and feminist standpoints are aligned in their point of view that women's perspectives are not respected or accorded equal importance with male viewpoints in contemporary discourse. Feminist philosophies inform feminist ethics perspectives of which there are several. While there is divergence related to certain aspects of the human condition, there is agreement that "moral decision-making must include an investigation of both hidden and overt power relationships implicit in ethical problems" (Grace, 2005, p. 105). Feminist ethics explorations have broadened to include oppression of other marginalized groups such as those who are poor, minorities, undocumented, or disabled. As noted in the Grace framework, feminist ethics adds to ethical analyses by asking us to consider how power relationships may play into decision-making. "Questions to pose from a feminist perspective… include: What are the power structures – social, institutional, or interpersonal? Is there an imbalance? Who has an interest in keeping the imbalance? How is this affecting the patient or the decision-making? How can we change the focus of power or empower the person who is the primary focus of the issue?" (Grace, 2018, p. 29).

Narrative ethics is another contemporary way of looking at ethical problems in healthcare. A narrative is a written or orally communicated story about connected events or experiences (Adams, 2008). A basic definition of narrative is a story that is being told that may have a discernable purpose, or a subconscious purpose. Narrative ethics, then, by definition is a story being told or elicited for the purpose of some sort of 'good'. Thus, what constitutes narrative ethics depends on purpose and setting. One may be using a narrative to: demonstrate a point to students, elicit different meanings and perspectives, understand better a patient's context and circumstances, resolve a conflict among persons and so on. Importantly there are no specific criteria for determining the 'moral' of a story. This makes narrative ethics somewhat amorphous as a method for resolving conflict and dilemmas (Charon et al., 2002) but can help gain clarity about the meaning the situation holds for the different players. In clinical ethics consults, narrative ensures that the perspective of each person is sought."Narrative approaches to ethics consultation deepen dialogue and stakeholders' engagement to reveal important values, preferences, and beliefs that may prove critical in resolving care challenges" (Childress et al, 2020).

What narrative ethics does, however, in the context of nursing practice, is focus on the patient and on eliciting and listening to the meaning of the present circumstance for the patient. Nurses actually use narrative without perhaps knowing what this is or what they are doing. Exploring a situational narrative means that we seek to include how each person who is involved views what is going on. "Narratives are stories of people's lives or situations told with rich detail and often from different perspectives" (Grace, 2018, p. 29). Eliciting a patient story means that we have to be careful not to impose our meaning on what the patient is saying but rather, reflect back as necessary what we think we heard. Narratives are not necessarily linear in process they often go back and forth. But deep listening with an intentional focus on what is the meaning that this situation holds for the person in question and perhaps associated persons, is the role of the elicitor. Narrative ethics is also used in teaching, and you will find it used throughout the book to facilitate understanding of aspects that might not have initially been considered. In teaching ethics we find that when students elaborate on why they are thinking a certain way, it allows their colleagues to broaden their moral horizons by trying to see the problem from their perspective.

One final perspective is that of virtue ethics. The idea behind virtue ethics is that persons who cultivate good habits will as a rule act well. It is beyond the ability of this book to describe virtue ethics in detail. However, we will be emphasizing how to develop characteristics that will enable us to be 'good nurses' wo can effectively advocate for the wellbeing of our patients. Chapters 2, 4 and 7 provide more discussion on how to develop the characteristics that lend themselves to habitual good actions.

3.5 Decision-Making Frameworks

Frameworks are available to assist nurses in their ethical decision-making whether this is a problem of everyday practice, a complex situation, or an ethical dilemma encountered by a nurse who is serving as a member of an ethics committee. These are best viewed as heuristics rather than progressing in a rigid linear fashion. While there is not always a good starting point, one way to begin is to recognize a situation that is worrying in some way. Exploring assumptions that are being made by the various stakeholders then allows one to see what is needed in the way of facts or questioning. In *Chapter 6, Models of Ethics Deliberation and Consultation*, several frameworks are discussed in enough detail that the reader can choose which is best to use for a particular issue that arises in practice.

3.6 Summary

Foundational to understanding the contemporary nature and tools of ethical decision making, we provided a sketch of how applied ethics for healthcare and for nurses developed from the discipline of philosophy. The most important takeaway from this chapter is the idea that the reason-for-being, goals, and perspectives of nursing provide the focus for navigating obstacles to good practice. Having this foundation, and developing one's comfort with the language and tools of ethics in addition to utilizing one's clinical knowledge permits effective communication of patient needs. It facilitates needed interdisciplinary collaborations when these are needed to overcome obstacles to good care.

3.7 Discussion Questions

The following questions are constructed to provide a foundation for facilitating self-reflection, reflection on prior and ongoing practice and in identifying needed ethics education and other resources that enable good healthcare and in practice and for society.

1. What are your prior preconceptions/assumptions about the scope and boundaries of your professional responsibilities to a) patients, b) communities and societies and how aligned are they with the ideas in this chapter.

2. In what ways does biotechnology improve and/or hinder your ability to provide good patient care (for example, do high tech monitoring devices shift attention away from viewing the patient as a complex individual.

3. What prevalent values about health, healthcare and the nursing profession exist in your country? Which ethical perspectives and/or principles are likely to be prioritized and why these?

4. In general, how confident are you and the nurses you know in their ethical decision-making skills and ability to advocate for a patient's perspective in team meetings and/or interdisciplinary settings?

5. Can you articulate the meaning of each of the ethical principles, exemplifying with practice examples?

6. Which areas of ethical decision-making are the most problematic for you and how would you go about remedying these areas?

References

Adams, T. E. (2008). A review of narrative ethics. *Qualitative Inquiry, 14*(2), 175–194. https://doi.org/10.1177/1077800407304417

Askitopoulou, H., & Vgontzas, A.N. (2018). The relevance of the Hippocratic Oath to the ethical and moral values of contemporary medicine. Part I: The Hippocratic Oath from antiquity to modern times. *European Spine Journal, 27*(7): 1481–1490.

Beauchamp, T. L., & Childress, J. F. (2009). *Principles of biomedical ethics* (6th ed.). Oxford University Press.

Beauchamp, T. L., & Childress, J. F. (2019). *Principles of biomedical ethics* (8th ed.). Oxford University.

Blacksher, E. (2002). On being poor and feeling poor: Low socioeconomic status and the moral self. *Theoretical Medicine and Bioethics* . https://doi.org/10.1023/A:1021381616824

Charon, R., & Montello, M. (Eds.). (2002). *Stories matter: The role of narrative in medical ethics.* Taylor and Francis/Psychology Press.

Childress, A., Lee, S. W., Matsler, J. S., & Farroni, J. S. (2020). Clarifying and expanding the role of narrative in ethics consultation. *Journal of Clinical Ethics, 31*(3), 241–151.

Donaldson, S. K., & Crowley, D. M. (1978). The discipline of nursing. *Nursing Outlook, 26*(2), 113–120.

Faria M. A. (2015). Neolithic trepanation decoded—A unifying hypothesis: Has the mystery as to why primitive surgeons performed cranial surgery been solved? *Surgical Neurology International, 6*, 72. https://doi.org/10.4103/2152-7806.156634

Fleischacker, S. (2009). Kant's Theory of Punishment. *Kant–Studien, 79*(1–4). https://doi.org/10.1515/kant.1988.79.1-4.434

Flexner, A. (2015). Is social work a profession? *Proceedings of the National Conference of Charities and Correction, 581*, 584–588, 590. Retrieved April 5, 2020 from: https://pages.uoregon.edu/adoption/archive/FlexnerISWAP.htm

Gilligan, C. (2014). In a different voice: Women's conceptions of self and morality. In *Feminist Social Thought: A Reader* (pp. 549–582). Taylor and Francis. https://doi.org/10.4324/9780203705841-42

Gilligan, C. (2011). *Joining the resistance.* Polity Press.

Godfrey-Smith, P. (2003). Theory and reality: An introduction to philosophy of science. IL: University of Chicago Press.

Grace, P. J. (2005). Ethical issues relevant to health promotion. In C. Edelman & C. L. Mandle (Eds.), *Health promotion across the life span* (6th ed) (pp. 100–125). Elsevier/Mosby.

Grace, P, J. (2018). Nursing ethics and professional responsibility in advanced practice (3rd Ed.).

Grace, P. J. & Zumstein-Shaha, M. (2019). Using Ockham's Razor to Redefine 'Nursing Science'. *Nursing Philosophy.* https://doi.org/10.1111/nup.12246https://doi.org/10.1111/nup.12246

Greenstone, G. (2010). The history of bloodletting. *British Columbia Medical Journal, 52*(1), 12–14.

Hellegers, A. (1971). Bioethics center formed. *Chemical and Engineering News* (11 October): 7.

Holm, S., & Williams-Jones, B. (2006). Global bioethics — myth or reality? *BMC Medical Ethics, 7*, E10. https://doi.org/10.1186/1472-6939-7-10

Jones, W. H. S. (2004). Introduction in T. E. Page (ed) *Hippocrates: The Oath* (vol 1), (pp. 291–297). Cambridge, MA: Harvard University Press - Loeb Classical Library, vol 1.

Jonsen, A. R. (1998). *The birth of bioethics.* Oxford University Press.

Jonsen, A. R., Siegler, M., & Winslade, W. J. (2015). *Clinical ethics: A practical approach to ethical decisions in clinical medicine* (8th ed.) McGraw-Hill.

Kant, I. (1967). Foundations of the metaphysics of morals. In A. I. Melden (Ed), *Ethical theories : A book of reading* (pp. 317–366). Prentice-Hall (Original work published 1785).

Keiner, E. (2002). Education between academic discipline and profession in Germany after World War II. *European Educational Research Journal, 1*(1), 83–98.

Kepler, M. O. (1981). *Medical stewardship: Fulfilling the Hippocratic legacy.* Greenwood.

Kohlberg, (1981). *Essays on moral development, Vol. I: The philosophy of moral development* Harper & Row. ISBN 978-0-06-064760-5.
Kopelman, L. M. (2009). Bioethics as public discourse and second-order discipline. *Journal of Medicine and Philosophy, 34*(3), 261–273.
Kuhse, H., & Singer, P. (2006). *Bioethics an anthology* (2nd ed.). Blackwell.
Lange, M. (1999). Why are the laws of nature so important to science? *Philosophy and Phenomenologic Research,* LIX(3), 625–652.
McCullough, L. B. (1998*) John Gregory and the invention of professional medical ethics and the profession of medicine.* Dordrecht, The Netherlands: Kluwer Academic Publishers.
Mill, J. S. (1967). *Mill's ethical writings.* (Edited with an introduction by J. B. Schneewind.) Macmillan. (Original work published in 1861).
Moreno, J. D. (2015). How national security gave birth to bioethics. *The Conversation, June 8.* Accessed April 10, 2020 from: https://theconversation.com/how-national-security-gave-birth-to-bioethics-40528
Nagel, T. (1987). *What does it all mean.* Oxford University Press.
Pellegrino, E. D., & Thomasma, D. C. (2004). The good of patients and the good of society: Striking a moral balance. In Boylan, M. (Ed.), *Public health policy and ethics* (pp. 17–37). Springer.
Powers, M., & Faden, R. (2006). *Social justice: The moral foundations of public health and health policy.* Oxford University Press.
President's Commission for the Study of Ethical Problems in Medicine and Biomedical and Behavioral Research (1982). *Making health care decisions* (33. PB83236703). U.S. Government Printing Office.
Rawls, J. (1971). *A theory of justice.* Harvard University Press.
Reich, W. T. (1994). The word "bioethics": Its birth and the legacies of those who shaped it. *Kennedy Institute of Ethics Journal, 4*(4), 319–335. https://doi.org/10.1353/ken.0.0126
Reich, W. T. (1995). The word "bioethics": The struggle over its earliest meanings. *Kennedy Institute of Ethics Journal, 5*(1), 19–34.https://doi.org/10.1353/ken.0.0143
Scher, S., & Kozlowska, K. (2018). The rise of Bioethics: A historical overview. In *Rethinking Health Care Ethics* (pp 31–44). Palgrave Pivot. Published online March 3, 2018. https://doi.org/10.1007/978-981-13-0830-7_3
Stanford Encyclopedia of Philosophy (2014). The history of utilitarianism. Accessed April 13, 2020 from: https://plato.stanford.edu/entries/utilitarianism-history/
Tai, M. C. T. (2013). Western or Eastern principles in globalized bioethics? An Asian perspective view. *Tzu Chi Medical Journal, 25*(1), 64–67. https://doi.org/10.1016/j.tcmj.2012.05.004
The Belmont Report (1979). National Commission for the Protection of Human Subjects of Biomedical and Behavioral Research. Retrieved from http://www.hhs.gov/ohrp/regulations-and-policy/belmont-report/
Truog, R. D., Mitchell, C., & Daley, G. Q. (March 23, 2020). The toughest triage: Allocating ventilators in a pandemic. *New England Journal of Medicine .* https://doi.org/10.1056/NEJMp2005689
Varden, H. (2017). Kant and women. *Pacific Philosophical Quarterly, 98*(4), 653–694.
Whitehouse, P. J. (2003). The rebirth of bioethics: Extending the original formulations of Van Rensselaer—Potter. *American Journal of Bioethics, 3*(4), W26–W31. https://doi.org/10.1162/152651603322614751
WHO. (2019). Accessed April 3, 2020 from: https://www.who.int/news-room/q-a-detail/q-a-coronaviruses
WMA. (2020). International Code of Medical Ethics. Accessed 4/5/20: https://www.wma.net/policies-post/wma-international-code-of-medical-ethics/
Windt, P. Y. (1989). Introductory essay. In P. Y. Windt, P. C. Appleby, M. P. Battin, L. P. Francis & P. M. Landesman (Eds.), *Ethical issues in the professions* (pp. 1–24). Prentice Hall.

Part II
Essential Knowledge and Skills for Ethical Deliberations

Chapter 4
Effective Communication—Improving Communication Skills

Ben Benjamin, Aimee Milliken, and Pamela Grace

Abstract This chapter focuses on providing the reader with ways to improve or refine their communication skills. It differs somewhat from other chapters in the book in that it explains a system, SAVI® that has proven useful in a variety of settings for facilitating direct, clear, and purposeful communication and for assisting parties to hear each other, be heard and be understood. In this chapter, we highlight the ethical importance of good communication. Then, the components of the SAVI system are described in detail. The chapter provides opportunities for the reader to practice skills individually or with a group of colleagues. We realize that it may be a little difficult to make the adaptation if your first language is not English and there is a cultural difference in communication. However, we have found that even among our colleagues for whom English is a second language, the themes are relevant. To find a Certified SAVI Trainer in Europe see SAVICommunications.com

4.1 Introduction: The Ethical Importance of Good Communication

Language is frequently cited as the greatest intellectual achievement of the human race. We use language every day, for a wide variety of purposes—from buying a newspaper to transacting a business deal to expressing our deepest feelings. In the field of nursing, verbal communication has a tremendous impact on patients, as well

---

SAVI® is a registered trademark of SAVI Communications LLC
© SAVI Communications LLC 2022

B. Benjamin (✉)
The Benjamin Institute, Cambridge, MA, USA
e-mail: drben@benbenjamin.com

A. Milliken · P. Grace
William F. Connell School of Nursing, Boston College, Chestnut Hill, MA, USA
e-mail: aimee.milliken@bc.edu

P. Grace
e-mail: Gracepa@bc.edu

as interdisciplinary dynamics. Yet all too often, the ways we communicate don't quite work and this is an ethical problem, as discussed in Chapter 3, if it means that we are unable to meet the goals of good patient care. The aim of this chapter is to introduce you to strategies that foster good communication.

All of us at times have conversations that end badly, for reasons we don't fully comprehend. Even when we recognize our habitual patterns of communicating—noticing, perhaps, that we seem to have the same kind of arguments over and over again—we're often unable to change them. When we think we know what's going wrong, we frequently conclude that the problem lies with the other person. Not only is this conclusion usually wrong, but it leaves us helpless to improve the situation until that person changes somehow, which is not particularly likely.

SAVI (the System for Analyzing Verbal Interaction) is a communication model that facilitates improved professional communication and thus allows us to work toward meeting mutually held health care goals of the various professions. SAVI allows us to collect relevant pieces of evidence—our communication behaviors—and use them to objectively and systematically analyze what happened. In this way we can work to improve our communication (Agazarian, 1968).

Communication behaviors are specific, discrete types of verbal expression, such as a Question, Answer, Opinion, Paraphrase, Yes-But, Blame, and so on. A key concept in understanding communication is the distinction between what we say (our content) and how we say it (the verbal behaviors and voice tones we use to communicate that content). Whether we communicate successfully depends more on the how than on the what.

With this understanding of how communication works—how each type of verbal behavior tends to affect a conversation—we can pinpoint where things start to go wrong and devise strategies for achieving different outcomes. The goal of our investigation is not to find fault, but to find alternative ways of behaving that improve our chances of being understood.

In addition to providing insights after we've run into trouble, studying SAVI helps us prepare for future conversations to prevent problems from occurring in the first place. Building on information theory (Shannon & Weaver, 1964) has led to guidelines that can help us navigate more successfully in conversation. By learning about these guidelines, we can improve the ways we communicate with both patients and colleagues.

4.2 Foundations of SAVI

In the sections that follow, we'll examine the general principles and reasoning that underlie the SAVI communication system.

4.2.1 The Challenge of Communicating: Noise

Before looking at how SAVI analyzes communication, it is helpful to clarify just what communication is. One of the simplest, broadest, and most useful definitions is "the transfer of information." SAVI focuses on verbal communication—the transfer of information through words and the associated voice tone.

Using this definition, communicating successfully means that a message gets transmitted accurately. The problem is that transmitting information accurately is not as simple as it may seem. Often the message that's received is quite different from the message that the speaker meant to send. This is because how we say something (the communication behaviors we use) strongly affects what the listener hears. Some behaviors, and patterns of behaviors, convey messages quite clearly; others, however, add "noise"—distracting or confusing interference. This noise acts like static on your radio or cell phone, making it more difficult for a message to get through. When messages aren't communicated clearly, members of the healthcare team may be frozen by conflict, resulting in potential ethical challenges or moral distress. SAVI identifies three sources of noise: contradiction, ambiguity, and redundancy.

Often, noise is introduced through voice tone, when the tone contradicts the words. Voice tone is a very powerful, yet often overlooked, factor in the success or failure of a communication. You can't tell what communication behaviors people are using just by reading the words they've said. When said with different voice tones, the same words may constitute very different behaviors and, therefore, have widely varying effects on a conversation. For example, consider the statement, "I am not angry." The effect of these words will be quite different depending on the voice tone that's used—whether the person is stating, "I am not angry" in a calm, neutral manner or screaming, "I am NOT angry!!!" The latter is a clear example of contradiction: while the words say, "I am not angry," the tone says, "I am absolutely furious!".

Contradiction is a major source of noise in communication. An example of a communication behavior that introduces contradiction is a righteous question. Consider an interaction in which a charge nurse is talking to one of the floor nurses about administering a patient's medication. If the charge nurse says, "How could you not give this patient their medication on time?!" Her words are asking a question, but her tone is making an attack. Whenever two contradictory messages are sent at the same time—one through words, and a different one through voice tone—it is significantly less likely that information will get through and be available for solving problems or making decisions.

Contradiction between words and tone isn't the only way noise creeps into our messages. Information also gets lost when we make comments that are ambiguous. For instance, if the physician says that a specific test has been ordered and the nurse responds with, "That's an interesting decision," without further elaboration it is not clear why the nurse said that and whether there is information she has that might change the physician's decision. Moreover, if she does not think it is a good decision she needs to ask for clarification and rationale. This ambiguity makes it less likely that what she really meant will be understood and the response appropriate. Ambiguous communication is risky for patients, at worst it could put them at risk for harm, which is an ethical problem. Even when it does not, it may result in suboptimal care.

The third source of noise in our communication is redundancy—being so repetitious that the listener tunes you out. One kind involves repeating the same content, even with different words over and over again. Another kind is replicating the same behavior patterns like Complaint-Proposal-Complaint-Proposal.

An understanding of the impact of noise goes a long way toward knowing why some conversations work well and others do not.

4.2.2 Understanding SAVI: The Shift from Analyzing People to Analyzing Behavior

When people try to figure out why a conversation went badly, they often refer to the personal characteristics of the other person—their motivations, hidden agendas, personality traits, and so forth. This involves a great deal of speculation, as it is difficult to know what someone else is thinking or feeling. In contrast, SAVI focuses on the actual observable behaviors people use as they communicate. This descriptive approach makes the job of analyzing, understanding, and intervening in difficult conversations a whole lot easier.

4.2.3 The Structure of SAVI

The SAVI grid identifies various distinct types of communication behaviors (see Fig. 4.1 SAVI Grid Overview). These behaviors fit into nine squares arranged in the grid below. The sections that follow discuss the Rows and Columns of the SAVI grid in more detail.

The Rows: Red, Green, and Yellow

We use the metaphor of a stop light to talk about the three SAVI Rows. The color of each row suggests its impact on the flow of information.

4.2.3.1 Red Light

Red light behaviors tend to hinder the transfer of information. They maximize noise in the communication.

Let's consider how Red-light behaviors may relate to conversations that are going badly. Think about a recent dialogue that didn't work well, and try to recall the types of things that were said. Now, take a look at the Red-light row, and see if you find any matches to the behaviors in your own challenging interaction. Did you find some? When we ask this question in SAVI workshops, most people recognize that in

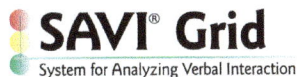

	Personal	Factual	Orienting
RED Light	**1 FIGHTING** Attack/Blame Righteous Question Sarcasm Self Attack/Defend Complaint	**2 OBSCURING** Mind-Reading Negative or Positive Prediction Gossip Joking Around Thinking Out Loud Social Ritual	**3 COMPETING** Yes-But Discount Leading Question Oughtitude Interrupt
YELLOW Light	**4 INDIVIDUALIZING** Personal Information Current Personal Information Past Personal Opinion/Explanation Personal Question	**5 FINDING FACTS** Facts & Figures General Information Narrow Question Broad Question	**6 INFLUENCING** Opinion Proposal Command Social Reinforcement
GREEN Light	**7 RESONATING** Inner Feeling Feeling Question Answer Feeling Question Mirror Inner Experience Affectionate Joke Self Assertion	**8 RESPONDING** Answer Question Clarify Own Answer (with data) Paraphrase Summarize Corrective Feedback	**9 INTEGRATING** Agreement Positives Build on Other's Ideas or Experience Work Joke

Silence, Laughter, Noise

SAVI® is a registered trademark of SAVI Communications LLC
© SAVI Communications LLC 2022. All rights reserved.

Fig. 4.1 Complete SAVI grid

their difficult conversations they Blame others, Yes-but, Complain, or Mind read. A conversation that is upsetting is more likely than not to contain Red light behaviors.

4.2.3.2 Green Light

These behaviors give evidence that information has been transferred. They minimize noise in a communication.

Most people report that these behaviors grease the wheels of communication, enabling information to flow back and forth more easily. Examples of Green light behavior in a conversation are Answering questions, Paraphrasing/Mirroring messages to check for accurate understanding, building on other's ideas instead of dropping them, and expressing feelings and wants in a non-blameful, non-complaining manner. The behaviors in the Green light row are necessary to help increase morale and productivity.

4.2.3.3 Yellow Light

These types of behaviors introduce unsolicited information into a conversation.

We use Yellow light behaviors to give information and nonjudgmental opinions or to solicit information from others. When you look at this row, you'll see that this is where we give our Facts and our Opinions, make our Proposals, talk about our preferences, and ask others for Facts or for their Opinions, wants, or ideas.

The effect of Yellow light behaviors on the transfer of information is a bit tricky to explain. It's important to recognize that introducing information is not the same as transferring it to someone else—and soliciting information doesn't mean that we'll get an answer. In other words, talking in the Yellow light row is different from communicating. Sometimes you may think you're communicating, when actually you're just talking to yourself, even though there are others in the room who look like they're listening to you.

A typical situation where conversation consists primarily of Yellow light behaviors is an unproductive staff meeting, in which each person gives new information, but nobody responds to anyone else's input. Each time new Facts, Opinions, Proposals, or Questions are introduced they seem to disappear like stones thrown into a lake, without leaving a ripple. At the end of such meetings, those involved have no evidence that anyone else understood what they said let alone whether they agreed or disagreed. This Yellow light pattern is why so many meetings feel so frustrating. It may often feel as though they're going in circles—and from a SAVI standpoint, that's exactly what's happening; the conversation is going around and around in Yellow light (see Fig. 4.2).

When stuck in a frustrating situation, many people's first instinct is to introduce even more Facts, Opinions, and Proposals, or to repeat what they've already said more loudly. However, when a communication system is already overloaded, putting in more information doesn't help; it just continues to feed the repetitive yellow light cycle. What *does* help is to make use of what's already on the table by shifting to communication behaviors that process that information—that is, Green light behaviors. For participants in a staff meeting, such behaviors might include: Answering questions that have previously been asked (Square 8); Building on someone else's

Fig. 4.2 Yellow light interactions

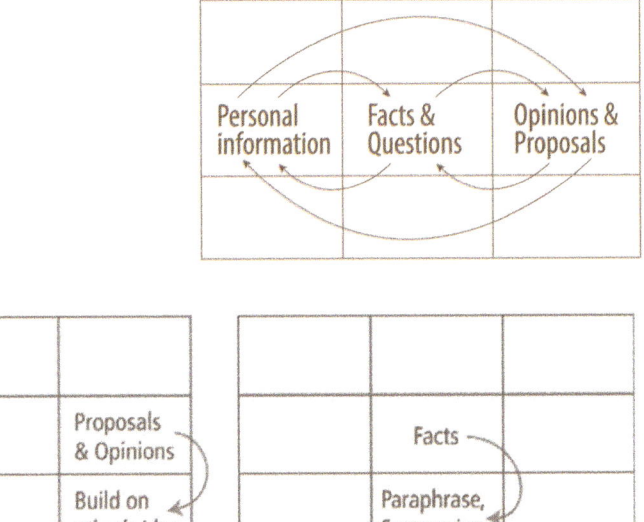

Fig. 4.3 Moving from yellow to green

ideas (Square 9); or Paraphrasing or Summarizing what's been said so far (Square 8). (See Moving From Yellow Light to Green Light) (Fig. 4.3).

4.2.4 Moving from Yellow Light to Green Light

A Yellow-Green information climate increases the chances that noise will be reduced and that new information will be transferred and processed. In a staff meeting, this means that the participants are much more likely to meet their goals and solve the problems they're trying to tackle.

Giving information is no guarantee that it will be used productively. In an all-Yellow communication climate, it doesn't get used at all. In other cases, Yellow light information does get used, but in a way that's counterproductive. For instance, in a Yellow–Red climate, your information may just provide more ammunition to fight with. This is what's happening when you find that everything you say gets Yes-Butted, Discounted, Attacked, or Complained about, or that the subject gets changed by Joking around or Gossip. In that type of communication climate, giving more Facts, Opinions, or Proposals is more likely to provoke competition or start an argument than to help in problem solving. For problems to get solved, some Green light behaviors need to be used—and probably by you, if you're the only one in the conversation with the skills to do that. It's within a Yellow-Green communication climate that Yellow light information is used to make decisions and generate creative solutions.

A key takeaway message here is that whenever you use a Yellow light behavior, it's the behaviors that follow which help determine the likelihood that your information will be used productively. If you're trying to get new information across, watch carefully to see which types of behaviors follow your input. If they are part of a Yellow-Green sequence, it's safe to continue. If they are Yellow-Yellow or Yellow–Red, it probably won't be helpful to bring more new facts or ideas into the conversation.

4.2.5 Using the Rows in Conversation

To highlight the distinctions between the three rows, let's look at how the same topic might be discussed in each row. Take the example of a nurse who's talking with a colleague about a patient who doesn't seem to be getting any better. The colleague may respond with Red light, Yellow light, or Green light behaviors. As you read through the various responses listed in the box below, think about how you'd feel if you were on the receiving end of each of these comments:

The nurse says: "I'm feeling upset and at a loss—my patient is refusing to get out of bed, despite me explaining why it's so important that he does."

Red Light Responses:
Attack: "You must not have asked him properly why he is refusing."
Discount: "Don't worry some patients are like that… that's his problem."
Yes—But: "Yeah, but most of your patients are doing great."

Yellow Light Responses:
Personal Information Past: "The last time this happened to me, I talked to the charge nurse."
Proposal: "You could try asking his wife to talk to him."
Question: "What have you tried? What's keeping you from asking for help?".

Green Light Responses:
Paraphrase: "I'm hearing that you're very concerned about this patient because although you've given him the appropriate information he is not doing what is best for him."
Feeling Question: "Are you worried that there is something else you ought to be doing to persuade him or that he is going to be harmed and does not seem to understand this?".

4 Effective Communication—Improving Communication Skills

4.2.6 The Columns: Personal, Factual, Orienting

So far we've been looking at the Rows of the Grid; now let's switch to thinking about the Columns. There are three Columns in the Grid, and these reflect the focus of the information carried in the communication.

Column 1: Personal behaviors—focus on the person part of the message (See Fig. 4.4 SAVI Grid-Column Two Personal)
Column 1 contains Personal behaviors. These are the behaviors we use to talk about ourselves, invite our listeners to talk about themselves, talk about our relationship, or express our feelings and impulses. The primary information they give is about the emotional state of the person speaking or the relationship between the people having the conversation. As we've seen from the discussion of the Rows, you can express Personal information using behaviors in the Red, Yellow, or Green light rows, and these will yield quite different effects (Fig. 4.4).

For example, if you're feeling angry, you could express that emotion directly:

I'm angry at my colleague for not showing up on time and not calling to let me know. (Square 7—Inner-feeling)

Or you can express it indirectly: "That nurse is such a jerk." (Square 1 of this column—Attack)

You can also express your wants or preferences directly: "I want to work no more than four eight-hour shifts a week." (Square 4—Personal information current)

Or, again, you can express it indirectly: "How do they expect us to keep up with this staffing, taking care of so many complex patients?" (Square 1—Complaint)

Column 2: Factual—focus on data (See Fig. 4.5 SAVI Grid—Column Two Factual)
The behaviors in Column 2 relate to Factual information that may be needed to solve problems. We use Factual behaviors to process, provide, or avoid concrete information about the world. One of the most common ways we avoid getting factual data is by giving Negative predictions (Square 2 of column two): "Once you hear the topic of tonight's lecture, you're not going to want to come with me."

We can get information into the conversation by introducing Facts and asking Questions (Square 5 of column two): "Tonight's lecture is by Dr. Jones. He's going to talk about the side-effects of antidepressant medications. Have you heard about his new research?".

Once we've been given Facts or asked Questions, we can process that information by giving direct responses (Square 8 of column two): "Yes, I have. I've read his latest paper." (Answering a question).

Column 3: Orienting—focus on directing the flow of what is being talked about (Fig. 4.6)
Column 3 behaviors influence the direction in which a conversation is moving. They orient listeners toward or away from the current discussion or change the subject by giving new Opinions or Proposals.

Personal	
1 FIGHTING Attack/Blame Righteous Question Sarcasm Self Attack/Defend Complaint	*Avoiding direct meaningful feeling information*
4 INDIVIDUALIZING Personal Information Current Personal Information Past Personal Opinion/Explanation Personal Question	*Giving or soliciting new information about the self that is not deeply personal*
7 RESONATING Inner Feeling Feeling Question Answer Feeling Question Mirror Inner Experience Affectionate Joke Self Assertion	*Sharing or soliciting meaningful feelings or authentic experience*

SAVI® is a registered trademark of SAVI Communications LLC
© SAVI Communications LLC 2022. All rights reserved.

Fig. 4.4 SAVI grid—Column one personal

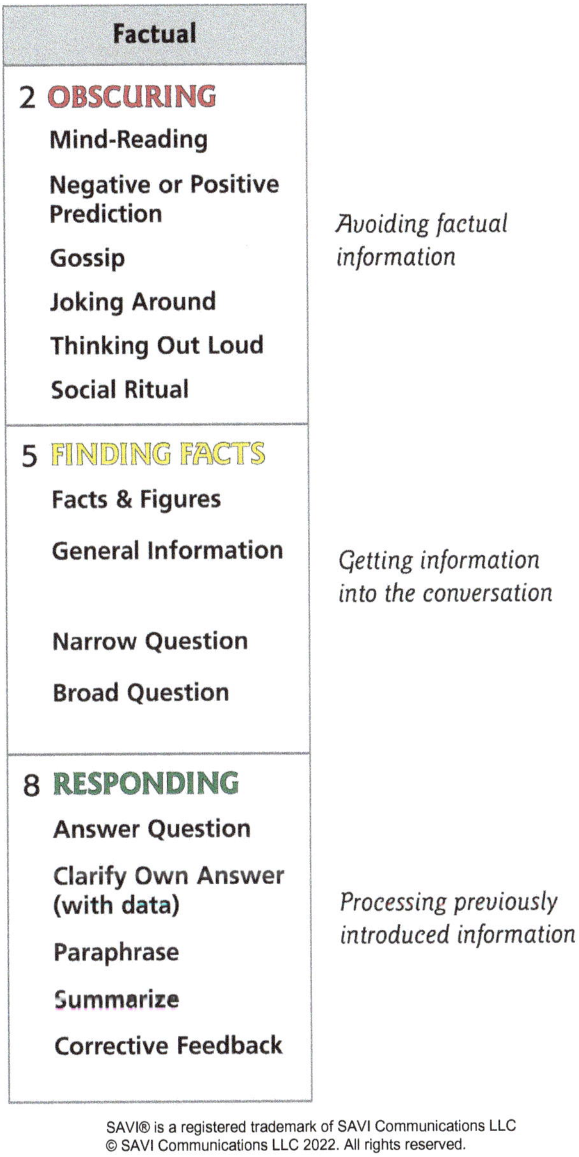

Factual	
2 OBSCURING Mind-Reading Negative or Positive Prediction Gossip Joking Around Thinking Out Loud Social Ritual	*Avoiding factual information*
5 FINDING FACTS Facts & Figures General Information Narrow Question Broad Question	*Getting information into the conversation*
8 RESPONDING Answer Question Clarify Own Answer (with data) Paraphrase Summarize Corrective Feedback	*Processing previously introduced information*

SAVI® is a registered trademark of SAVI Communications LLC
© SAVI Communications LLC 2022. All rights reserved.

Fig. 4.5 SAVI Grid column two—Factual

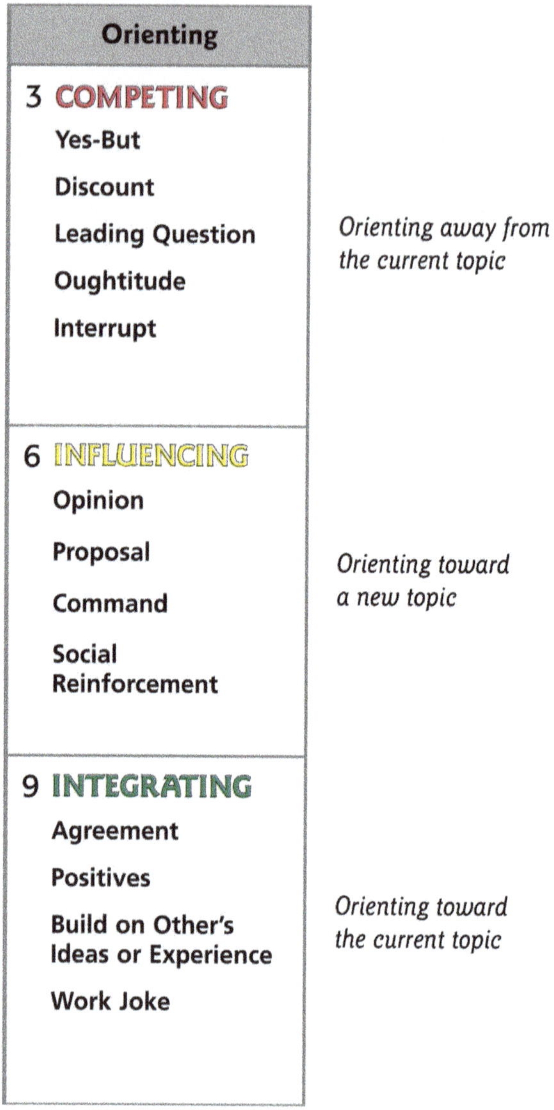

Orienting
3 COMPETING Yes-But Discount Leading Question Oughtitude Interrupt
6 INFLUENCING Opinion Proposal Command Social Reinforcement
9 INTEGRATING Agreement Positives Build on Other's Ideas or Experience Work Joke

Orienting away from the current topic (COMPETING)

Orienting toward a new topic (INFLUENCING)

Orienting toward the current topic (INTEGRATING)

SAVI® is a registered trademark of SAVI Communications LLC
© SAVI Communications LLC 2022. All rights reserved.

Fig. 4.6 SAVI Grid column three—Orienting

When we introduce new topics, it's often in the form of Opinions (Square 6 of column three): "I think all health insurance plans should cover mental health services."

Once a topic has been introduced, we can orient toward that topic—for example by expressing Agreement and Building (Square 9) on a previously mentioned idea: "I agree. That would make mental health services accessible to many people who couldn't otherwise afford it."

Alternatively, we can orient away from that topic. This is frequently done in the form of a token agreement followed by a different idea (a "Yes-But," Square 3): "Yes, but then the insurance companies would go broke."

Now let's finish our tour of the Grid by looking at each of the nine Squares. Then we'll bring all this information together to explore how we can apply SAVI skills to real-life conversations, both with patients and families as well as in interdisciplinary team contexts.

4.2.7 The Squares

The impact of the Rows and Columns on our communication becomes clearer when we see how they intersect in the nine Squares (See Fig. 4–1: Complete SAVI grid). For example, consider the intersection of Column 1 (Personal) with Row 1 (Red Light). If you think about a bad argument you've had with someone close to you, you'll probably have first-hand knowledge about the behaviors that belong in this Square. Square 1's label, "Fighting," says it all. Square 1 behaviors, such as Attack, Self-Attack, Sarcasm, and Complaint all belong in the Personal column because they give very important information about the speaker's feelings. Think back to the argument you had: chances are, you are both talking about something that provoked strong feelings in you. The problem with Square 1 is that the emotions in the message are conveyed indirectly. For instance, we may express anger through Attack ("You're so irresponsible when you borrow my things"); sadness or frustration through Self-Attack ("I'm just lousy at all the details"); or apprehension through Complaining ("Integrating new nurses into our team is always so stressful") and so forth. These important emotional messages can be transferred with less noise by being direct, in Square 7 (e.g., "I'm annoyed that you didn't return my stuff when you said you would"; "I'm feeling discouraged because I can't seem to get things organized"; or "When I think about this new person joining our team I feel nervous."). Expressing our feelings directly makes it much more likely that our listener will hear what we're trying to say and respond effectively to our concerns.

Each of the Squares has its own distinctive character. To illustrate, let's look at some concrete examples of behaviors from each one. The examples address a variety of situations: Let's see how comments on this topic would sound from all nine Squares.

Square 1: Fighting
The behaviors of this Square are put-downs of the self or others through content or voice tone.

Attack: "That scrub top you wore yesterday was totally unprofessional." Righteous question: "Don't you have any sense of how a care professional should dress?!" (Fig. 4.7).

Square 2: Obscuring
The behaviors of this Square include assumptions presented as fact; statements that are ambiguous in topic, content, or source; and stories or jokes that distract for better or worse away from the flow of a conversation.
Gossip: "Did you hear that Paul got fired because he was having an affair with one of the doctors"
Positive prediction: "In 10 years, nurses will be able to practice fully independently without any doctor's oversight?"
Mindread: "I just know my coworkers think I'm too novice and not good at my job." (Fig. 4.8).

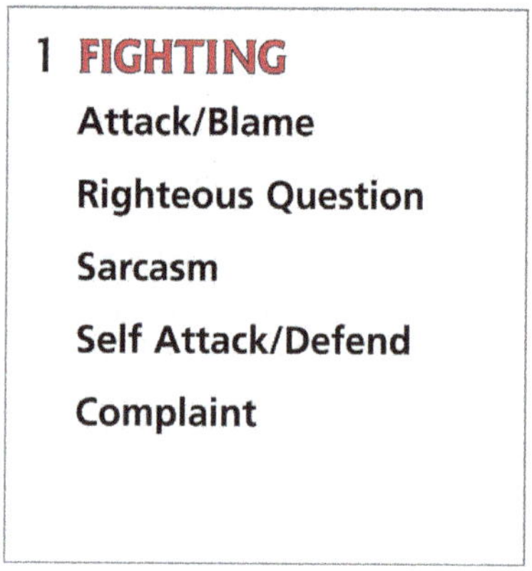

Fig. 4.7 Square 1—Fighting

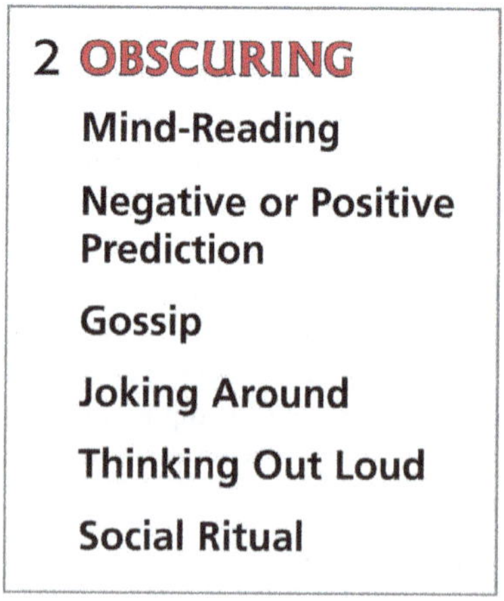

1 FIGHTING
Attack/Blame
Righteous Question
Sarcasm
Self Attack/Defend
Complaint

Fig. 4.8 Square 2—Obscuring

2 OBSCURING
Mind-Reading
Negative or Positive Prediction
Gossip
Joking Around
Thinking Out Loud
Social Ritual

Square 3: Competing

Square 3 behaviors express opinions that directly or indirectly contradict or interrupt the input of others.
Yes-But: "It's all well and good to want safe staffing but the nursing staff also needs to understand that resources aren't infinite."
Leading question: "Don't you think the doctors would take us more seriously if we were more direct in our communication?" (Fig. 4.9).

Square 4: Individualizing

Square 4 behaviors express information, opinions, or questions about one's social self that are not deeply personal.
Personal information past: "Where did you go to nursing school?"
Personal question: "What type of unit are you most comfortable working on?" (Fig. 4.10).

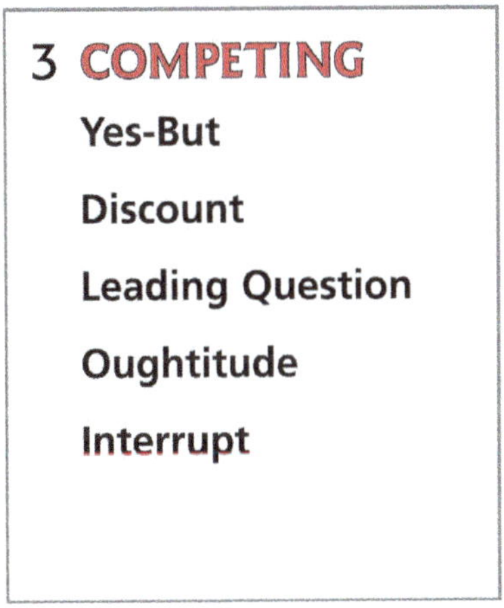

Fig. 4.9 Square 3—Competing

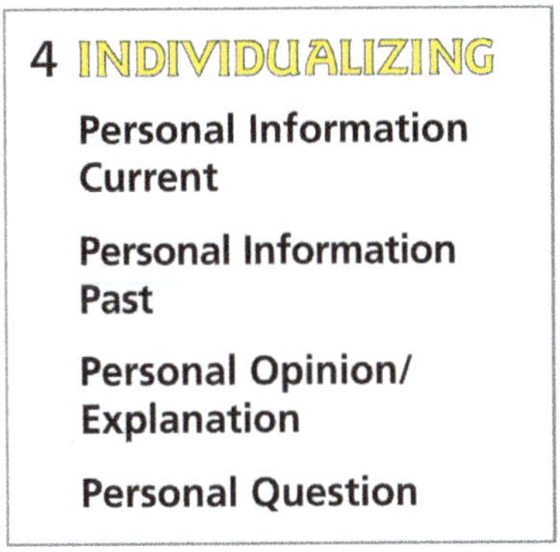

> **3 COMPETING**
> Yes-But
> Discount
> Leading Question
> Oughtitude
> Interrupt

Fig. 4.10 Square 4—Individualizing

> **4 INDIVIDUALIZING**
> Personal Information Current
> Personal Information Past
> Personal Opinion/ Explanation
> Personal Question

Square 5: Finding Facts
Square 5 behaviors either give information verifiable by observation and public data or ask questions that seek such information from others.
Facts & figures: "According to one survey, 70% of nurses in hospitals have their bachelor's degrees."
Narrow question: "Do you typically work day shifts or night shifts?" (Fig. 4.11).

Square 6: Influencing
Square 6 behaviors convey the speakers' opinions and orientation about what is being discussed.
Opinion: "I think working in the ICU is more exciting than working on a MedSurg unit."
Proposal: "Let's do a survey and see what types of units most nurses prefer." (Fig. 4.12).

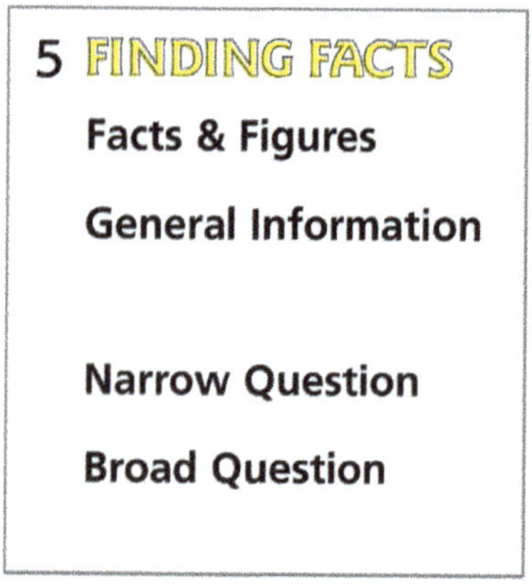

Fig. 4.11 Square 5—Finding facts

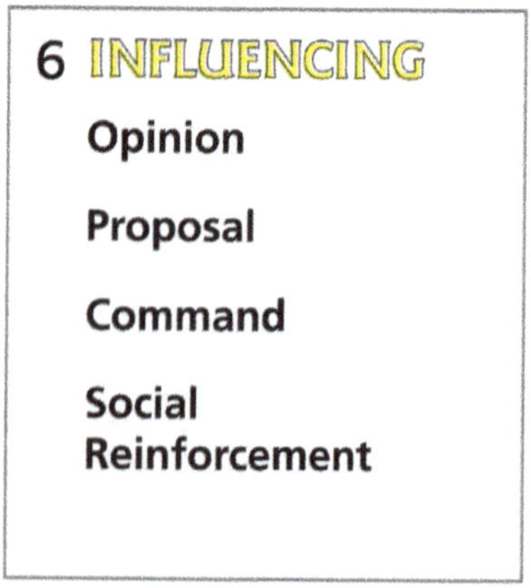

5 FINDING FACTS

Facts & Figures

General Information

Narrow Question

Broad Question

Fig. 4.12 Square 6—Influencing

6 INFLUENCING

Opinion

Proposal

Command

Social Reinforcement

4 Effective Communication—Improving Communication Skills

Square 7: Resonating

Square 7 behaviors communicate information that is emotionally meaningful to the speaker or to others. They frequently involve a sense of taking a risk or going out on a limb.
Feeling question: "Were you upset by that comment I made earlier on rounds about the patient you are taking care of?"
Answers feeling question: "Yes, I was really upset when you said that." (Fig. 4.13).

Square 8: Responding

Square 8 behaviors express direct responses to others' input or otherwise give evidence that input has been processed or received.
Answer to a question: "In answer to your question I think the doctors would take nurses more seriously if we were more direct in our communication."
Paraphrase: "What I heard you say is that your dad would want to be comfortable at the end of life." (Fig. 4.14).

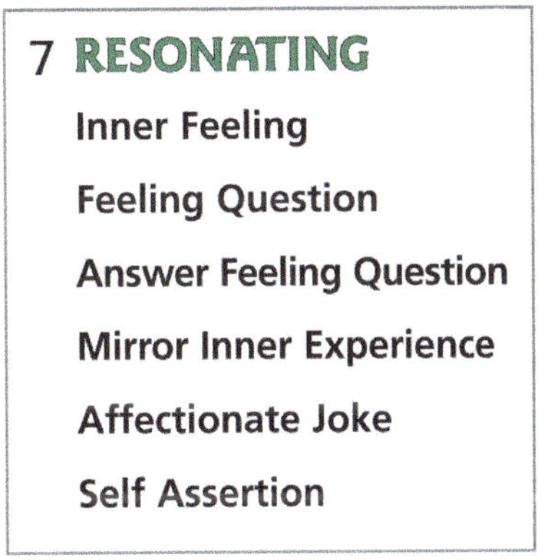

Fig. 4.13 Square 7—Resonating

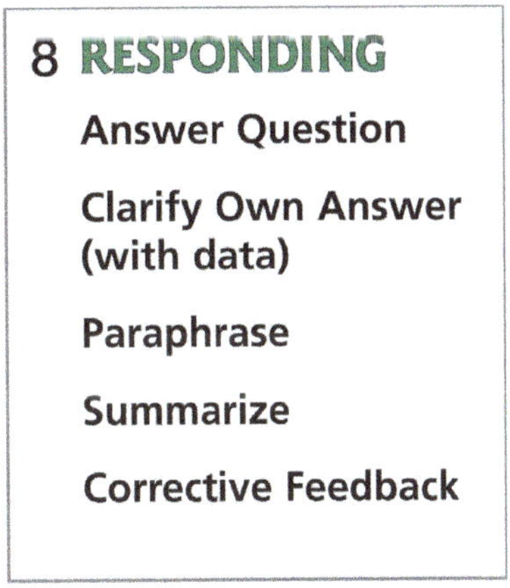

7 RESONATING

Inner Feeling

Feeling Question

Answer Feeling Question

Mirror Inner Experience

Affectionate Joke

Self Assertion

Fig. 4.14 Square 8—Responding

8 RESPONDING

Answer Question

Clarify Own Answer (with data)

Paraphrase

Summarize

Corrective Feedback

Square 9: Integrating

Square 9 behaviors are cooperative acts that integrate by explicitly valuing or building upon someone else's communication.

Agreement: "I agree with what you said earlier—that is the best plan for my patient."

Positives: "I like how you dealt with that patient's family, you were clear about your boundaries as well as compassionate." (Fig. 4.15).

Squares in Action: Building a Yellow-Green Climate

Imagine that a patient tells the nurse that his friend's doctor has been prescribing immunotherapy to many of his patients, and the following conversation takes place:

Family member: "Don't you think my mother might be getting better faster if we tried immunotherapy?".

Nurse: (said with irritation) "If I thought it would be better for your mother, don't you think we'd be using it?".

Here's what happened:

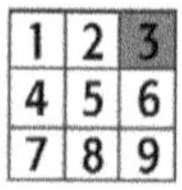

1	2	**3**
4	5	6
7	8	9

Family member: "Don't you think my mother might be getting better faster if we tried immunotherapy?" (Leading question)

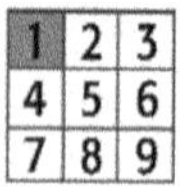

1	2	3
4	5	6
7	8	9

Nurse: (said with irritation) "If I thought it would be better for your mother, don't you think we'd be using it?" (Righteous question)

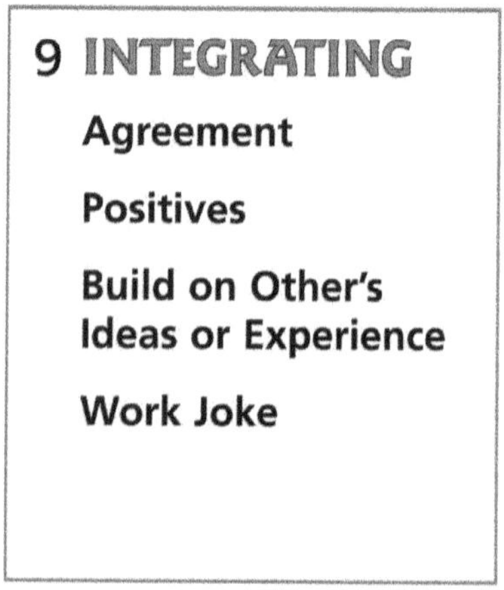

Fig. 4.15 Square 9—Integrating

9 INTEGRATING

Agreement

Positives

Build on Other's Ideas or Experience

Work Joke

If the nurse thought back on this interaction, she could notice that the family members' comment was a Leading question, a Red light behavior, and she might remember the pull she felt to join the client up in Red. The next time a family member asks a question of the "Don't you think ..." variety, the nurse can choose among various Yellow or Green light alternatives. For example:

Expressing Agreement (Square 9):
"I'm glad you feel free to ask me questions about something that is of concern to you."

Giving a Paraphrase (Square 8) and checking it out with a Narrow question (Square 5):
"I'm hearing you tell me that your friend told you about immunotherapy and you're wondering whether that treatment would be helpful for your mother, too. Is that right?"

Asking a Broad question (Square 5):
"Why are you thinking that immunotherapy would be good for your mother?"

Asking a Personal question (Square 4):
"Is there something about your mother's treatment that's concerning you?"

4.2.8 Putting it All Together: A Dynamic Systems Perspective

Until now we've been talking about communication by focusing on specific, isolated behaviors: Green light behaviors that carry a minimum of noise, Red light behaviors that carry lots of noise, and Yellow light behaviors that bring in unsolicited information.

However, since every conversation is a dynamic system, no single behavior can determine how that conversation will evolve. Communication is like a chess game: we can't understand what's happening by looking at an individual "move." For example, a pawn moved onto a certain square may be a winning move in one game and a losing move in another. In chess, we need to examine the sequence of moves to get a sense of what's going on. Looking at the big picture is essential in determining how to make a useful next move. Likewise, to understand why a conversation is going well or going poorly, we need to look at the sequence of communication behaviors. Analyzing the sequence of behaviors is the direct route to making useful decisions about what behaviors to use next.

Looking at a conversation as a dynamic system, it becomes clear that no particular communication behavior is good or bad in and of itself; the effect of any behavior depends on the sequence of interactions that have been happening (which we've called the "communication climate"). As we saw in the section on Yellow light behavior, in Yellow-Green communication climates, new information contributes usefully to problem solving and decision making, but in Red- Yellow climates, that same input can make the problem worse. Consider, for example, the situation in which a colleague has been complaining about his or her working conditions for months. You've tried to be helpful by listening and making suggestions (Proposals), and every time the response is to complain more about why your proposal won't work.

> *Nurse manager*: I'd like you to take this new admission, it's a complicated case.
> *Nurse*: My assignment is too busy to take the new admission. (Complaint)
> *Nurse manager*: What about if Susie takes one of your patients (Proposal)
> *Nurse*: No, these patients are way too complicated, she would not be able to get caught up. (Complaint)
> *Nurse manager*: Well, I guess I can just give Susie the new admission. (Proposal)
> *Nurse*: Well Susie is a new nurse, she wouldn't know how to handle a complex patient like this admission. (Complaint)
> *Nurse manager*: Well, how about…etc. etc. (Proposal)

It's clear that this dialogue is going nowhere. So what's the problem? In a word: redundancy. Earlier, we talked about redundancy as the third source of noise in a communication system (in addition to contradiction and ambiguity). Redundancy makes it more difficult for a message to get through because we tune out when we hear the same thing repeated over and over again. We intuitively know that redundancy makes us tune out when it is the content that gets repeated; we get bored hearing about someone's vacation for the umpteenth time. What may be less obvious is that a repetitious pattern of communication behaviors can also be redundant and cause us to stop listening. The "New admission" dialogue illustrates how we can get caught in a spin cycle of repeating behaviors: (Fig. 4.16).

Behavior A is followed by
behavior B followed by
behavior A followed by
behavior B, etc.

No matter what person A says, person B will respond predictably, and then A will try again with the same behavior, maybe louder, only to be met by B's typical response.

From a SAVI perspective, there's nothing inherently wrong with a single use of any behavior. What's causing the problem in our dialogue is not the use of a Complaint or a Proposal; rather, it is the ineffective jointly created pattern of redundant verbal behaviors (Complaint/Proposal/Complaint/Proposal, etc.).

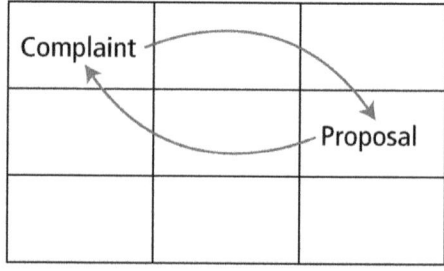

Fig. 4.16 Repeating behaviors

Examples of other common noisy, redundant patterns are:
Yes-But/Yes-But/Yes-But

Nurse: You need to stop eating so much fast food so we can get your Diabetes under control.
Patient: But it takes so long to cook.
Nurse: I understand, but if you don't change your diet, I worry that you will begin to experience complications from your high blood sugar.
Patient: Yes, but I already work sixteen hours a day and it's hard to do all that shopping and cooking.
Nurse: But if you don't then you might not be around very long to see your kids grow up.
Patient: But...

Try putting yourself in the place of either the patient or the nurse. How does it feel to be involved in this redundant pattern? Can you predict how the conversation might proceed from there?

Narrow Question/Answer/Narrow Question/Answer

Nurse: How much do you smoke?
Patient: A pack a day.
Nurse: Can you stop smoking altogether?
Patient: No, not really.
Nurse: You need to quit. Have you tried a nicotine patch?
Patient: No, I'm not interested in that.

If you were the patient in this dialogue, how would you be feeling toward the nurse at this point? How would you feel if this pattern of questions and responses were to continue for several more minutes?

Question/Non-Answer/Question/Non-Answer

Patient: When will I start to feel better?
Nurse: Well, you know these things take time.
Patient: Can you give me a range?
Nurse: You know, if I had a nickel for every time I've been asked that question, I'd be rich.
Patient: Well, are we talking weeks or months or years? Etc.

Again, put yourself in the patient's place. What could the patient do differently when the nurse didn't answer the question for a second time? Consider how the redundant pattern might change if the patient switched to using Personal information current, Square 4, and Narrow Question, and switched to Square 5: "I notice you're not answering my question. Is there a reason?" Likewise, putting yourself in the nurse's place, think about how you'd feel inside this redundant loop, and then compare that with how you'd feel if you switched behaviors (e.g., "You're asking me a question that I don't have an answer for. That's frustrating to me because I'd like to be able to give you a real number.").

Attack/Attack/Attack

The nurse for the next shift arrives an hour late and the nurse waiting to go home says:

Nurse 1: Where have you been?! You're late!
Nurse 2: Traffic is really bad and you were late yesterday.
Nurse 1: We're not talking about me. You do this all the time.
Nurse 2: You know I'm going through a hard time and you don't even care.
Nurse 1: You should never let your personal issues get in the way of doing your job.
Nurse 2: That's easy for you to say, you only work part time because your husband makes so much money.

It's clear that some strong negative emotions are coming up for both nurses. If this Red light, indirect pattern of discharging their emotions were to continue, would you expect them to feel better or worse?

The good thing about spotting redundant patterns is that it gives us a chance to change them. Since we're talking about sequences of behaviors, noisy redundant patterns can be "fixed" by anyone in the conversation by means of trying a different behavior. Let's see how this might happen. Think back to the Complaint/Proposal dialogue. In this example, either speaker could interrupt the redundant pattern by trying a different sort of behavior. For instance, the person giving Proposals could switch to:

Asking a Personal question, Square 4 (e.g., "What do you think we ought to do with this new admission?" or "What kind of help would you like from me in order to take the new admission?") or Giving a Command, Square 6 (e.g., "Tell me what you think might help to work this out.").

Or your colleague (the person Complaining) could switch to active problem solving by making a Proposal of his own:

"Is there a supervisor available that could just check on Susie to help her if she has any trouble with the new admission?"

As we realize that it's patterns (sequences of behaviors)—not just individual behaviors—that make or break conversations, it also becomes clear that no individual ever has sole responsibility for the failure of a communication. Even if one person uses noisy behaviors such as Attack, Sarcasm, or Yes-Buts, that alone does not cause a conversation to fail. In any dialogue, patterns of communication evolve through input from both parties, so both have the ability to influence how things are going. Even in habitual, repeated conversations that always seem to end in a stalemate, one person can help move the conversation toward a satisfying outcome for both by altering her or his own side of the dialogue. This empowering realization is at the heart of SAVI training.

4.3 SAVI IN PRACTICE

At this point you've learned a lot about the SAVI Grid, from its theoretical underpinnings to the nuts and bolts of rows, columns, and squares and how they interact in dynamic conversations.

"So what?" you may be tempted to ask. "I can't possibly track every single behavior I use!" And you'd be absolutely right. The good news is that SAVI is not meant to be used all the time. But, like a hammer or a paint brush, it's a great tool to have on hand for those occasions when you need it. The most useful time to "think SAVI," that is, to think about the verbal behaviors you're using, is when you're in a conversation that makes you uncomfortable or that doesn't seem to be going well. For example, if you're in the midst of a conflict of opinion with a physician and realize you need to take a break to calm down, you can use SAVI instead of just counting to ten. Often, just spotting the color of the communication behaviors being used enables you to start figuring out what's going wrong and how to make things work better. Even if you can't take a break in the middle of the conversation, you can try to find time in the hours or days that follow to consider what you might do differently in the future.

Since our communication habits are deeply ingrained, we may have difficulty recognizing our own communication blind spots. If you are lucky enough to know someone who can talk these ideas over with, by all means use her or him as a resource. The people we live, work, and play with often know more about our behaviors than we do. They may have feedback and suggestions that would not have occurred to us.

If you do invite feedback, you may be surprised by what you learn. One person who took a SAVI workshop brought the ideas home to share with her family and put a SAVI Grid up on the refrigerator. From then on, her kids pointed out whenever she was "Yes-Butting" them, which she was doing much more than she had realized. In exchange for putting up with her own behavior being monitored, she had a tool to help her deal better with her children's "You did"/ "No I didn't"/ "Yes, you did"/ "No I didn't" never-ending battles.

4.4 Summary and Case Examples

As described, effective communication is an essential component of good (ethical) patient care. When we are unable to convey our messages clearly, teamwork is hampered, and patient care is compromised. Developing and practicing the skills of effective communication, using tools like SAVI, can ensure that ethical issues are identified and addressed.

After reading these case examples answer the questions posed in the exercise below.

Case Examples

1. Mrs. Smith is a 55 year old woman who received a heart transplant in 2016. Her recovery has been complicated by end stage renal disease, recurrent GI bleeding, and respiratory failure for which she has had a tracheostomy placed. She has been readmitted to the cardiac intensive care unit (CICU) from a rehabilitation setting multiple times since her transplant. She has not been home in over a year.

   During this admission, Mrs. Smith has been febrile, hypotensive requiring vasopressors (drugs that help maintain a sufficient blood pressure to oxygenate important organs), and has had a decline in her mental status. She has not been following commands and has not been able to engage with the physical therapist and improve her mobility and daily functioning. Despite this, Mrs. Smith's husband, Jim, believes she will get better. He wants the team to "do everything" for Mrs. Smith.

   The nursing staff worry that Mrs. Smith will not improve and feel as though they are "torturing" her with routine care. They feel like they "know where this is headed" and that the team should talk to Jim about redirecting Mrs. Smith's goals of care to comfort.

   The Cardiology doctors seem to disagree with the nursing staff and continue to say there is a "chance" Mrs. Smith will improve enough to be able to return to a rehabilitation setting. They do not want to involve the Palliative Care service or to have a discussion about what the ultimate possible goals for Mrs. Smith would be at this time, saying it is premature.

2. Jane is a nurse caring for Mr. H, a patient in an intensive care unit (ICU). Mr. H recently had a cerebrovascular stroke for which he received tissue plasminogen activator (TPA) a drug designed to dissolve clots that are responsible for ischemic strokes and which requires close monitoring for at least 24-h. While the usual 24-h monitoring period is complete, Mr. H remains quite agitated. The neurology and ICU physicians want to transfer him to the neurosurgical floor now that he has "no ICU needs." Jane is worried that he will be at risk for falling or injuring himself if he moves to the floor, as the staffing ratios are quite different than in the ICU (1 nurse for 4 patients versus 1 nurse for 1–2 patients). She wants to communicate her concern to the team but isn't sure how to do this without seeming to be confrontational or obstructionist.

3. Tim is a new nurse on a medical-surgical floor. He has three patients assigned to him and is very busy and behind on his documentation and medication administration. His charge nurse comes to him to tell him he will be taking the next admission. He feels overwhelmed as it is, and worries that with a fourth patient he will be spread so thin that mistakes could happen. He is not sure how to communicate this concern to his charge nurse, and wants to be a team player.

4.5 Exercises

For each of the cases, answer the following questions:

1. Using Green-light techniques, how might the nurse involved frame their concern?
   a. In what way is the concern ethical in nature?
2. What communication techniques should the nurse use, and why?
3. What is an example of a "Red light" response the nurse may receive?
   a. How should the nurse respond? Which communication techniques should they use? Why?

SAVI was developed in the 1960s by Anita Simon and Yvonne Agazarian (Agazarian, 1968; Simon & Agazarian, 2000) as a tool to study the effects of verbal behavior in educational, therapeutic, and organizational settings. The groundbreaking theory of information transfer had originally been investigated by Claude Shannon at Bell Labs (Shannon & Weaver, 1964) to determine what got in the way of accurately transmitting electronic messages in Morse code. Yvonne Agazarian and Gantt (2000) adapted and modified that work to apply to human verbal communication.

References

Agazarian, Y. M. (1968). *A theory of verbal behavior and information transfer.* Dissertation submitted at Temple University, Philadelphia.
Agazarian, Y. M., & Gantt, S. P. (2000). *Autobiography of a theory.* Jessica Kingsley.
Shannon, C. E., & Weaver, W. (1964). *The mathematical theory of communication.* University of Illinois Press.
Simon, A., & Agazarian, Y. M. (2000). SAVI—The system for analyzing verbal interaction. In A. P. Beck & C. M. Lewis (Eds.), *The process of group psychotherapy: Systems for analyzing change* (pp. 357–380). American Psychological Association.

Chapter 5
Models of Ethics Deliberation and Consultation

Aimee Milliken, Settimio Monteverde, and Pamela Grace

Abstract In this chapter, we describe the origins of institutional healthcare ethics consultation services and the development of healthcare ethics committees in the US, Switzerland and elsewhere. We discuss some of the landmark situations, cases and macro-political and social frameworks that have contributed to their genesis. Next, we describe common models of ethical decision-making. While this list is not meant to be exhaustive, it covers approaches to ethical decision-making that are commonly used in clinical ethics, and which also can be found in the nursing ethics literature. We examine the roles that healthcare ethics committees fill in some hospitals in the US, including collaborative and consultative functions for clinical ethics issues and organizational ethics questions. We all note that in other countries ethics deliberations are not necessarily carried out only this way, for example in Switzerland. Also noted is the role that nurses with advanced education and ethical expertise can play in supporting and empowering point of care nurses and other clinicians to address moral distress as discussed in other chapters. Finally, we describe preventive ethics, and the critical role of nurses in the early recognition of emerging problems and calling attention to them before they escalate to intractable conflict.

A. Milliken (✉) · P. Grace
William F. Connell School of Nursing, Boston College, Chestnut Hill, MA, USA
e-mail: aimee.milliken@bc.edu

P. Grace
e-mail: Gracepa@bc.edu

S. Monteverde
Department of Health Professions, Bern University of Applied Sciences, Murtenstrasse 10, C3008 Bern, Switzerland
e-mail: settimio.monteverde@bfh.ch

University Hospital of Zurich, Gloriastrasse 31, C8091 Zurich, Switzerland

5.1 History of Healthcare Ethics Committees and Consultation

While questions about what is "right" or "good" have existed for as long as people have relied on others for assistance with their health care needs, ethics committees and clinical ethics services did not formally exist in the US until the late 1970s and early 1980s. The development of clinical ethics services and resources in Europe occurred more recently (Schildmann et al., 2010). According to Tapper (2017) and as discussed in earlier chapters, the advent of organ replacement therapy and intensive care in the 1960s were two major drivers in the development of clinical ethics consultation services, followed by increasingly common and complex issues of scarce resources, in the light of these technological advances and other socioeconomic conditions. As technology has continued to advance, so has the complexity of the ethical questions clinicians are faced with answering. Indeed, it is the increasing complexity of healthcare and the socio-political context in which healthcare services are developed, funded, and provided that brought "strangers" to the bedside (Rothman, 1991). Rothman recounts the move by healthcare professionals to include members of other disciplines, such as lawyers, philosophers, sociologists, theologians, and clergy, including those specially trained to work with patients, in deliberations about value-laden and at times fraught questions that go beyond diagnostic reasoning to decisions of existential import to individuals, the family, and sometimes the broader community.

5.1.1 Landmark Cases

Contemporary ethical frameworks have been influenced by several historical developments, and in fact are always embedded in historical developments or innovations and resulting questions about what we should do or how we should live. A basic reference system can be seen in the law. Although ethics and law may be based in similar concepts or principles (e.g., justice, duties or rights) and case law may even refer to ethical principles, it is important to distinguish ethical arguments (i.e., arguments on what constitutes good medical and nursing practice) from legal considerations; not all ethical problems require adjudicating in law, and sometimes what the law requires may actually cause ethical problems for a particular person. However, these two frameworks are often aligned, especially when serious new problems caused by our biotechnological advancements arise. Thus, there are seminal legal cases that have guided the framing of contemporary ethical challenges and the origins of healthcare ethics committees (HECs), especially in the US. In Europe and elsewhere the interconnection between the legal system, case law and the settling of healthcare ethics questions may be weaker. However, the arguments underlying case law decisions have had an influence on healthcare ethics thinking also outside the US. In particular, two major legal cases in the US court system provided influential decisions about the permissibility of withholding and/or withdrawing life sustaining treatment.

In 1976, the case of Karen Ann Quinlan provoked questions about the legal and ethical permissibility of ventilator withdrawal. Philosophical arguments support that there is no valid distinction between not starting a life-saving intervention and discontinuing an intervention once started, although studies in moral philosophy have pointed to the fact that human beings are more emotionally affected by the latter. These studies provide insights into why the Quinlan case became so notorious. After an accidental overdose, Karen was left ventilator-dependent in a persistent vegetative state. Up to this point, the ethical and legal permissibility of terminal extubation was unclear. Terminal extubation is the permanent removal of an endo- or naso-tracheal tube from someone who is not expected to survive without such respiratory support. Ultimately, the New Jersey Supreme Court ruled that the ventilator could be disconnected (Annas, 1990). Due to the discomfort of some in the healthcare team with this plan, Karen was slowly weaned off the ventilator and subsequently continued breathing on her own due to the presence of autonomic reflexes. She survived for nearly ten more years while being sustained through artificial nutrition and hydration (Beauchamp & Childress, 2013; Tapper, 2017).

This ruling provided precedent to justify the removal of life-sustaining treatments, including ventilation, regardless of whether the person would be able to sustain their respirations. The ruling was affirmed in the US in 1983, when the President's Commission for the Study of Ethical Problems in Medicine and Biomedical and Behavioural Research published *"Deciding to forgo Life-Sustaining Treatment"* which reiterated the right of a patient with decision making capacity, or their surrogate, to refuse resuscitative measures including the authority to consent to the removal of life sustaining treatments (LST) that are already in place (Shelstad, 2005). Importantly, the Quinlan case also served as the impetus for the development of HECs in the US, as the court in this case recommended the formation of hospital-based "ethics committees" to facilitate resolution of difficult cases that may arise (Aulisio et al., 2004).

A second major US court case took place in 1990, when the family of Nancy Cruzan challenged the Missouri Department of Health in an effort to discontinue tube feedings for Nancy, who was in a persistent vegetative state after a car accident. Even though it had become more acceptable to discontinue 'extraordinary' LST under certain conditions, the question arose whether nutrition and hydration could be considered 'extraordinary measures.' Nancy did not require a ventilator for respiratory support, but she did receive nutrition and hydration via feeding tube. The family argued she would not want to live in her current clinical state (Annas, 1990) and asked that the feeding tube be removed. The courts again supported a person's right to refuse LST (or to have a surrogate do so on their behalf), however this time introduced the requirement of "clear and convincing evidence" that the person would not want this type of treatment (Shelstad, 2005).

Under case law in other countries including Canada and the United Kingdom, courts have similarly established that LST may be withdrawn if the treatment is not determined to be in the patient's best interests, however legal oversight and consent requirements vary by location (Downar et al., 2016; The General Medical Council, 2010). Similarly, in European countries under common law, the courts have repeatedly confirmed the right to self-determination in end-of-life situations (for Germany see Grimm & Hillebrand, 2009). At the level of the European Court for Human Rights, the 'right to life' at the *end of life* has repeatedly been formulated as a right to 'private' life, encompassing respect for the sphere of autonomy in decision-making of competent people to forgo treatment (Hendriks, 2019), with many national jurisdictions sharing this line of thought (For the recent French case of Vincent Lambert, a male nurse in a persistent vegetative state after an accident in 2008, whose nutrition and hydration were suspended following his wife's appeal to Vincent's will and against the parents' wishes, see Hendriks, 2019).

Fundamentally, these court rulings have been ethically justified by the principle of autonomy, or an individual's right to self-governance and the ability to act in accordance with a plan of their choosing (Beauchamp & Childress, 2013; Gedge et al., 2007). These situations represent a shift in perspective away from healthcare professionals' obligation to preserve life as being the singular critical principle, towards the recognition that patients' reasoned actual or previously expressed decisions, where known or knowable, should be honoured. But for those patients who lack decision-making capacity and/or whose likely wishes cannot be determined, the courts in the US and Europe have also confirmed the necessity of careful weighing of professional obligations. In these cases, ethical principles other than autonomy have been evoked to determine professional duties. Among these duties are the professional responsibility of providing beneficial treatments, limiting harms and suffering, carefully balancing means and ends, and providing justification for the use of (increasingly scarce) resources. Careful decision-making has been explicitly called for in "medically stable" situations, especially when the means applied to preserve life were not seen as disproportionately burdensome or expensive to reach reasonable ends, e.g., patients with brain injuries needing in medically stable situations needing long-term care (Grimm & Hillebrand, 2009; Hendriks, 2019).

5.1.2 The Evolution of HECs

During these developments, and for the reasons given above, clinical ethics services and hospital ethics committees (HECs) have continued to expand their presence both in the US and elsewhere. In the early 1980s, only 1% of US hospitals had an ethics committee of any kind. More recently, that number has increased and 100% of hospitals with over 400 beds (Fox et al., 2007; Tapper, 2017) have an on-site ethics resource or committee. While the US, Canada, and several European countries were amongst the first to introduce HECs, other regions, including the Eastern Mediterranean and South-East Asia have followed suit in establishing such services (Hajibabaee et al., 2016).

Research in the US, where HECs have existed for the past 40 to 50 years, has indicated a general trend towards increased utilization of HECs and an increased variety in the reasons consults are requested (Aulisio et al., 2009; Gorka et al., 2017). Hospital ethics committees have also gained an increasing presence in Europe. Their establishment follows a complex dynamic and formally began in the late 1980s (Pfafflin et al., 2009). Unlike the US, the linguistic and cultural framework conditions in Europe, historical developments, but also—as in the case of Switzerland—the tradition of direct democracy and decentralized governance result in complex dynamics which affect the way in which these committees have been established (Barazzetti et al., 2014). In Germany, important triggers were the recommendation issued in 1997 by the Catholic and Protestant Hospital Federation, whose institutions were among the first to introduce structures of ethics consultation (Frewer, 2012) and in 2006 by the recommendation of the Central Ethical Committee of the German Medical Association to build HEC capacities. Of particular importance was the case of Marion Ploch, a young woman, brain dead after an accident in 1992, whose pregnancy was continued, but the foetus died in the 17th gestational week. According to Frewer (2012), this case can be considered the "paradigm case" for clinical ethics in Germany (p. 8). It caused public doubt or indignation about "secret machinations" of physicians in the context of medical options not yet known to the larger public. A similar phenomenon was also described in Switzerland after the first successful heart transplant in 1969 (Hofmann, 2016). These public perceptions show that a major driver for the development of HEC in European countries was not only the *normative* function of facilitating orientation or giving advice, but the *expressive* function of giving full account of medical decisions before the public in order to foster transparency and trust in medicine (Holm, 2007). The early integration of healthcare ethics committees into the hospital certification requirements in Germany is another circumstance that triggered the rapid development of these structures. However, this also made it challenging to obtain reliable data on the number, functioning and quality of such structures (Frewer, 2012).

What could have been the reasons for this public scepticism and for the "delayed" adoption of HEC structures in Germany and Switzerland (see Schildmann et al., 2010)? A comparison of developments in the US, Germany, and Switzerland reveals a complex dynamic with at least two distinctive features. In Germany, after World War II, the attempt of society to process the ineffable atrocities against humanity under Nazi medicine can be seen as one roots of societal scepticism toward medical innovations (e.g., in the field of organ transplantation or reproductive medicine). The fear of treating people's lives as "not worth living" resulted in resistance and reluctance to openly and/or publicly address ethically sensitive issues of medical progress, even under the conditions of democracy, rule of law and civil rights (Krones, 2006; Schöne-Seifert & Rippe, 1991). In Switzerland, on the other hand, the call for public accountability for what goes on "behind the walls" of the hospital also had additional cultural roots. These are characterized by an understanding of direct democracy and civic participation, in which questions of life and death cannot simply be left to a panel of experts behind closed doors. This demand for transparency was accompanied by a willingness of citizens to actively participate in discussions regarding the common good, a pronounced mistrust towards "experts," the fear of bureaucratisation and centralisation of decision-making powers, but also the fears of the medical profession itself of losing their decision-making responsibilities (see also Fournier, 2015). Compared to the US, the latter circumstances were additional reasons for the delayed introduction of HECs, clinical ethicists, and other structures of clinical ethics support in Switzerland (Barazzetti et al., 2014; Hurst et al., 2008).

An important driver for the formation of such structures was the Swiss Academy of Medical Sciences (SAMS). In 1979, the academy established the Central Ethics Committee. One task of the committee is to issue medical-ethical guidelines for various areas of medical practice including the declaration of death, dementia care, coercion in medicine, research with humans or critical care. The law governing the medical profession refers to these guidelines, making them binding for medical practice. In 2012, the SAMS issued the medical-ethical guidelines "Ethics Support in Medicine" (SAMS, 2012). This moment not only gave an opportunity to assess the state of development of these structures, but also to formulate basic standards.

The first clinical ethics committee was established in Switzerland in 1988 (Hurst et al., 2007). In 2003, 18% of hospitals in Switzerland reported to have clinical ethics structures with a variety of methodologies and structures, ranging from committees and so-called "Ethics Forums" to clinical ethicists (Hurst et al., 2007, 2008). Ackermann et al. reported in 2016 that 42% of all healthcare institutions have clinical ethics structures with an increasing number of clinical ethicists compared to 2006 and a broad portfolio, the most common structure being a committee.

A recent review of international research studies synthesized the most common reasons for ethics consult requests, including: conflicts around do-not-attempt-resuscitation orders, questions about decision-making capacity, withholding or withdrawing life-sustaining interventions, and surrogate or proxy-decision-making questions (DeSante-Bertkau et al., 2018). Studies have also demonstrated that a majority of clinical ethics consult requests come from critical care units (Bruce et al., 2011; Wasson et al., 2016) where many of the aforementioned issues arise relatively frequently. These categories reflect contemporary challenges that healthcare providers face in practice, and while legal and/or professional society guidance exists, the application of these standards to the individualized situation is not always clear. The contextual aspects surrounding determining and enacting what is best for a particular patient can pose challenges for all involved.

Critiques of the goals, purposes and functions of ethics committees or consultation services, regardless of type and member qualifications, exist. These critiques include such issues as: a focus on behaviour in individual cases rather than changing the ethical culture of the institutions (Kuczewski, 1999); a lack of clarity about the goals (Carter et al., 2018; Garrett, 2016; Schwab, 2016); that they only deal with the few difficult cases that are brought to their attention (Garrett, 2016); inconsistent knowledge, education, and skills of members (Kopelman, 2009); and that they protect the interests of institutions rather than those of patients and their families. The American Society for Bioethics and Humanities (ASBH) has recently developed a credentialing exam for ethics consultants in the US to try to address some of these issues (ASBH, 2014, 2015).

Helen Kohlen's (2009) research findings on the work of HECs in the US and Germany resulted from a qualitative analysis of literature, observation of committee meetings at various institutions and interviews. She notes that while the need for such committees is generally attributable to technological advances and associated complexity, economic and socio-political influences have also played a part in their evolution. Germany, among other countries, has tended to follow the lead of the US in developing institutional ethics committees.

5.2 Healthcare Ethics Committees Description and Functions

Ideally, HECs address three major functions within hospitals and healthcare systems: ethics consultation, ethics education, and policy development (Hester & Schonfeld, 2012). While the HEC's role in each of these categories may vary by location and institution, it is generally accepted that HECs should have a role in addressing each function in order to facilitate the ethical climate of an institution and improve the quality of patient care.

5.2.1 Clinical Ethics Consultation

Clinical ethics consultation is defined as "a set of services provided by an individual or group in response to questions from patients, families, surrogates, healthcare professionals, or other involved parties who seek to resolve uncertainty or conflict regarding value-laden concerns that emerge in health care" (ASBH, 2011, p. 2). Ethics consultation can be conducted by full committee, by an individual, or in a team-based model (Tarzian, 2013). Often, ethics consultants comprise a sub-group of the larger HEC who have additional skills or training in ethics consultation. Committee make-up is discussed in a subsequent section. When consults are conducted by individuals or teams and not the full committee, post-hoc case review is sometimes conducted by the full committee as a mechanism of education and peer review. In some instances, cases that are particularly fraught or challenging may be brought before the full committee even in institutions where individual or team models of consultation predominate.

The general goals of clinical ethics consultation are to "improve the quality of health care through the identification, analysis, and resolution of ethical questions or concerns" (Tarzian, 2013, p. 4). Ethics consultations may address a broad scope of issues, including questions about end-of-life care, beginning of life care, privacy and confidentiality, professionalism, resource allocation, shared decision-making, and research, among others (Tarzian, 2013). Generally, clinical ethics questions that may benefit from ethics consultation relate to questions about what is "right" or "good" for a particular patient when this is either not clear, or what is right or good is being disputed by a team member, family member, or proxy decision-maker. In the US ethics consultation recommendations are advisory and are not medical orders or clinical determinations (American Medical Association, 2019). Specific models of ethics deliberations are discussed in a following section.

5.2.2 Ethics Education

Another major function of HECs often includes ethics education at the individual, group, or institutional level. For example, in England, HECs have been structured to focus on educational activities and policy development as opposed to a strict focus on case consultation (Pfafflin et al., 2009). Similarly, education about institutional priority setting has been identified as a major function of HECs in Norway (Magelssen et al., 2017), and is recommended as a core competency by ASBH in the US (ASBH, 2015).

Education can be conceptualized in several ways. Some HECs provide formalized education to hospital employees through bedside rounds, lecture series, or newsletters. Ethics consultants also provide ethics education to all parties involved in the context of specific ethics consultations. Others have described the role of the ethics consultant as that of a "coach" whose goal is to "assist and support another individual or group striving to achieve excellence" (Kockler & Dirksen, 2015, p. 25). In other words, the act of ethics consultation can "help transform clinical skills and applied knowledge... into professional caregiving practices" (Kockler & Dirksen, 2015, p. 25). In this way, ethics education can help nurses and other clinicians develop the skills necessary to begin to identify and address ethical issues that arise in their practice.

5.2.3 Ethics Policy Development

A hospital's policies are important drivers of the ethical climate (Hester & Schonfeld, 2012). Thus, a crucial function of HECs is the writing and/or evaluation of hospital policy, especially policies that are overtly ethical or have ethical dimensions to them. This is also an organizational ethics function; we say more about organizational ethics in relation to ethics committees in a later section. For example, some policies may directly relate to issues that are within the purview of the HEC, including policies about surrogate decision making, organ donation, or the withdrawal of LST. Others may have ethical considerations related to social justice and patient rights, such as policies about access to certain services. Both can benefit from review by an HEC, which often consists of an interdisciplinary group with some degree of ethical training and a variety of perspectives.

A 2017 study found that institutional "priority setting" was a major function of HECs in Norway, specifically when it came to questions about resource allocation (Magelssen et al., 2017). Other authors have described the increased role HECs have had in policy development in the UK (Doyal, 2001; McLean, 2007). In addition, a well-run HEC should have policies specific to the committee itself, related to the desired structure, process, and outcomes (ASBH, 2011).

5.2.4 Healthcare Ethics Committees: Composition

It is recommended that HECs are multidisciplinary in nature and include a wide variety of perspectives and disciplines (Hester & Schonfeld, 2012). In the US, it is common for one or two community members, who do not have ties to the hospital or clinic, to be included in a HEC. However, these members need to be educated about the critical importance of respecting the confidential nature of committee discussion. It is also important that at least one or two members have advanced skills and training in ethics, when possible, to help frame the ethical issues and guide the discussion (ASBH, 2011; Hester & Schonfeld, 2012). That said, in the US at least, participation on HECs and in ethics consultation is often a voluntary activity undertaken in addition to one's professional activities (Fox et al., 2007). The lack of adequate institutional financial support can significantly limit available consultation resources.

5.2.5 Access

Historically, in many places, access to HECs and ethics consultation was limited to physicians or required a physician order to initiate (Gordon & Hamric, 2006; LaPuma et al., 1988). Anecdotally, and from her work in a variety of critical care units, hospitals, and states during the 1980s and 1990s, the third author (P.G.) notes that physicians tended to control when an ethics consult could be requested and were often reluctant to involve consultants. Her experiences are supported by research during that era (Davies & Hudson, 1999). A study by Gaudine et al. (2011) categorizes reasons why healthcare professionals may fail to consult an ethics committee, including fear of reprisals from colleagues such as physicians.

While this may still be the case in certain areas, particularly where there is a deeply entrenched hierarchy, in recent years there have been efforts made to ensure open access, meaning nurses, patients, families, and other members of the healthcare team can request ethics consultation. The ASBH, for example, recommends that requests from non-physician parties, including nurses, be accepted by matter of policy, and that HECs and ethics consult services are available in all healthcare institutions (ASBH, 2011). Nevertheless, despite these recommendations, access to ethics consultation, and even the existence of hospital-based HECs, is far from universal (Fox et al., 2007) and perhaps especially in pediatric institutions and settings (Kesselheim et al., 2010).

5.3 Ethical Frameworks and Consultative Approaches

Approaches to clinical ethics consultation may vary according to local practice, as may the ethical framework used for deliberation. Goals of consultation typically include "clarifying the situation and/or providing recommendations, ensuring effective communication among diverse groups" and "empowering clinical staff to assess and address ethical issues themselves" (Hester & Schonfeld, 2012, p. 3). An important future role as discussed later is that of supporting the point-of-care professionals to recognize emerging problems and address these before they reach the dilemma stage. This requires good communication skills as discussed in Chapter 4. It is generally accepted that many serious or intractable conflicts emerge from poor or inconsistent communication (Benjamin et al., 2012; Pavlish et al., 2011).

In most places, ethics consultations are conducted using one of three models: consultation by full HEC committee, by an individual consultant, or by a small team. An ethics consultation, whether facilitated by an individual, team, or full committee, tends to involve a formal meeting with all involved parties, a series of meetings with the involved parties, or a combination of both. Hearing the perspectives of all stakeholders is an essential component of the consultation process, to ensure all moral viewpoints have been considered.

In the US, a "facilitation" approach to consultation is recommended by ASBH. In this approach, the consultant(s) aim to accomplish two major tasks: (1) to analyse the nature of the value uncertainty and (2) to facilitate the building of a principled ethical resolution (ASBH, 2011; Dubler & Liebman, 2004; Tarzian, 2013). The facilitation approach involves, for example, hearing the perspectives of the medical team, nursing staff, and patient's family, listening for areas of shared interest, and recommending a plan that can achieve shared goals, despite apparent conflict.

The facilitation approach stands in contrast to the "authoritarian approach" and the "pure consensus approach" (ASBH, 2011; Tarzian, 2013). In the authoritarian approach, the ethics consultant(s) serve as the sole decision maker. While this may facilitate quick decision-making, it runs the risk of overlooking or undervaluing important points of view, particularly from those whose voices might be less powerful, and fails to account for the possibility of personal bias on the part of the decision-maker.

In the pure consensus approach, the focus of the consultation is on achieving agreement amongst all parties. This approach has the benefits of pleasing the involved, however there is a risk that the consensus may be problematic or in contrast to ethical standards. The consensus model also risks overpowering those with less powerful voices (Wilkinson et al., 2016). The facilitation approach avoids both extremes and their associated problems. This model is widely used in the US, and has been used with increasing frequency in Europe (Pfafflin et al., 2009).

5.3.1 Practical Approaches to Ethical Deliberation

There are other approaches to ethical decision making, which may be used by ethics consultants or by individual clinicians, including nurses, looking to work through ethically complex cases. What follows is a description of these models.

Jonsen et al. (2010) have described the "four quadrants" approach. In this approach, the clinician navigates four "quadrants" that relate to the clinical situation, the patient's preferences, the patient's quality of life, and the context of the case. Each quadrant relates to an ethical principle or principles. This approach is widely used by clinicians in the US and in parts of the UK (Sokol, 2008). The four quadrants, and their associated questions are as follows:

- The Clinical Situation (Beneficence and Nonmaleficence)
  - What is the patient's diagnosis and prognosis?
  - What are the possible treatment options and the likely outcome of each option?
- The Patient's Preferences (Autonomy)
  - What is the decisionally capable patient's choice?
  - If the patient is not decisionally capable, are there any advance directives?
  - If there are no advance directives, what do surrogates think the patient would want?
  - If there are no surrogates (or no information to them), what is in the best interest of the patient?
- The Patient's Quality of Life (Beneficence and Nonmaleficence)
  - What among the choices for intervention (or decline of intervention) would seem to be the best option from the perspective of
    - The patient
    - The family
    - The physicians
    - The nurses
    - Other moral stakeholders
- The Context of the Case (Justice/Fidelity)
  - What are the influences of family dynamics?
  - Are there financial considerations to be considered?
  - Are there significant cultural or religious issues?
  - Are there relevant legal precedents? (Jonsen et al., 2010, p. 8)

Other authors have recommended the **FESOR** framework (McCormick-Gendzel & Jurchak, 2006). In this framework, nurses begin by considering the **F**acts, the **E**thical questions, relevant **S**takeholders, brainstorming about **O**ptions, and concluding with a **R**ecommendation, or **R**e-evaluation the options if the recommendation needs revising. FESOR is a helpful acronym to help remember the critical steps in the process and can be applied in a wide range of circumstances.

Lo (2015) recommends the following stepwise process to thinking through cases:

1. *In plain terms, what is the problem or dilemma?*
2. *What are the medical facts and issues?*
3. *What are the concerns, values, and preferences of the [clinicians]?*
4. *What are the concerns, values, and preferences of the patient?*
5. *What are the ethical issues?*
6. *What ethical guidelines are at stake?*
7. *What practical considerations need to be addressed?* (Lo, 2015, p. 7)

Grace has explicated the following ethical decision making framework (Table 5.1), developed for use by nurses in difficult situations (Modified from Grace, 2018, pp 64–65):

Table 5.1 Nurse ethical decision-making in difficult situations

Steps (non linear)—considerations	Questions
Identify the major problem(s)—relate these to professional goals	• Discern facts: clinical, social, environmental? • What implicit assumptions are being made? • Pertinent ethical principles or perspectives? Egs: questionable autonomous decision making, conflicting values among stakeholders. Economic/Expediency vs. Patient good • Power imbalances? What or who has the control?
Identify information gaps	• Do you need more information? Exploring assumptions provides a start • From whom or where can info. be gained?
Determine who is involved	• Who is the main focus? Is there more than one person? Who has (or thinks they have) an interest in the outcome (relatives, staff, other)? Who will be affected by the outcome?
Decide what the prevalent values are Determine if an interpreter is necessary (for cultural or language issues) Who would be the most appropriate interpreter (knowledgeable and neutral)?	• Values held by patient, staff, institution • Value conflicts? Interpersonal, interprofessional, personal vs. professional, patient vs. professional • Cultural perspectives? Who can help with these?
Identify possible courses of action and probable consequences	• Which course of action is likely most beneficial & the least harmful to those involved, including you? • Can safeguards be envisioned for unforeseen consequences?
Implement the selected course of action Conduct an ongoing evaluation	• Does the actual outcome correlate with the anticipated outcome? What was unexpected? Was this foreseeable given more data? • Do similar problems keep reoccurring? If so, why (requires a look at underlying environmental or societal issues perhaps)? Does this point to the need for policy changes or development at the site, institution, or societal level? What further actions might be needed? • Are there continuing staff provider education needs related to the issue?
Engage in self-reflection, reflection on practice (individually, in an interdisciplinary group debriefing session, or in a specialty group forum)	• Could you have done things differently? What would you have liked to understand better? • Would a consultation with colleagues or an ethics resource person have altered your conception of the issue or the course of action taken? • What valuable insights did you gain that should be shared with others and may be applicable to the approach used for future problems?

Grace, P. J. Nursing Ethics and Professional Responsibility in Advanced Practice (3rd ed.). Copyright 2018: Jones and Bartlett Learning, Burlington, Ma. WWW.jblearning.com. Reprinted with permission

Pfafflin and colleagues (2009) describe a hybrid-approach used at a hospital in Germany, combining the Nijmegen approach, the Basel method, and a framework from Leuven. In this approach, "medical, nursing, religious, and social aspects are assessed" (p. 408) first, followed by a clarification of communication problems or misunderstandings. Potential options are identified, along with their pros and cons, and the group works towards achieving a majority agreement. Minority dissenting views are also recorded, and a recommendation is made based on the agreements in the meeting. These recommendations are then documented in the patient's chart (Pfafflin et al., 2009).

The aforementioned frameworks and decision-tools aim to help the nurse consider relevant factors in navigating ethically challenging decisions. There is no one gold standard, some frameworks are better for intractable dilemmas and others for issues encountered in daily practice. For very complex cases it is often helpful to engage with local ethics resources or the local ethics consult service or HEC.

5.4 Organizational Ethics Consultative Models

Organizational ethics involves attention to the moral questions that arise in the actions of healthcare systems (Goold et al., 2000) and is concerned with the ethical issues faced by hospital leadership, and the impact of organizational decisions on patients, hospital employees, and the broader community (Suhonen et al., 2011). The question may be less about *what* the right action is, but more about *how* the right action gets accomplished within the system (Goold et al., 2000). Increasingly, these questions are addressed by HECs in many organizations, although some organizations have developed specific "organizational ethics committees" to answer these sorts of questions.

Wlody (2007) describes four general categories of organizational ethical tensions that can arise in the intensive care unit (ICU) environment. She identifies the locus of tension as stemming from: nursing/patient care, resource allocation/financial issues, physician, ICU leadership, or healthcare organizational leadership. For example, a nursing-focused challenge may relate to staffing, patient transfers, or unanticipated admissions. Resource allocation challenges may include increasing costs, limited resources (including beds and staff), and billing issues (Wlody, 2007). While the types of questions may vary by organization, the major distinguishing factor between organizational ethics and clinical ethics is the focus on the obligations of the organization itself, rather than the particularities of an individual patient's case.

Despite an increase in literature describing the ethical obligations of healthcare institutions or organizations there remains a paucity of research about what sorts of organizational ethics programs or resources exist, or which institutions have a separate venue for discussing these (Suhonen et al., 2011). There are shared problems that institutions face regardless of country such as ensuring quality, cost effectiveness, and managing scarce resources. But there are also ethical conflicts that are specific to a particular region or country's healthcare funding mechanism, social setting and cultural influences. Nevertheless, several models have been introduced to assist organizations in understanding their responsibilities to the patient population and in identifying and addressing systemic ethical issues.

For example, Goold et al. (2000) were concerned with developing a process that would identify steps to resolve thorny problems faced by an institution. The case they use to discuss the model is a peculiarly US one caused by a fragmented system where seamless care transitions are often not available or easily accessed. However, the following model is applicable to institutional ethics analyses regardless of healthcare system. The steps involve questioning:

1. *Who deliberates?*
2. *What is the problem?*
    a. *Who are the organizational and individual actors with dominant roles in the case?*
3. *What should happen (or what should have happened) in this case?*
4. *What organizational policies, procedures, or structures could have prevented, ameliorated, or catalyzed the case? What system features might have prevented such a problem and perhaps prevent future problems? What recommendations does the committee or individual have for changes in organizational policies, procedures, or structures that are feasible?*
5. *Which individuals need to be contacted with these recommendations? Who will have the responsibility for writing these recommendations and to whom should copies of these recommendations be sent?* (Goold et al., 2000, p. 76)

In this model, the authors encourage engaging content experts who may be of assistance in working through the problem, including administrative experts from external organizations, legal expertise, social workers, clinicians, and community representatives.

Winkler and Gruen (2005) propose a model based on four principles: provide care with compassion, treat employees with respect, act in a public spirit, and spend resources reasonably. In "providing care with compassion" (p. 109) the authors argue that healthcare organizations should: ensure competence by setting high standards; ensure compassion and kindness through formal and informal rules and rewards; develop trust between patients and providers by providing individualized care; and use a shared decision-making framework that entails patients and caregivers jointly deciding on treatment. "Treating employees with respect" involves treating employees fairly, facilitating empowerment, and participation. In order to "act in a public spirit," the organization should promote the optimal health of the community it serves. Finally, organizations should "spend resources reasonably" by ensuring the process for limit setting is deliberate, fair, and transparent (Winkler & Gruen, 2005).

5.4.1 Organizational Ethics: Case Examples

5.4.1.1 Veterans Health Administration

One organization in the US that has a robust commitment to organizational ethics is the Veterans Health Administration (VHA). The VHA services nearly 6 million patients annually at more than 1500 locations in the United States (Fox et al., 2010). It provides integrated life-long healthcare services to eligible military veterans. Since 2008, the VHA has implemented an Integrated Ethics® (IE) model, an evidence-informed model with a goal to "support, maintain, and improve ethics quality in health care" (Department of Veterans Affairs, 2018, p. 1).

The organization defines ethics quality in health care as "practices throughout a healthcare organization that are consistent with widely accepted ethical standards, norms, or expectations for the organization and its staff" and these practices are aimed at three levels: decision and actions; systems and processes; and environment and culture (Department of Veterans Affairs, 2018, p. 1). Ethics consultation addresses ethics quality at the level of decisions and actions, preventive ethics addresses ethics quality at the level of systems and processes, and ethical leadership addresses ethics quality at the level of environment and culture (Fox et al., 2010).

To this end, the VHA uses ISSUES, a systematic quality improvement approach to identify and address ethics quality gaps. The steps in the ISSUES approach are: (1) Identify an issue, (2) Study the issue, (3) Select a strategy, (4) Undertake a plan, (5) Evaluate and adjust, (6) Sustain and spread. The organization also uses a preventive ethics (PE) approach, aimed at reducing variation in ethical practices by "identifying and intervening in aspects of an organization's systems and processes that contribute to ethics quality gaps" (Department of Veterans Affairs, 2018, p. 6). Preventive ethics will be discussed in greater detail in the next section. In addition, the IE model requires that VHA organizations have an IE Council. This council is tasked with oversight of the IE program.

5.4.1.2 Harvard Pilgrim Health Care

Harvard Pilgrim Health Care (HPHC) is another organization with a well-developed organizational ethics program. HPHC is a not-for-profit health insurance company in the North East United States, serving over one million members (Sabin & Cochran, 2007). The organization has an "Ethics Advisory Group" (EAG), founded on the premise that "virtually all HPHC activities have implications for the ethical quality of care and service our members receive" (Harvard Pilgrim Health Care, 2019). The EAG includes HPHC employees, members, purchasers, brokers, and physician leaders, in addition to members from the community. EAG meetings occur quarterly, and the group typically deliberates about cases where a request for consultation has been made by HPHC leaders or managers who "desire consultation about the values associated with a particular business decision or activity for which they are responsible" (Harvard Pilgrim Health Care, 2019). As with most HECs, these recommendations are advisory in nature and not meant to serve as the final word or decision on the issue at hand (Sabin & Cochran, 2007).

James Sabin, MD, former co-chair of the HPHC EAG, recommends four developmental steps for any HEC that chooses to take on questions of organizational ethics. First, he recommends educating the HEC about the organization's broader administrative functions, including finance, law, human resources, etc. Second, he suggests cultivating links to administrative leadership. Third, there should be broad membership on the committee in accord with the expanded purview. This involves including key stakeholders in the organization and the community. Finally, he recommends starting slowly and using a "try-it-fix-it" approach. This may require pilot-testing ideas and collecting data to measure effectiveness (Sabin, 2016).

Sabin (2016) also suggests three potential methodologies for "doing" organizational ethics. One approach is via quality improvement, similar to the model described at the VHA. A second option is through the support of a mission, which may be appropriate at, for example, a faith-based organization. A third method is using stakeholder analysis, which is the model used at HPHC (Sabin, 2016).

5.5 Preventive Ethics

Both clinical and organizational ethics consultation should be aimed at fostering a preventive ethics approach. Preventive ethics is a proactive, rather than reactive, approach to managing ethical issues that includes identifying possible sources of ethical conflict before they develop into intractable problems (Epstein, 2012). This has also been called "proactive ethics" (Pavlish et al., 2013). A major assumption in preventive ethics is that ethical conflict is predictable, and that sources of conflict can be identified (Epstein, 2012; Forrow et al., 1994). Preventive ethics has been described as akin to a "preventive medicine" approach, where the focus is on identifying and addressing the factors that give rise to conflict, rather than the conflicts themselves (Forrow et al., 1994).

Preventive ethics efforts may be focused at an organizational level by implementing policies and procedures to mitigate possible conflict (McCullough, 2005), or may identify recurring "triggers" in a particular area of practice. For example, in an intensive care unit, "triggers" of potential ethical conflict may include: unrealistic expectations about the prognosis, infrequent visits or contact with the health care team, lack of social support, or cultural beliefs that are unfamiliar to the providers (Epstein, 2012). In contrast to a reactive-ethics approach, where conflict has already occurred, a preventive ethics approach aims to prevent escalation of conflict by addressing it early.

5.5.1 Models of Preventive Ethics

Pavlish and colleagues (2013) propose a stepwise framework for managing potential ethical conflict in a proactive way. Their model begins with "primary prevention" strategies, including education, policy development, ethics guidelines, and ethical work environments. These strategies are aimed at deterring the occurrence of ethical conflict. Next, the model progresses to "secondary prevention," or "risk reduction." This step is aimed at modifying risk factors for conflict, such as the "triggers" previously mentioned. Finally, "tertiary prevention" is aimed at repairing relationships when ethical conflict has already occurred. These cases are where ethics consultation is typically involved in mediating conflict and helping parties achieve a resolution.

As described, preventive ethics is an integral part of the VHA's IntegratedEthics® model. The organization describes preventive ethics as "activities performed by an individual or group on behalf of a healthcare organization to identify, prioritize, and address systemic ethics issues" (Foglia et al., 2012, p. 15). Their system recommends that preventive ethics functions include: someone to coordinate the function (a coordinator), staff to carry out the preventive ethics activities, an organizing structure (such as a team), and a specific, systematic approach. At the VHA, the ISSUES approach (previously described) is used (Foglia et al., 2012).

Palliative care services, while not always thought of as being a preventive ethics resource, are often able to defuse emerging conflict that interferes with providing optimal care to a person. Barriers to optimal care may include difficulty in determining what is best for the person in question or blocks that person in some way from receiving what is needed to relieve their suffering. As discussed earlier, pressures from family members may lead to ethical conflict as the person accedes to the desires of that person or tries to make peace among various factions. The availability of a palliative care team, composed of a team of experts from diverse professions can, by meeting the comprehensive needs of patients and their families, prevent ethical conflicts from arising or escalating. They can help support family members charged with surrogate decision-making and who are experiencing decisional conflict (Allen et al, 2008). Good communication is especially important in reducing decisional conflict around serious illness can help resolve differing opinions about the goals of care (Smith-Howell et al., 2016).

5.5.2 Palliative Care, Nursing, and Preventive Ethics

The term palliative care was coined in the early 1970s, by Canadian physician Balfour Mount who had taken the idea of hospice from Dame Cicely Saunders and adapted it to encompass more than terminal care of a patient at end-of-life (Lynch et al., 2013). His idea was to provide quality care for those with life threatening illnesses, not solely those imminently dying. Efforts have been made since then to settle on a definition of palliative care that captures its essential aspects. However, as a relatively new specialty healthcare practice research on qualitative outcomes remains scarce. Nevertheless, various aspects of activities and intentions such as evaluating the person's physical, psychological and contextual needs have been shown to improve the quality of care in cases of life-threatening illness or severe and seemingly intractable symptoms (Ferrell et al., 2018). In the US, the 4th Edition of the National Consensus Project Clinical Practice Guidelines for Quality Palliative Care Guidelines (Ferrell et al., 2018), recognizes the need "to improve access to quality palliative care for all people with serious illness regardless of setting, diagnosis, prognosis, or age" (p. 1684). Moreover, the guidelines affirm that recognizing the need for palliative care is an obligation of all who provide care to the seriously ill. Nurses are often the ones in hospital settings who are the first to recognize that a patient would benefit from a palliative care consult or evaluation. However, there may be hurdles to surmount including that palliative care can be associated with hospice. This association can lead patients and family members to believe the team has given up treating an underlying condition. Indeed, even some clinicians may be reluctant to engage palliative care given this misconception about the specialty's purpose.

Nurses can play a pivotal role in ensuring a patient's voice, preferences and values are honored in palliative care settings, especially when the team focuses more on the medical needs than psychological, contextual, and spiritual. Moran and colleagues' (2021), integrative review revealed that nurses were not always heard, and their 'hidden' work not always recognized. The "values of nursing; care, compassion and commitment … while depicted within descriptions of practice …were not articulated (seen but not heard)." The authors worried, in an era where evidence-based practice rules, that nurses' work becomes invisible and discounted. Thus, palliative care nursing contributions may risk being too vague and devalued unless nurses learn how to articulate what is their value-added role in the palliative care team (Moran et al., 2021). The World Health Organization's (WHO, 2020) latest definition of palliative care and patient's rights to access, perhaps unintentionally, highlights the potential role of nurses whether in non-palliative or palliative care setting.

> Palliative care is an approach that improves the quality of life of patients (adults and children) and their families who are facing problems associated with life-threatening illness. It prevents and relieves suffering through the early identification, correct assessment and treatment of pain and other problems, whether physical, psychosocial or spiritual. (WHO 2020)

Palliative care teams focus on alleviating suffering regardless of type and are usually available to provide support to family members or significant others. Because the focus is about helping relieve the person's suffering, a comprehensive approach utilizing the input of various professionals is warranted. Team members vary based on the complexities and areas of a person's needs; however, nurses are invariably involved in various ways. Chapters 1, 2, 3, and 4 provide the rationale, strategies and tools enabling nurse moral agency. As a reminder that is the ability to articulate their concerns related to patients and palliative care in interdisciplinary collaborations. Far from being unimportant, the nursing perspective is one of humanizing the healthcare environment and we need to find ways to articulate this for the purpose of fulfilling nursing goals and to prevent potential ethical issues from escalating into conflicts.

5.5.3 Advance Directives and Advance Care Planning

As the aforementioned landmark cases highlight, decision making at the end of life can be rife with ethical challenges. Ideally, some of these difficulties can be mitigated by adopting a preventive-ethics approach, as described. One such intervention involves the completion of advance directives and the related activity of advance care planning.

5.5.3.1 Advance Directives

In the United States, The Patient Self Determination Act (PSDA) was passed in 1990 with the goal of promoting the use of advance directives as a way for people to exercise autonomy and self-determination regarding end-of-life care (Dobbins, 2007). The law was also supposed to encourage education and "communication about end-of-life issues" (Grace, 2004, p. 314). It was also supposed to ensure that upon entering a healthcare institution a person would be informed of their right to accept or refuse treatment. Regardless of whether there are laws in a given country supportive of advance care planning, it is widely recognized as an ethical autonomy-supporting right in those countries where human rights are honored. Recently a International Advanced Care Planning Society (ACP-I, 2021) was formed to further the goals of helping people determine what they would want in the event that the ability to articulate their wishes were lost. Advance directives typically involve two components: (1) a living will, which is a document stating preferences regarding end-of-life decisions, and (2) the appointment of a surrogate decision maker tasked with making decisions on behalf of the patient should they lose decision-making capacity.

Studies over the past several decades have extensively examined the effectiveness of the PSDA in the United States, and advance directives more broadly to evaluate their usefulness in guiding end-of-life care. One early landmark study in the United States found that, even with the advent of the PSDA, most patients had not completed advance directives. When they had, the study found that advance directives did not significantly impact the plan of care and resuscitation efforts (The SUPPORT Principal Investigators, 1995).

Multiple studies since the SUPPORT Intervention have indicated that advance directives have limited effectiveness, and some authors assert that advance directives have failed entirely (Burt, 2005). Research continually suggests that only a minority of patients have completed advanced directives. In the instances where an advance directive has been completed, a surrogate decision maker may be appointed, however this does not guarantee that the surrogate has discussed end-of-life preferences with the patient (Murray & Jennings, 2005).

Advance directives themselves contribute to the problem. Living wills are either overly vague or overly specific, and do not predict every possible situation (Hickman et al., 2005). For example, directives may state "do not keep me alive on machines" or "let me die if I am a vegetable." On the other hand, they may specify directives only in specific situations, such as "if in a vegetative state" (Hickman et al., 2005, p. S27). This leads to surrogates having to make decisions based on presumed patient preference, which may be very difficult to infer.

Advance directives also tend to be static unless discussed with the patient by healthcare providers during healthcare visits. Once they are completed, they do not typically get readdressed (Hickman et al., 2005). Preferences may change over time and with variation in a patients' condition, but these changes may not get readdressed in the directives (Fagerlin & Schneider, 2004). This can be a source of concern for surrogates, who worry that if they follow the directives they aren't truly making a decision that their loved one would have made in that moment. Further, evidence has shown that surrogates are barely better than chance at accurately predicting what their loved one would choose (Shalowitz et al., 2006; Torke et al., 2014).

In addition, advance directives are oriented more towards defining what medical treatments a patient would refuse. Patients typically do not receive much assistance in defining what outcomes they do want from treatment (Hickman et al., 2005). If goals and values go unaddressed, the advance directive provides the surrogate with very little guidance for decision-making.

5.5.3.2 Advance Care Planning

In reaction to the limitations posed by advance directives, advance care planning has been suggested as a process to improve the utilization and effectiveness of advance directives. Advance care planning is more comprehensive than merely appointing a proxy-decision maker or having a written document and should allow patients to express "wishes about medical care, placement, or related financial and legal issues to cover times of future incapacity" (Perkins, 2007). It should take place over time and be an evolving discussion between provider and patient (Hickman et al., 2005). The surrogate should be actively involved in the process.

Advance care planning uses advance directives to document a person's preferences, but is a more fluid process that does not end with the completion of the living will or written document (Messinger-Rapport et al., 2009). Typically performed on an outpatient basis, providers should assess the level of understanding that their patients and families have about their condition. A values assessment can be performed, which helps to identify what the patient values and considers important in their quality of life. This helps guide what treatments would be considered acceptable and not acceptable. Ensuring the named surrogate decision maker has a good understanding of these values can aid in future decision making (Messinger-Rapport et al., 2009), and realistic goals can be formulated. Goals can then be readdressed in the case of illness exacerbations or other deteriorations in condition (Lynn & Goldstein, 2003). Patients and families should also understand the limitations of the advance directive itself; it is not an omnipotent document and cannot predict every situation (Perkins, 2007).

Involving not only surrogates but other family members as well is paramount in these discussions (Perkins, 2007). Ensuring that everyone involved with the patient's care understands the patient's wishes will help minimize conflict and improve the surrogate's ability to advocate for the patient (Perkins, 2007). Families should also be emotionally prepared when a patient already has an illness (Lynn & Goldstein, 2003). Preparing patients and families for what to expect when the disease worsens helps to minimize conflict with decision-making as well.

Another key element of advance care planning is ensuring that advance directives are readily available in all healthcare situations. Having the document present ensures that patients' wishes are made known to providers and facilitates surrogate decision-making. In the US, one tactic for accomplishing this, especially for those with serious chronic and/or life-threatening conditions is to request a form to be completed in concert with one's physician. The form is titled Physician Orders for Life-Sustaining Treatment (POLST) (Hickman et al., 2010). This takes the form of a brightly-colored document that translates patient preferences into physician orders and follows patients regardless of institution (Hickman et al., 2010). One study utilizing POLST found that patients were more likely to have their preferences respected and were less likely to receive intravenous fluids or be hospitalized (in accordance with their wishes) (Hickman et al., 2010). The use of electronic medical records has also been suggested as a promising way to ensure their portability. (Collins et al., 2006).

Advance care planning also requires that clinicians be more involved with patients throughout the continuum of their journeys with illness. Clinicians involved in advance care planning should be readily accessible in time of crisis to the patient and to the family to help reiterate decisions that were made (Perkins, 2007). A 2010 study in Australia found that advance care planning led to decreased symptoms of post-traumatic stress disorder (PTSD) in surrogates and increased reports of satisfaction in family members surrounding end of life care (Detering et al., 2010). The study also found that, in 92% of cases where the patient's wishes were known, they were respected.

Hickman et al. (2005) summarize the goals of advance care planning. It should focus on defining "good care" for each patient. Wishes, goals, plans and the person identified as the surrogate should be identified and documented. The advance care plan forms should be standardized so that they are portable across institutions. Advance directives should be revisited periodically so that the wishes documented reflect the most recent desires of the patient. Finally, advance care plans should be built into policy and incorporated across all parts of the healthcare system. Comprehensive advance care planning programs, such as "Five Wishes," "Let Me Decide," and "Respecting Choices," exist and can be used to facilitate this process (Hickman et al., 2005). See Appendix A for an example.

5.6 Summary

The structure and function of healthcare ethics committees (HEC) and consultative services vary based on region and country. However, the main focus of them all is on addressing ethical conflict in inpatient care and in some countries on determining social policies that support the ethical treatment of the population related to healthcare. HECs can focus specifically on issues of clinical ethics, or more broadly on organizational ethics. Nurses play a pivotal role in identifying issues where ethics consultation may be helpful. They are likely to be most effective in this role when they have a strong grounding in the goals and perspectives of their profession, an understanding of their professional responsibilities to provide good patient care, and the skills and knowledge to overcome barriers to good care. This involves developing confidence in their ethical decision-making skills, having a basic grasp of ethical principles, and the presence of a supportive environment. Moreover, nurses are critically important members of ethics committees. They are the professionals in most frequent, sustained, and intimate contact with patients and their families and thus can advocate for the perspectives of patients and their family members to be heard. Finally, preventive ethics is an approach to preventing ethical conflict by identifying common potential sources, and then developing interventions aimed at addressing them.

Appendix A: Example Discussing Advance Care Planning With a Patient

What follows is a hypothetical example of the nurse's role in discussing advance care planning with a patient.

Amina Jordan is a Registered Nurse at a community primary healthcare center in a small Massachusetts town. Prior to her marriage she had worked as a critical care nurse in a busy academic medical center in the North East United States. She was familiar with the problems and conflicts that could arise when patients lost their decision-making capacity (either permanently or temporarily) and it was not known what their values and preferences were related to life sustaining treatments (LST).

Among her practice responsibilities now is educating the practice population about the importance of advance directives for preserving patient's autonomy even after ability to express values and preferences is lost. To facilitate this Amina completed a continuing education course focused on advance care planning that provided her with the basic knowledge and skills for having such conversations. She also persuaded the practice to allow her to provide classes on the topic for members of the community. This brief presentation demonstrates how Amina introduces the topic to a healthy recently retired patient who just moved into the community. She is married and her husband is also healthy. They have no family in the immediate area. At Clara Darnbrough's first visit as part of the data-gathering by the Nurse Practitioner she is

5 Models of Ethics Deliberation and Consultation

asked whether she has completed an advanced directive or has appointed a surrogate decision-maker in the event of her inability to express her wishes. She says she has not and always thought her husband would know what to do but was open to discussing this further. An appointment is made for her to talk with Amina. The following is a re-enactment of the discussion.

Amina (who has prepared the room so that she is sitting facing Clara with some space but no barriers between them): Welcome Ms. Darnbrough. I'm Amina Jordan, a Registered Nurse here at the practice. My only purpose today is to learn what you know about advance directives and help you to think through what your wishes might be for future healthcare interventions if you became unable to tell people yourself. The staff at this clinic asks every new patient over the age of 18 years whether they have an advance directive and we revisit this every year to see if anything has changed. We believe that having an advance directive is the best way for our patients to exercise their autonomy even when they have lost the ability to express what they want in the way of medical interventions. I am wondering how you would like me to address you today (Clara or Miss, Mrs, Ms. Darnbrough?).

Clara Clara is fine.

Amina OK Clara it is, Perhaps a good place to start is to ask you what you know about advance care planning?

Clara Well I am not sure ... I have heard about living wills? I have heard that people who are very sick should probably think about what they want in terms of the doctors 'doing everything' to keep the person alive or not. But since I have always been healthy, I thought I would just deal with that at the time. I suppose no-one likes to think about such possibilities especially as one gets older. My hope has always been that death would be fast and I would not be aware of it happening (*laughs* ... I suppose that could also be called me avoiding thinking about it).

Amina Yes that is understandable and you are certainly not alone in thinking that. However, as a nurse who used to work in critical care settings, I have seen many situations where people become sick so quickly they do not have time to tell people what they do and don't want. Then their loved ones are faced with trying to figure it out at a time when they themselves are stressed and may not have a good understanding of the medical situation or options. So in a way you are both trying to make sure that you do not receive the type of treatment that you would not want, and that you *do* receive the type of treatment you *would* want. So having thought about this beforehand, you can empower the person who is having to make decisions for you and reassure them that they are choosing what you would want.

There are four main areas of advance care planning – you need not remember them ... we can revisit this after you have had time to think about what you want and discuss it with others. I will also give you some information to take home:

- Deciding who you want to make decisions for you if you become unable – this may or may not be your spouse or partner (it may be too big a burden for them to take on), it may be someone you trust to carry out your wishes.
- Thinking about what courses of action (treatments/interventions) you would find acceptable and under which conditions
- Talking things over with others such as your loved ones, your physician/nurse practitioner, a knowledgeable nurse who can walk you through different scenarios
- Documenting what you would want (most like a living will)

It is important to know that whatever you decide, even if written and witnessed, *can be changed by you any time you want to make revisions perhaps as your situation changes*—advance directives—your written or spoken wishes, are not permanent.

Clara That is good to know. I would hate to think I had committed myself to something I think I want now and that I might not want later.

Amina Yes it can be very tricky to sort through everything that could possibly happen and what that would mean and envision what you want. We can talk again after you have had time to discuss with your husband and other family members or friends. You can also bring him or her to our next meeting if you think that would be helpful. Think about what kinds of activities are most important to you, and use those to guide your decision-making. For example perhaps time spent interacting with family is something that brings you joy, and if you were ever in a state where this was not possible, this would not be an acceptable quality of life for you.

There is an easier way of thinking about what you would want that has been prepared by the *Aging with Dignity* organization. It is in the form of five questions to consider and is called the Five Wishes. Instead of trying to describe what you would want in a range of possible situations the organization has come up with questions to ask oneself. They developed this as a result of their founder's experiences working in Mother Teresa's homes for the dying. They wanted to "ensure that every person who was facing problems at the end of life, or with changed circumstances, is given the opportunity to talk about what matters most, and to ensure that their wishes are known:" (https://fivewishes.org/) I will give you some more information on this to take home with you and we can talk a little more about them now and after you have had time to consider what you want.

The first wish is about deciding who you would like to make decisions for you if you lost ability. We talked a little about this earlier. Perhaps think about whether your husband would be the best person or someone else. You could also think of a second person who can support your husband. It is best to have someone who knows you well and is able to put their own worries and needs to the side so they can determine what you would most likely want.

The second wish has to do with what kind of medical treatment you would or would not want. It is often helpful to think about how long you would be okay with certain treatments as well. For example, some people would consider it alright to be on a ventilator to help their breathing for a short time (say, a few weeks) especially if they thought this would allow them to recover enough to do the things they normally like to do. However, they might not want to be on a ventilator for months or years. If you recover your ability to make your wishes known, at any point you can change your mind about what you find acceptable and you have a right to stop the treatment or intervention. The person you appoint to make your decisions only does so for the amount of time that you cannot communicate what you want and your reasons for wanting it.

Third, you can think about how comfortable you would want to be, and in what setting you would be most comfortable. Is being at home very important? Would you be OK with some discomfort if it would allow you to be at an important life event for a loved one (a marriage say, or the birth of a grandchild)? For example, some medications used to treat cancer can weaken you and cause side effects but might extend your life. Or would you prefer to have your pain treated with medications, such as morphine, that provide comfort but do not extend life? Would you be okay being cared for in a facility, if necessary?

This relates to the fourth wish, which has to do with how you want people to treat you. What matters most to you in your care? What would you want your providers to know about you, your values and preferences.

Finally, the fifth wish is about what you want your loved ones to know. What do you want to make sure they are aware of, in the event that you are no longer able to tell them?

Clara Well, this has certainly given me a lot to think about. I like the idea of talking about the Five Wishes with my family.

Amina That is a great place to start. Here's some information to help you and some internet resources that you can use. Call the office when you are ready to talk more and think about whether you would like me to help you discuss this with your family. It is something that the people in your life should also be thinking about if they haven't already.

References

Ackermann, S., Balsiger, L., Salathé, M. (2016). Ethikstrukturen an Akutspitälern, Psychiatrischen Kliniken und Rehabilitationskliniken der Schweiz. Dritte, erweiterte Umfrage der Schweizerischen Akademie der Medizinischen Wissenschaften. *Bioethica Forum, 9*(2), 52–59.
Advanced Care Planning International Society. (2021). https://www.acp-i.org/society/

Allen, R. S., Allen, J. Y., Hilgeman, M. M., & DeCoster, J. (2008). End-of-life decision-making, decisional conflict, and enhanced information: Race effects. *Journal of the American Geriatrics Society, 56*(10), 1904–1909. https://doi.org/10.1111/j.1532-5415.2008.01929.x

American Medical Association. (2019). Ethics committees in health care institutions. Retrieved from Code of Medical Ethics Opinion 10.7 website: https://www.ama-assn.org/delivering-care/ethics/ethics-committees-health-care-institutions

American Society for Bioethics and Humanities (ASBH). (2011). *Core competencies for healthcare ethics consultation* (second). American Society for Bioethics and Humanities.

American Society for Bioethics and Humanities (ASBH). (2014). Code of ethics and professional responsibilities for healthcare ethics consultants. *Improving competencies in clinical ethics consultation: An education guide.*

American Society for Bioethics and Humanities (ASBH). (2015). *Improving competencies in clinical ethics consultation: An education guide* (Second). American Society for Bioethics and Humanities.

Annas, G. (1990). Nancy Cruzan and the right to die. *New England Journal of Medicine, 323*(10), 670–673.

Aulisio, M. P., Chaitin, E., & Arnold, R. M. (2004). Ethics and palliative care consultation in the intensive care unit. *Critical Care Clinics, 20*(3), 505–523. https://doi.org/10.1016/j.ccc.2004.03.006

Aulisio, M. A. R. K. P., Moore, J., Blanchard, M., Bailey, M., & Smith, D. (2009). Clinical ethics consultation and ethics integration in an urban public hospital. *Cambridge Quarterly of Healthcare Ethics, 18*(4), 371–383. https://doi.org/10.1017/s0963180109090574

Barazzetti, G., Bondolfi, A., Hurst, S., & Mauron, A. (2014). Switzerland (entry). In H. ten Have & B. Gordijn (Eds.), *Handbook of global bioethics* (pp. 1537–1557). Springer.

Beauchamp, T. L., & Childress, J. F. (2013). *Principles of biomedical ethics* (7th ed.). Oxford University Press.

Benjamin, B., Yeager, A., & Simon, A. (2012). *Conversation transformation*. McGraw-Hill.

Bruce, C. R., Smith, M. L., Hizlan, S., & Sharp, R. R. (2011). A systematic review of activities at a high-volume ethics consultation service. *Journal of Clinical Ethics, 22*(2), 151–164.

Burt, R. (2005). The end of autonomy. *Improving End of Life Care: Why Has It Been So Difficult? Hastings Center Report Special Report, 34*(6), S9–S13.

Collins, L., Parks, S., & Winter, L. (2006). The state of advance care planning: One decade after SUPPORT. *American Journal of Hospice and Palliative Medicine, 23*(5), 378–384.

Carter, B., Brockman, M., Garrett, J., Knackstedt, A., & Lantos, J. (2018, June). Why are there so few ethics consults in children's hospitals? *HEC Forum, 30*(2), 91–102.

Davies, L., & Hudson, L. D. (1999). Why don't physicians use ethics consultation? *Journal of Clinical Ethics, 10*(2), 116–125.

Department of Veterans Affairs. (2018). *IntegratedEThics*. https://www.ethics.va.gov

DeSante-Bertkau, J., McGowan, M., & Antommaria, A. (2018). Systematic review of typologies used to characterize clinical ethics consultations. *Journal of Clinical Ethics, 29*(4), 291–304.

Detering, K., Hancock, A., Reade, M., & Silvester, W. (2010). The impact of advance care planning on end of life care in elderly patients: Randomized controlled trial. *British Medical Journal, 340*, 1–9.

Dobbins, E. (2007). End-of-life decisions: Influence of advance directives on patient care. *Journal of Gerontological Nursing, 33*(10), 50–56.

Downar, J., Sibbald, R. W., Bailey, T. M., & Kavanagh, B. P. (2016). Withholding and withdrawing treatment in Canada: Implications of the Supreme Court of Canada's decision in the Rasouli case. *CMAJ, 186*(16), E622–E626.

Doyal, L. (2001). Clinical ethics committees and the formulation of health care policy. *Journal of Medical Ethics, 27*(SUPPL. 1), 44–49. https://doi.org/10.1136/jme.27.suppl_1.i44

Dubler, N., & Liebman, C. (2004). *Bioethics mediation: A guide to shaping shared solutions* (second). United Hospital Fund of New York.

Epstein, E. G. (2012). Preventive ethics in the intensive care unit. *AACN Advanced Critical Care, 23*(2), 217–224. https://doi.org/10.1097/NCI.0b013e31824b3b9b

Fagerlin, A., & Schneider, C. (2004). Enough: The failure of the living will. *Hastings Center Report, 34*(1), 30–42.

Ferrell, B. R., Twaddle, M. L., Melnick, A., & Meier, D. E. (2018). National consensus project clinical practice guidelines for quality palliative care guidelines (4th ed.). *Journal of Palliative Medicine, 21*(12), 1684–1689. https://doi.org/10.1089/jpm.2018.0431

Foglia, M. B., Fox, E., Chanko, B., & Bottrell, M. M. (2012). Preventive ethics: Addressing ethics quality gaps on a systems level. *Joint Commission Journal on Quality and Patient Safety, 38*(3), 103–111.

Fournier, V. (2015). Clinical ethics: Methods (reference work entry). In: H. ten Have (Ed.), Encyclopedia of global bioethics. Springer. https://doi.org/10.1007/978-3-319-05544-2

Forrow, L., Arnold, R., & Parker, L. (1994). Preventive ethics: Expanding the horizons of clinical ethics. *The Journal of Clinical Ethics, 4*(4), 287–294.

Fox, E., Bottrell, M. M., Berkowitz, K. A., Chanko, B. L., Foglia, M. B., & Pearlman, R. A. (2010). Integratedethics: An innovative program to improve ethics quality in health care. *Innovation Journal, 15*(2), 1–36.

Fox, E., Myers, S., & Pearlman, R. A. (2007). Ethics consultation in United States hospitals: A national survey. *American Journal of Bioethics, 7*(2), 13–25. https://doi.org/10.1080/15265160601109085

Frewer, A. (2012). Klinische Ethik und Ethikberatung. In A. Frewer, F. Bruns, & A. May (Eds.), *Ethikberatung in der Medizin* (pp. 8–18). Springer.

Garrett, J. R. (2016). The poverty of value clarification: Using ethical theory to critique and transcend the "Givens" of Clinical Ethics Consultation. *The American Journal of Bioethics, 16*(9), 48–51.

Gaudine, A., Lamb, M., LeFort, S. M., & Thorne, L. (2011). Barriers and facilitators to consulting hospital clinical ethics committees. *Nursing Ethics, 18*(6), 767–780.

Gedge, E., Giacomini, M., & Cook, D. (2007). Withholding and withdrawing life support in critical care settings: Ethical issues concerning consent. *Journal of Medical Ethics, 33*(4), 215–218. https://doi.org/10.1136/jme.2006.017038

Goold, S., Kamil, L., Cohan, N., & Sefansky, S. (2000). Outline of a process for organizational ethics consultation. *HEC Forum, 12*(1), 69–77.

Gordon, E., & Hamric, A. (2006). The courage to stand up: The cultural politics of nurses' access to ethics consultation. *Journal of Clinical Ethics, 17*(3), 231–254. http://search.ebscohost.com/login.aspx?direct=true&db=cin20&AN=105950423&site=ehost-live.

Gorka, C., Craig, J., & Spielman, B. (2017). Growing an ethics consultation service: A longitudinal study examining two decades of practice. *American Journal of Bioethics, 8*(2), 116–127. https://doi.org/10.1080/23294515.2017.1292327

Grace, P. J. (2004). Ethics in the clinical encounter. In S. K. Chase (Ed.), Clinical judgement and communication in nurse practitioner practice (pp. 295–332). F. A. Davis.

Grace, P. J. (2018). *Nursing ethics and professional responsibility in advanced practice* (3rd ed.). Jones and Bartlett.

Grimm, C., & Hillebrand, I. (2009). Sterbehilfe. Rechtliche und ethische Aspekte. Freiburg, Karl Alber.

Hajibabaee, F., Joolaee, S., Cheraghi, M. A., Salari, P., & Rodney, P. (2016). Hospital/clinical ethics committees' notion: An overview. *Journal of Medical Ethics and History of Medicine, 9*, 1–9.

Harvard Pilgrim Health Care. (2019). The Harvard Pilgrim Health Care Ethics Program. https://www.harvardpilgrim.org/public/the-harvard-pilgrim-health-care-ethics-program

Hendriks, A. C. (2019). End-of-life decisions. Recent jurisprudence of the European Court of Human Rights. *ERA Forum, 19*(4), 561–570.

Hester, M., & Schonfeld, T. (2012). *Guidance for healthcare ethics committees.* Cambridge University Press.

Hickman, S., Hammes, B., Moss, A., & Tolle, S. (2005). Hope for the future: Achieving the original intent of advance directives. *Improving End of Life Care: Why Has It Been So Difficult? Hastings Center Report Special Report, 34*(6), S26–S30.

Hickman, S., Nelson, C., Perrin, N., Moss, A., Hammes, B., & Tolle, S. (2010). A comparison of methods to communicate treatment preferences in nursing facilities: Traditional practices versus the physician orders for life-sustaining treatment program. *Journal of the American Geriatrics Society, 58*(7), 1241–1248.

Hofmann, S. (2016). Umstrittene Körperteile. Eine Geschichte der Organspende in der Schweiz. Bielefeld, transcript.

Holm, S. (2007). Policy-making in pluralistic societies. In B. Steinbock (Ed.), *The Oxford handbook of bioethics* (pp. 153–174). Oxford University Press.

Hurst, S. A., Reiter-Theil, S., Perrier, A. et al. (2007). Physicians' access to ethics support services in four European countries. *Health Care Analysis, 15*, 321–225.

Hurst, S. A., Reiter-Theil, S., Baumann-Hölzle, R., Foppa, C., Malacrida, R., Bosshard, G., Salathé, M., & Mauron, A. (2008). The growth of clinical ethics in a multilingual country: Challenges and opportunities. *Bioethica Forum, 1*(1), 15–24.

Jonsen, A. R., Siegler, M., & Winslade, W. J. (2010). *Clinical ethics: A practical approach to ethical decisions in clinical medicine*. McGraw-Hill.

Kesselheim, J. C., Johnson, J., & Joffe, S. (2010). Ethics consultation in children's hospitals: Results from a survey of pediatric clinical ethicists. *Pediatrics, 125*(4), 742–746.

Kockler, N. J., & Dirksen, K. (2015). *Competencies required for clinical ethics consultation as coaching*. https://www.chausa.org/docs/default-source/hceusa/kockler---formatted.pdf?sfvrsn=12

Kohlen, H. (2009). *Conflicts of care: Hospital ethics committees in the USA and Germany*. Campus Verlag.

Kopelman, L. M. (2009). Bioethics as public discourse and second-order discipline. *Journal of Medicine and Philosophy, 34*(3), 261–273.

Krones, T. (2006). The scope of the recent bioethics debate in Germany: Kant, crisis, and no confidence in society. *Cambridge Quarterly of Healthcare Ethics, 15*, 273–281.

Kuczewski, M. G. (1999). When your healthcare ethics committee "Fails to Thrive." *HEC Forum, 11*(3), 197–207.

LaPuma, J., Stocking, C. B., Silverstein, M. D., Dimartini, A., & Siegler, M. (1988). An ethics consultation service in a teaching hospital: Utilization and evaluation. *JAMA: The Journal of the American Medical Association, 260*(6), 808–811. https://doi.org/10.1001/jama.1988.03410060078031

Lo, B. (2015). *Resolving ethical dilemmas: A guide for clinicians* (5th ed.). Wolters Kluwer, Lippincott Williams & Wilkins.

Lynch, T., Connor, S., & Clark, D. (2013). Mapping levels of palliative care development: A global update. *Journal of Pain and Symptom Management, 45*(6), 1094–1106.

Lynne, J., & Goldstein, N. (2003). Advance care planning for fatal chronic illness: Avoiding commonplace errors and unwarranted suffering. *Annals of Internal Medicine, 138*(10), 812–818.

Magelssen, M., Miljeteig, I., Pedersen, R., & Førde, R. (2017). Roles and responsibilities of clinical ethics committees in priority setting. *BMC Medical Ethics, 18*(1), 1–8. https://doi.org/10.1186/s12910-017-0226-5

McCormick-Gendzel, M., & Jurchak, M. (2006). A pathway for moral reasoning in home for moral reasoning in home healthcare. *Home Healthcare Now, 24*(10), 654–661.

McCullough, L. B. (2005). Practicing preventive ethics—They keys to avoiding ethical conflicts in health care. *Physician Executive* (March/April), 18.

McLean, S. A. M. (2007). What and who are clinical ethics committees for? *Journal of Medical Ethics, 33*(9), 497–500. https://doi.org/10.1136/jme.2007.021394

Messinger, B., Baum, E., & Smith, M. (2009). Advance care planning: Beyond the living will. *Cleveland Clinic Journal of Medicine, 76*(5), 276–285.

Moran, S., Bailey, M., & Doody, O. (2021). An integrative review to identify how nurses practicing in inpatient specialist palliative care units uphold the values of nursing. *BMC Palliative Care, 20*, 111. https://doi.org/10.1186/s12904-021-00810-6

Murray, T., & Jennings, B. (2005). The quest to reform end of life care: Rethinking assumptions and setting new directions. *Improving End of Life Care: Why Has It Been So Difficult? Hastings Center Report Special Report, 34*(6), S52–S57. Report Special Report, 34(6), S14–S18.

Pavlish, C., Brown-Saltzman, K., Hersh, M., Shirk, M., & Nudelman, O. (2011). Early indicators and risk factors for ethical issues in clinical practice. *Journal of Nursing Scholarship, 43*(1), 13–21.

Pavlish, C., Brown-Saltzman, K., Fine, A., & Jakel, P. (2013). Making the call: A proactive ethics framework. *HEC Forum, 25*(3), 269–283. https://doi.org/10.1007/s10730-013-9213-5

Perkins, H. (2007). Controlling death: The false promise of advance directives. *Annals of Internal Medicine, 147*(1), 51–57.

Pfafflin, M., Kobert, K., & Reiter-Theil, S. (2009). Evaluating clinical ethics consultation: A European perspective. *Cambridge Quarterly of Healthcare Ethics, 18*(4), 406–419. https://doi.org/10.1017/S0963180109090604

Rothman, D. J. (1991). *Strangers at the bedside: A history of how law and bioethics transformed medical decision-making*. Basic Books.

Sabin, J. E. (2016). How can clinical ethics committees take on organizational ethics? Some practical suggestions. *The Journal of Clinical Ethics, 27*(2), 111–116.

Sabin, J. E., & Cochran, D. (2007). From the field—Confronting trade-offs in health care: Harvard Pilgrim Health Care's organizational ethics program. *Health Affairs, 26*(4), 1129–1134. https://doi.org/10.1377/hlthaff.26.4.1129

SAMS Swiss Academy of Medical Sciences. (2012). *Ethics support in medicine. Medical ethical guidelines*. SAMS. Retrieved January 28th, 2020 https://www.samw.ch/dam/jcr:af42a2d7-9fdd-44ae-a001-70d9bb11d980/guidelines_sams_ethics_support.pdf

Schwab, A. (2016). The ASBH code of ethics and the limits of professional healthcare ethics consultations. *Journal of Medical Ethics, 42*(8), 504–509.

Schildmann, J., Gordon, J.-S., & Vollmann, J. (2010). Introduction. In: J. Schildmann, J.-S. Gordon, J. Vollmann (Eds.), *Clinical ethics consultation: Theories and methods, implementation, evaluation* (pp. 1–7). Ashgate.

Schöne-Seifert, B., & Rippe, K. P. (1991). Silencing the singer: Antibioethics in Germany. *Hastings Center Report, 21*(6), 20–27.

Shalowitz, D. I., Garrett-Mayer, E., & Wendler, D. (2006). The accuracy of surrogate decision makers: A systematic review. *Archives of Internal Medicine, 166*(5), 493–497.

Shelstad, K. (2005). Landmark United States biomedical ethics cases. *Medical Reference Services Quarterly, 18*(2), 27–53. https://doi.org/10.1300/j115v18n02_03

Smith-Howell, E. R., Hickman, S. E., Meghani, S. H., Perkins, S. M., & Rawl, S. M. (2016). End-of-life decision making and communication of bereaved family members of African Americans with serious illness. *Journal of Palliative Medicine, 19*(2), 174–182. https://doi.org/10.1089/jpm.2015.0314

Sokol, D. K. (2008). The "four quadrants" approach to clinical ethics case analysis; An application and review. *Journal of Medical Ethics, 34*(7), 513–516. https://doi.org/10.1136/jme.2007.021212

Suhonen, R., Stolt, M., Virtanen, H., & Leino-Kilpi, H. (2011). Organizational ethics: A literature review. *Nursing Ethics, 18*(3), 285–303. https://doi.org/10.1177/0969733011401123

Tapper, E. B. (2017). Consults for conflict: The history of ethics consultation. *Baylor University Medical Center Proceedings, 26*(4), 417–422. https://doi.org/10.1080/08998280.2013.11929025

Tarzian, A. J. (2013). Health care ethics consultation: An update on core competencies and emerging standards from the American Society for Bioethics and Humanities' Core Competencies Update Task Force. *American Journal of Bioethics, 13*(2), 3–13. https://doi.org/10.1080/15265161.2012.750388

The General Medical Council. (2010). *Treatment and care towards the end of life*. Accessed February 22, 2022 https://www.gmc-uk.org/ethical-guidance/ethical-guidance-for-doctors

The SUPPORT Principal Investigators. (1995). A controlled trial to improve care for seriously ill hospitalized patients: The study to understand prognoses and preferences for outcomes and risks of treatment (SUPPORT). *Journal of the American Medical Association, 274*(20), 1591–1598.

Torke, A. M., Sachs, G. A., Helft, P. R., Montz, K., Hui, S. L., Slaven, J. E., & Callahan, C. M. (2014). Scope and outcomes of surrogate decision making among hospitalized older adults. *JAMA Internal Medicine, 174*(3), 370–377.

Wasson, K., Anderson, E., Hagstrom, E., McCarthy, M., Parsi, K., & Kuczewski, M. (2016). What ethical issues really arise in practice at an academic medical center? A quantitative and qualitative analysis of clinical ethics consultations from 2008 to 2013. *HEC Forum, 28*(3), 217–228. https://doi.org/10.1007/s10730-015-9293-5

World Health Organization (WHO). (2020). Palliative Care. https://www.who.int/news-room/fact-sheets/detail/palliative-care

Wilkinson, D., Truog, R., & Savulescu, J. (2016). In favour of medical dissensus: Why we should agree to disagree about end-of-life decisions. *Bioethics, 30*(2), 109–118. https://doi.org/10.1111/bioe.12162

Winkler, E. C., & Gruen, R. L. (2005). First principles: Substantive ethics for healthcare organizations. *Journal of Healthcare Management, 50*(2), 109–120. https://doi.org/10.1097/00115514-200503000-00008

Wlody, G. S. (2007). Nursing management and organizational ethics in the intensive care unit. *Critical Care Medicine, 35*(2 SUPPL.). https://doi.org/10.1097/01.CCM.0000252910.70311.66

Chapter 6
Cultural, Religious, Language and Personal Experiences: Influences in Ethical Deliberations

Annette Mendola, Pamela J. Grace, and Aimee Milliken

Abstract In this chapter we highlight the influences and roles of culture, religion, language, and personal experiences in ethical deliberations, whether these be in nurse-patient relationships or healthcare team deliberations. The importance of self-reflection about biases, prejudices and of striving for cultural sensitivity is emphasized in relation to realizing nursing goals. Additionally, we explore the role of traumatic past experiences in the ability and willingness of structurally disadvantaged groups to trust healthcare settings and healthcare professionals. Finally, we provide strategies to enhance communication when language and cultural differences present difficulties and hinder our ability to further nursing goals for individuals.

6.1 Introduction

It is well-established that respect for and responsiveness to diverse cultures are essential for ethical nursing practice. Cultural factors contribute to beliefs, practices, habits, and values related to health and health care. Illness and injury are not simply biomedical phenomena; they affect every dimension of a person's being. They threaten to disrupt a person's independence, financial situation, relationships, living situation—in short, the things that matter. Because of their roles and commitments, nurses have particular opportunities to integrate cultural factors into patient care. Moreover, there is an ethical responsibility to do so, as discussed in Chapters 2 and 3, based on the reasons nursing exists and the promises made to those served as articulated in

---

A. Mendola
Department of Medicine, The University of Tennessee Medical Center, Knoxville, TN, USA
e-mail: AMendola@utmck.edu

P. J. Grace (✉)
Brigham & Women's Hospital, Boston, MA, USA
e-mail: Gracepa@bc.edu

A. Milliken
William F. Connell School of Nursing, Boston College, Chestnut Hill, MA, USA
e-mail: aimee.milliken@bc.edu

its country-specific and international codes of ethics (American Nurses Association (ANA), 2015a; International Council of Nurses (ICN), 2012).

In one sense, culture refers to the norms, customs, laws, conventions, communication patterns, and other social behaviors associated with a particular group. For health care contexts, this description is incomplete; it calls attention to the external trappings of culture and obscures the role of culture in human lives. A more complete understanding of culture is "a shared framework of beliefs, values, and attitudes …the vessel through which personal identities and ideologies are created" (Carter & Klugman, 2001, p. 17). Cultural beliefs, values, practices, and so on provide structure and meaning to our lives, especially at emotionally charged, existentially threatening moments such as birth, death, and serious illness.

Some cultures are associated with race, some with national or geographic origin, some with religion; culture may be associated with several of these variables or none at all (Deaf culture, for example). Gender identity and sexual orientation aren't cultures per se but share attributes with cultures in that one's gender comes with norms, expectations, and values. Moreover, gender expression is profoundly affected by the other culture(s) in which the individual resides. Similarly, religion (discussed later in this section) shares affinities with culture and is affected by culture.

Some myths and misunderstandings about culture include that are addressed in this chapter include that:

- cultures are fixed, static institutions
- members of a culture all think, dress, and talk alike
- members of a culture all identify strongly as members of that culture
- if a belief or value is culturally embedded, it can't be morally wrong because it's "part of their culture"

Additionally, while patients and families are usually the most vulnerable parties in a healthcare encounter, it is important to remember that nurses and other care providers are vulnerable to bias and prejudice from patients and families. The health care environment must protect the well-being and autonomy of nurses and other members of the team as well as those of patients (Garran & Rasmussen, 2019).

6.2 Perspectives on Ethics and Culture

It is useful to distinguish between two spheres of cultural differences in health care: differences in what we think is *morally right* (values/ethics) and differences in what we think is *true about the world* (science/medicine). Of course, sometimes both kinds of differences are involved. Moreover, it is helpful when discussing ethics and culture to consider the three basic perspectives on the nature of ethics: Moral Subjectivism, Moral Relativism, and Moral Absolutism. *Moral Subjectivism* is the belief that ethics is completely subjective, like fashion. There are no ethically right or wrong answers; morality is simply a matter of taste. For example, slavery and genocide are deeply repugnant to *us*, but on this view, they are not *wrong* any more than wearing plaid with stripes. *Moral Relativism* is the belief that morally right answers and wrong answers in ethics depend on one's culture, like social norms. Individuals can be wrong (if their moral beliefs differ from those of their culture, for example) but whole cultures cannot be wrong. For example, from a relativist perspective, slavery is "wrong for us" but may not be wrong for others. *Moral Absolutism* is the belief that ethics is objective, like science or mathematics. From this perspective, there are universal moral principles—some fundamental rights and wrongs. That is, some values or moral beliefs are wrong, just like some scientific beliefs are wrong—even if embraced by a cultural group.

Moral absolutism seems, at first, to be an intolerant view. However, it does not mean that there is only one right answer to moral questions, or that it is permissible for one group to force their views on another. It *does* mean that there are some right and some wrong answers to moral questions. Moral progress requires the notion of moral truth; in order to make progress, we have to be moving toward something independent of human belief. Furthermore, the view that there are right and wrong answers to moral questions does not imply that we always *know* the right moral answers, just as the view that there are right and wrong answers to scientific questions does not imply that we know all the right answers to all scientific questions. It does mean that we can make moral progress by exchanging narratives in the spirit of a genuine desire for mutual understanding.

6.3 Culture, Value, and Meaning

6.3.1 Culture as a Vehicle for Meaning

Discussions of culture in health care often take the form of dilemmas: cases in which the culturally embedded beliefs and values of the patient are at odds with those of the care team. Such framing invites us to learn a set of facts about a culture and to devise "answers" to the "problems" that can occur in intercultural contexts. It also implies that culture is something other people have (i.e. not us—we're just normal) and obscures the fact that there is a culture associated with health care in general—and different health systems, specialties, and practice settings have their own subcultures. We should recognize, however, that there is no vantage point that is culture-free (Carter & Klugman, 2001). Every nursing encounter may be understood as an intercultural event, comprising the nurse's culture, the patient's culture, and the culture of the setting.[1]

There is certainly tremendous value in learning about the history, common experiences, and perspectives of other cultures in effort to understand their beliefs and values, especially when one's practice is in an area with high numbers of a specific

---

[1] Even when the nurse and patient appear to be members of the same culture, they are likely (as most of us are) to be members of multiple cultures and subcultures—a Lutheran, Generation X nurse from the American Midwest has at least four cultures influencing their worldview.

cultural group. However, more than differences in etiquette, diet, and rituals, culture is about what is significant to people: what matters, what is at stake, what it all means. Consider the case of Claude, a Haitian man with severe bone pain from metastatic cancer. Despite excruciating discomfort, he declined the use of pain medications because, as a devout Christian, he viewed suffering as "Christ-like." His wife supported him in this decision. To accept pain medication in this context would have been a moral lapse for Claude; accepting suffering with forbearance was meaningful to him. However, his decision was emotionally and morally distressing to the nurses caring for him, who felt they could provide "good" end of life care, if only he would accept medication to alleviate his discomfort.

When the patient and the health care team have different beliefs about the nature and scope of the illness, and/or different goals for treatment based on different values, careful consideration has to be given to the patient's perspective on her or his situation. What is genuinely meaningful to the patient takes precedence, as in the case of Claude. In such situations, nurses may need support to understand the patient's values and to manage their own discomfort in watching someone suffer physically when they know that suffering can be relieved. In Claude's case, a discussion with the hospital chaplain was very helpful for the nursing staff. While the patient and the team do not need to have exactly the same beliefs and values, they do need a shared understanding of *what is happening* and *what is desired.* Trust is essential for patient care and can be easily lost—or difficult to build—when the patient's beliefs and values are discounted.

There are several models for integrating the patient's cultural perspective with those of the health care team. One early model was developed by psychiatrist and medical anthropologist Arthur Kleinman (1988). Kleinman encourages asking questions in order to understand the patient's conception of her/his condition. This framework does not suggest the patient's understanding of the illness is right and the clinician's is wrong; rather, that each party has important knowledge that others don't have.

The Cultural Engagement model, developed by Michele Carter and Craig Klugman, comprises a series of questions to help patients/families and care providers exchange their explanatory models. The goal is to develop a shared explanatory model that can lead to shared goals and more satisfactory health outcomes , (Fig. 6.1).

6.3.2 Important Definitions

A plethora of terms have emerged to describe skills and approaches to incorporating culture into nursing care, including *cultural competence, cultural sensitivity, cultural humility, cultural awareness, cultural intelligence, cultural safety, cultural efficacy, cultural literacy,* and *culturally congruent care.* Several of these terms emerged in effort to respond to some of the problems that have been identified with overreliance on one of the earliest of these: cultural competence. The American Nurses Association (2015b) prefers the following:

Categories	Practitioner Interview	Patient Interview
Illness or Health Problem(s)	What are the patient's health problems?	What are your health problems?
	What has the patient told you about the health problems?	How have the problems affected your body and your life?
Causes or etiologies	What are the causes for each health problem?	What do you think caused these problems?
Treatment goals and concerns	What has been done for these health problems?	What have you done for these health problems?
	How can you help this patient?	What do you need in order to be helped? What can the doctor do for you?
	What is your concern or problem about the patient?	Who helps you make health decisions? Who should be told your medical condition?

Fig. 6.1 Interview questions for the cultural engagement chart (Carter & Klugman, 2001)

> Culturally congruent practice is the application of evidence-based nursing that is in agreement with the preferred cultural values, beliefs, worldview, and practices of the healthcare consumer and other stakeholders. Cultural competence represents the process by which nurses demonstrate culturally congruent practice. Nurses design and direct culturally congruent practice and services for diverse consumers to improve access, promote positive outcomes, and reduce disparities. (p. 31)

Cultural competence has been criticized as implying that the appropriate approach to culture in healthcare is to learn the relevant do's and don'ts about a cultural group and to apply these assiduously. That perspective, in turn, may suggest that culture is essentially a set of facts to master about a particular group of people. The objective of "competence" can foster unwarranted assumptions about individuals based on their membership in a cultural group. It can also inappropriately magnify the significance of culture in a situation. Mundane, universal situations can get wrongly framed as cultural, making individuals seem "exotic" and concealing the relevant aspects of a situation (Botelho & Lima, 2020).

6.3.3 Checking Assumptions—Avoiding Stereotypes

A key to avoiding the potential pitfalls of cultural competence is to handle assumptions about patients with care. To begin with, any assumptions we may have about a given culture should be checked, since cultures and subcultures change over time as people experience significant events and other influences. Moreover, members of any given culture adhere to aspects of that culture and identify with that culture to different degrees (and sometimes to different degrees at different times in their lives). It is easy to rely too heavily on our own beliefs about other cultures without treating patients as individuals, with their unique perspectives, preferences, and values. At the same time, skillful, patient-centered use of our knowledge of other cultures is an appropriate place to begin. The distinction between a stereotype and a generalization may be useful here. Stereotypes—fixed beliefs about other people, based on their group membership—are dangerous because they prevent us from understanding the patient as an individual. Generalizations—initial assumptions that are open to revision about other people based on their group membership—encourage us to ask culturally-sensitive questions.

For example, if a female patient presents wearing a hijab, it is a reasonable starting point to think she is Muslim and, as such, may prefer a female provider. In fact, it might be insensitive not to notice her hijab, not to make an initial assumption about her cultural background, and not to consider how that initial assumption, if true, might affect her values regarding her care. It would be a mistake, however, to take that assumption and act on it without asking the patient about her preferences.

In the United States at one time, race was routinely included in an initial presentation of a case (e.g. "The patient is a 52-year-old white female who presents with …"). This practice has been criticized as inviting bias and unjustified assumptions, particularly since some long-held assumptions about racial differences in medicine are poorly founded, and since there is no genetic basis for race. More recently, however, some argue for the inclusion of race because of the effect racism has on patients' physical and mental health. "Color-blind" health care may exacerbate the very problem it is meant to ameliorate.

6.3.4 Situate Responsibilities in Nursing Goals and Perspectives.

As a reminder, in Chapters 1 and 2 we emphasized how the goals of nursing were outlined in both the American Nurses Association's Code of Ethics (2015a) and the International Council of Nursing's Code of Ethics for Nurses. The goals are the same in both if expressed slightly differently. Here, we use the ICN (2012) definition due to the international scope of the book. "Nurses have four fundamental responsibilities: to promote health, to prevent illness, to restore health and to alleviate suffering. The need for nursing is universal" (p. 1). The perspective of nursing, or the central unifying focus of the discipline as identified from decades of nursing literature is that of humanizing the environment and facilitating "meaning, choice, quality of life, and healing in living and dying" (Willis et al., 2008, p. E28). These goals and perspectives underlie the scope of professional responsibilities. To fulfil these goals using our perspective on persons means that we have responsibilities to account for the cultural beliefs and values of our patients. However, this is not the same as saying we have to accede to cultural demands that ask us to engage in actions that are integrity shaking for us. For example, a nurse is not obligated to assist with a cultural practice such as infibulation (a ritual in some cultures where parts of female external genitalia are excised), although they may need to try and minimize harms associated with the practice. The issue of determining when it is ethically permissible to remove oneself from participation in interventions based on one's conscience is discussed shortly.

Accounting for individual needs, preferences and values inevitably means including pertinent aspects of a person's cultural beliefs. In turn, this may also mean that they do not make decisions in isolation from their family or community but rather decision-making is a group undertaking. Additionally, some patients may opt to defer decision-making to a loved one, as in the case of a woman who prefers her eldest son be given information about her likely cancer diagnosis and treatment options. This can be viewed as an extension of the patient's autonomy, so long that it is done willingly and not under duress.

6.3.5 Shared Trauma and Microaggression

Three concepts that have recently appeared in the psychology, mental health, and healthcare literature are 'shared trauma', 'historical trauma' and 'microaggression'. Since these have implications for how healthcare workers respond to their own situations and those of their patients, we discuss them briefly here.

6.3.5.1 Shared Trauma

The term 'shared trauma' appeared in the literature following the events of September 11, 2001 and the destruction of the World Trade Center towers an event now widely known as 9/11. It was a way to "describe the ramifications of the clinicians' direct and indirect exposure to collective trauma" (Tosone, 2012, para 1). For example, at the time of this writing, direct care providers worldwide are suffering from shared trauma related to the COVID-19 pandemic as has been widely documented (Ng et al., 2020). Initially, shared trauma applied to mental health clinicians who were caring for persons experiencing the same catastrophic events as they themselves were. Examples include devastation from hurricane Katrina in the US, the 2011 Tōhoku earthquake and tsunami in Japan, and populations displaced by war. Clinicians can feel a sense of personal disequilibrium, be worried about their safety, suffer guilt and grief as a result of shared trauma (Bell & Robinson, 2013). They may also carry a burden of responsibility for being the one who emotionally supports patients, friends, and family. In the COVID-19 pandemic, nurses and other health care professionals caring for patients worried about falling ill due to COVID-19 themselves—or infecting their families. "Health care professionals face the same stressors as those in the general population in addition to those tied to their professional roles" (Werner et al., 2020, p. 4). Supportive strategies for nurses related to this and other such difficulties are provided in the Social Justice chapter.

6.3.5.2 Historical Trauma

Historical trauma "is multigenerational trauma experienced by a specific cultural, racial or ethnic group. It is related to major events that oppressed a particular group of people because of their status as oppressed, such as slavery, the Holocaust, forced migration" (Administration for Children and Families, 2020). The violent colonization of native peoples in Australia, Canada, New Zealand, and the United States has also given rise to historical trauma. The damage from what happened becomes part of the 'who' of the person and is subsequently passed down to successive generations in various ways. So even family members who were not subjected to the harms caused may feel the effects and this can persist over generation [Walters et al., 2011]. One must be careful however, as noted earlier, not to generalize or assume that everyone within a given group is actually suffering the results of historical trauma. Rather, it is important to consider whether historical trauma is playing a role in a given situation; if so, it is necessary to be able to respond appropriately. Strategies for appropriate responses are provided after the next section. Persons who are suffering the aftermath of historical trauma are likely to distrust systems put in place by the perceived oppressors, including aspects of the healthcare system. In the United States for example, the many injustices perpetrated on African American, Native American, Hispanic, and Asian populations over several centuries have led many to distrust the healthcare system and healthcare providers. Examples include experimentation without consent, involuntary sterilization, inadequate pain control, and being refused treatment.

6.3.5.3 Microaggressions

Microaggressions are likely to have a different label in different languages, however, a general definition given by Sue (2010) is that it is the "constant and continuing everyday reality of slights, insults, invalidations and indignities visited upon marginalized groups" (p. XV). They are subtle and may not be noticed by those who perpetuate them. Indeed, this is part of their power, as they reflect unconscious biases. Examples of microaggressions include failing to pronounce names properly even after one has been corrected, telling someone from a minority culture that he or she is very articulate (as if it would be expected that they would not be), and failing to use the correct pronoun for a transgender or nonbinary person. This next section discusses in more depth how one can learn to avoid the effects of bias and prejudice in one's relations with others and in caring ethically for patients.

6.4 Reflection on Personal Beliefs And Values And The Role Of Bias, Implicit Bias, And Prejudice

As discussed in Chapter 2.6, an essential, but often-overlooked, component of ethical nursing practice is self-reflection. Developing a rich awareness of one's own cultural heritage, beliefs, values, and commitments permits the nurse to recognize when a patient's beliefs and values differ from her or his own, and to respond appropriately. A related duty involves being aware of gaps in one's understanding regarding culturally-congruent practice, particularly with the common cultures and subcultures in the region where one practices. This requires a commitment to the lifelong learning and character development needed to fill these gaps. Even nurses who have vast interest in and knowledge of other cultures will be challenged to respond ethically to patients as cultures develop, divide, and change. Cultures are not static! In addition to adding to one's cognitive understanding of cultural differences, this commitment includes continuous development of compassion and common ground with patients, families, and other providers who have different worldviews. This is sometimes easier when the other person is from a culture that one finds foreign and exotic than when the culture or subculture is closer to one's own.

Every person has issues they find difficult to deal with because of her or his own history and experiences. Bias is ubiquitous and inevitable, and it can be distressing to acknowledge our own lapses in this area (Weston, 2011). Nurses are not expected to be free from bias, but ethical nursing practice requires courage and self-compassion to discover bias in oneself and to work to overcome it.

Consider, for example, a case involving a family meeting planned for an African American family whose members are angry about the care their loved one is receiving. The nurse wonders if the hospital's security service should be made aware of when and where the meeting will be held in case they become disruptive, then recognizes that this family is not showing signs of violence; they are simply angry. She realizes this as an example of implicit bias and withdraws the suggestion. While this is a US specific case, the bias could just as easily be toward members of another marginalized group such as the Romani in Europe and an expectation by healthcare providers that interactions will be conflictual.

6.4.1 Conscientious Objection

In cross-cultural contexts, situations can arise in which a nurse feels that performing an expected duty would result in a serious violation of his or her personal moral commitments. In such situations, the moral harm to the nurse could compromise his or her ability to provide good care in future. *Conscientious objection* refers to the refusal to perform a task on the grounds that doing so would violate one's moral integrity. Wicclair (2011) notes that this means what one is being asked to do violates one's "core moral beliefs (ethical or religious and which is) ... perceived by the agent as an act of self-betrayal" (p. 5). It should be noted that refusing to provide care on the grounds of conscience is a serious decision, not to be taken lightly. Simply disagreeing with a practice or finding it incongruent with one's moral commitments is not sufficient grounds to invoke appeal to conscientious objection. Invoking conscientious objection is appropriate in situations in which participation in the aspect of patient care would be a true violation of one's moral code, the objection has a plausible moral or religious rationale, and the burdens to the patient and to colleagues is acceptably small (Lachman, 2014).

In such situations, a course of action that respects the rights and moral commitments of all involved must be found. Solutions most commonly involve the transfer of duties to another nurse who is more comfortable with the task in question. Nurses should take steps to ensure that their refusal does not jeopardize patient care (e.g. by informing their supervisors of their need for accommodation early and cooperating with the accommodation plan) and should refrain from discussing the conflicting beliefs and values with patients. Nurse Managers and other Nurse Leaders should develop and implement practices that foster seamless delivery of patient care while respecting the moral commitments of individual nurses. Finally, nurses should consider their moral commitments when choosing a work environment: for example, nurses who feel that elective abortion is morally wrong should avoid working in areas in which they are likely to be expected to assist with these procedures.

6.5 Religious and Spiritual Influences on Ethical Decision-Making

Religion and spirituality are closely related to culture. These phenomena, like culture, comprise practices, values, and beliefs that help us make meaning of the events of our lives. One's sense of personal identity and belonging may be profoundly connected to religion, whether in the form of an organized religion or a set of spiritual beliefs. While many cultures and subcultures are commonly associated with particular religions, it is important to remember that members of a culture may not practice the religion that is often associated with it.

Religious and spiritual beliefs can have a profound impact on ethical decision making in health care. Many religions have prescribed and proscribed practices regarding health, including rules regarding food and hygiene. Duties to the sick and duties of the sick (such as what care they should accept, or what they should not demand of others) may be grounded in religion; recall the case of Claude earlier in this chapter. Finally, religious and spiritual beliefs can inform what an illness means to a patient or family, as when illness is thought to be a punishment for wrongdoing and healing a sign of God's favor. Understanding what religious beliefs patients and families bring with them to the health care setting can help nurses provide comfort, demonstrate respect, and mitigate or avoid conflict.

6.5.1 Belief in Miracles and Effects on Patient 'Good'

A particularly challenging clinical situation occurs when a patient or family member chooses a course of action (often to ask for interventions the care team believes have low likelihood to achieve the patient's goals) because they are hoping for a miracle. One reason this is difficult is that the hope for a miracle generally appears when only a miracle will produce the hoped-for outcome: to go along with the hope for a miracle seems dishonest and likely to expose the patient to harmful interventions with no expectation of utility, but to quash the hope of a miracle feels cruel and heartless. The fact that patients' outcomes are sometimes far better than expected complicates this challenge; we have all witnessed recoveries that have seemed miraculous. The tasks for the health care team, then, are to practice good medicine, respect the patient's and family's beliefs, and retain appropriate humility in trying to understand the meaning that the situation holds for them.

Some best practices include exploring what "a miracle" means for this patient and family, negotiating appropriate compromises, setting time-limited trials, helping nurture a diverse set of hopes, and helping identify and address fears and the meaning infusing these fears (DeLisser, 2009; Feudtner, 2014).

6.5.2 Surrogate Acting Against Patient Preferences

As noted in earlier sections, not all patients and family members share a culture, and not all who do embrace all of the dimensions of their culture in the same way or to the same degree. This is true of religion as well. The task of a surrogate decision maker is to make health care decisions according to their truest understanding of the patient's values, preferences, and commitments. This task is notoriously hard, both cognitively and emotionally. When a patient and surrogate have different religious commitments, there is fertile ground for conflict. Such situations are further exacerbated when the patient and surrogate once shared a religious tradition, and the surrogate feels that the patient has been unfaithful or "needs to come back into the fold".

Consider the case of Annie, who was one of Jehovah's Witnesses for much of her life and whose family are Jehovah's Witnesses, but who no longer practices that faith. As a result of complications from surgery, her hematocrit and hemoglobin were dangerously low. Her daughter was uncomfortable acting as her mother's surrogate, as she did not want to be in a position of having to either authorize something her mother would have chosen but went against her own religious principles or staying true to her beliefs but going against her mother's wishes. After careful consideration and discussion with the health care team, she abdicated the role of decision maker to a close family friend.

Another facet of this issue involves children whose parents' religious beliefs are working against the medical best interests of the child. Examples include refusal of medical care for life-threatening conditions by Christian Scientists and requests for genital cutting by members of some African Muslim sects. In these cases, many factors come into play, including the age of child and degree to which they can participate in decision making, and the degree to which the request threatens their health. The importance of preserving a child's right to an "open future" in which they are able to choose their own commitments may limit the scope of authority of a parent to make medical decisions for their child. Nurses have an important role in these situations given their commitment to family-centered care. It is vitally important that these situations are navigated in such a way that trust in the health care system and family relationships is preserved to the degree possible—an enormous challenge to be sure. Nurses are well-positioned to help generate compromises where these are possible, thereby communicating respect to families even when some of their requests cannot be honored.

6.5.3 Conflicts of Conscience

As discussed in more detail in Sect. 6.5.1, situations can arise in which the care needs of the patient conflict with the ethical commitments of the nurse. When such situations involve a nurse's religious commitments, the nurse's distress may be even more acute. Some conflicts engender moral discomfort, while others rise to the level of conscientious objection. An important strategy involves the nurse's discernment regarding what is causing the moral discomfort to ascertain whether there is enough common ground between the nurse's beliefs and the patient's requests that the nurse can participate in the care. The American Nurses Association (2015c) has a position statement on *Risk and Responsibility in Providing Nursing Care* that can guide the nurse in deciding what to do.

6.6 Language and Interpretation Difficulties

To provide ethical health and nursing care, effective communication is essential. However besides difficulties of understanding different cultures and cultural practices, situations in which a patient does not speak or is not fluent in the language of the setting makes good communication difficult. In many countries interpreters who are specially trained to interpret medical information are available and regulations exist to support patient rights to these services and their accessibility. The International Medical Interpreters Association (IMIA) is a relatively new organization with

Chapters in 13 countries. They are bound by a code of ethics and offer resources such as information and training (IMIA, 2006). However, in some countries so many different languages or dialects exist that it would be impossible to access a trained interpreter and an informal interpreter must be used. Bezuidenhout and Borry (2009) note that "(I)deally, professional interpreters must understand the ethics of the situation, control the flow of the session, correctly use healthcare terminology and understand the impact of culture on the patient's decision-making process" (p. 159). Thus, they act as culture brokers and are more 'visible' in the interaction than someone who directly translates the language (Bezuidenhout & Borry, 2009). The interpreter has an active part to play in the interaction. When an interpreter is available, it is critically important that the nurse and clinical team (if possible) brief the interpreter about the facts of the situation and the goal of the impending conversation, so that the interpreter can be prepared and can relay any potentially important cultural considerations to the team.

Even when interpreter services exist, and the particular language or dialect can be accommodated, convenience often leads to the use of family members or friends as interpreters for patients. This is probably fine for such things as food preferences or other daily activities but for evaluative, diagnostic, or informed consent to treatment activities there are several reasons why official interpreters should be used where they are available. Where they are not available, an appropriate informal interpreter can be used as long as certain safeguards are in place.

6.6.1 Risks to Patients and Family

6.6.1.1 Risk to Patient

Informal interpreters may pose a risk to patient care if they do not convey information to and from the patient accurately. Nurses should be aware of the possibility that a family member or partner serving as informal interpreter may consciously or unconsciously modify information. Just as any message is vulnerable to being modified in the repeating, messages relayed by untrained interpreters are susceptible to being altered. This is especially problematic if there is a power differential, and the dominant partner is recounting the information. For example, in situations where there is human trafficking or inter-partner violence the perpetrator is likely to distort the information either to hide the cause of violence or to prevent the clinician from recognizing that the person is essentially enslaved.

Family members may have cultural or emotional reasons to alter the information and may also find it very difficult to convey bad news, particularly if they are having difficulty processing it themselves. Another potential problem is that patients may withhold or modify information when it has to be relayed through an interpreting family member, because of the secret or intimate nature of a problem or the circumstances leading up to the need for medical care.

Given these potential problems nurses may need to find ways to validate the information in either direction: what the patient is saying and what is being told to the patient. For example, asking the family member to tell you what they think is going on, asking her or him to explain what they told the patient, and checking in with the interpreting family member about their comfort level in that role.

6.6.1.2 Risks to Children and Adolescents

The temptation to use a patient's child as an interpreter should be considered carefully. As an example of possible problems, we use a modified case from the Hastings Center Report (2004). In this case of an immigrant family from China whose native language is Cantonese, the fifteen-year-old daughter is most fluent and acculturated although there are also two older sons. Her father was admitted with serious cardiac problems, neither he nor his wife speaks very much English. An interpreter would not be available until after the weekend at which point the attending cardiologist would have gone on vacation and she was worried that her replacement was not experienced enough to handle the problem. She wondered whether she could use the daughter.

In addition to possible risks to the patient as discussed above, interpreting in this context would be a heavy burden for the daughter. She would have to convey bad news to the rest of the family while trying to process it herself. She may not understand the nuances of the medical situation and its meaning, which will add additional stress. Moreover, her acting in this role would likely disrupt family dynamics, as important and upsetting news is being conveyed to the family by one of its most junior members. Therefore, we need to keep in mind that over-reliance on a child can be harmful to them. If used, attention to their emotional well-being is essential.

6.6.2 Appropriate Nurse Actions

Given an understanding of the potential problems related to interpretation and patient and family rights to information and support there are several actions nurses can take to facilitate best care under sub-optimal circumstances.

1. Educate themselves about interpreter resources in their settings or country and best practices in working with them.
2. Consider the nuances and context of the situation. Are there reasons to suppose the patient will not get an accurate interpretation from the family member or accompanying person?
3. Does the patient seem to be in danger from the accompanying person (human trafficking, interpersonal violence situations)?
4. What burdens may exist by using a family member—either for the family member or on the patient.

5. If a trained interpreter is not available, who other than the patient might be available to assist? Preferably someone with medical knowledge and who can be neutral while still recognizing patient concerns.
6. When doubts exist about veracity, ask the interpreter to tell you what they told the patient and what the response was.

6.7 Strategies for Nurses to Use

6.7.1 Improving Sensitivity to Cultural Differences and Language Difficulties

Among the strategies for nurses to use is self-reflection on biases and prejudices. While one can do this on one's own, there is reason to believe that group discussion in a safe and open moral space can raise one's awareness of hidden or subconscious biases, microaggression tendencies, and subtle problems associated with language difficulties (Lee et al., 2019; Walker, 1993). In institutional settings it can be helpful to have short educational unit meetings with experts, such as interpreters, ethicists and persons from cultures most often encountered.

Another strategy is to work with unit or ward managers and organize 'ethics rounds' where recent difficult cases are discussed in order to develop guidelines and resources for future similar cases. In our work educating nurses and other healthcare professionals on ethical aspects of care, we have found that constructing a case and then asking people to play different roles can be helpful for perspective-taking about what a situation might be like for the other.

6.7.2 Virtues of Biomedical Ethics

As discussed in Chapter 2, one of Rest's components of moral action is moral character. Virtues are the character traits, or moral habits, that are grounded in moral principles. Some suggest that "doing the right thing" comes more naturally when one cultivates good moral habits, such as trustworthiness, integrity, and so on, than by considering abstract moral principles or provisions in a Code of Ethics.

The five focal Virtues of Bioethics are Compassion, Discernment, Trustworthiness, Integrity, and Conscientiousness (Beauchamp & Childress, 2019). While each of the virtues is important in the realm of culture and nursing practice, virtues that are especially germane in this realm are discernment, integrity, and conscientiousness.

Discernment is the ability to choose ethically-sound decisions without being unduly influenced or distracted by "moral noise", personal fears and preferences, or outside pressure.

- *Ask: How does this patient's cultural perspective make me feel? Am I stuck in my own perspective? Have I fallen into unconscious bias? Am I overcompensating in effort to avoid being prejudiced? Am I checking my assumptions about what will make this patient most comfortable?*

Integrity involves the willingness to act consistently on one's moral commitments, even when uncomfortable or in the presence of personal risk.

- *Ask: Am I living up to my own standards for myself? Am I hiding from conflict in order to "get along" or because it's easier than expressing my concerns?*

Conscientiousness requires us place the appropriate weight on the competing duties in a situation. Conscientious people have a sense of when to compromise and when to insist on a course of action. They try to do the right thing for the right reasons, without getting caught up in the letter of the law.

- *Bullet Ask: Am I looking for solutions that respect everyone's interests? Am I giving in when I should be standing up—or being rigid when I should be flexible?*

This trifecta of virtue is especially helpful in navigating situations in which cultural practices and commitments are not merely different from one's comfort zone but have the potential to endanger someone or to interfere with someone's human rights.

6.7.3 Principles of Shared Decision Making

"Shared decision making is a *collaborative process* that allows patients, or their surrogates, and clinicians to make healthcare decisions together, taking into account the best scientific evidence available, as well as the patient's values, goals, and preferences" (Kon, et al., 2016, p. 190; emphasis added). Shared decision making requires providers to learn the values, hopes, and fears of the patient/family, to explain relevant medical information and options in language that is easily understandable, and to facilitate decision making that makes use of each person's sphere of knowledge. It also involves providers discerning their own values, fears, and hopes, as lack of awareness of our own biases and values can lead to *unconscious* fact-framing (vs. framing choices in light of patient values). This approach acknowledges the inherent power and knowledge difference between providers and patients (and their families), and channels it in service of the patient (Brody, 1992). Nurses especially contribute to shared decision making when they help elicit patient and family goals, hopes, and fears, when they help check for their understanding of the patient's condition, prognosis, and options.

Part of shared decision making is the recognition that people do not make decisions the way economists think they do; they do not dispassionately consider the facts of the matter according to their values and make rational, self-interested decisions. Facts play a role in decision making, but so do spirituality, identity, history, and hope. Patients and families rely on providers to explain the situation in a way that is both cognitively and existentially understandable. Key features of shared decision making in cross-cultural contexts include becoming aware of the preferences of the patient and family *multicultural individuals*, being responsive to the need for translators and "cultural brokers", being sensitive to the likely short- and long-term consequences of the decision for patient and community and being aware of one's own multiculturally-informed beliefs, experiences, and values.

6.8 Summary

Understanding the cultural perspectives of patients and families is a dimension of nursing practice that is gaining recognition, owing to the increasing diversity in many communities and the growing awareness of the connection of culture, meaning, and health care. Responsiveness to patients' culturally informed experiences, perspectives, and values aligns nursing goals with patient goals, increasing trust and improving outcomes. A lifelong commitment to learning about the history, common experiences, and perspectives of other cultures serves nurses well in their quest to provide excellent care.

References

Administration for Children and Families. (2020). *Trauma: What is historical trauma*. Resource guide to trauma informed family services. Retrieved February 16, 2021 from https://www.acf.hhs.gov/trauma-toolkit/trauma-concept

American Nurses Association. (2015a). *Code of ethics for nurses with interpretive statements*. Author. https://www.nursingworld.org/practice-policy/nursing-excellence/ethics/code-of-ethics-for-nurses/

American Nurses Association. (2015b). *Nursing: Scope and standards of practice* (3rd ed.). Nursesbooks.org.

American Nurses Association. (2015c). *Risk and responsibility in providing nursing care*. https://www.nursingworld.org/~4ad4a8/globalassets/docs/ana/riskandresponsibility.pdf

Beauchamp, T., & Childress, J. (2019). *Principles of biomedical ethics* (8th ed.). Oxford University Press.

Bell, C. H., & Robinson, E. H., III. (2013). Shared trauma in counseling: Information and implications for counselors. *Journal of Mental Health Counseling, 35*, 310–323. https://doi.org/10.17744/mehc.35.4.7v33258020948502

Bezuidenhout, L., & Borry, P. (2009). Examining the role of informal interpretation in medical interviews. *Journal of Medical Ethics, 35*(3), 159–162.

Botelho, M. J., & Lima, C. A. (2020). From cultural competence to cultural respect: A critical review of six models. *Journal of Nursing Education, 59*(6), 311–318. https://doi.org/10.3928/01484834-20200520-03 PMID: 32497232.

Brody, H. (1992). *The healer's power*. Yale University Press.

Carter, M. A., & Klugman, C. M. (2001). Cultural engagement in clinical ethics: A model for ethics consultation. *Cambridge Quarterly of Healthcare Ethics, 10*(1), 16–33. https://doi.org/10.1017/s0963180101001049 PMID: 11326783.

DeLisser, H. M. (2009). A practical approach to the family that expects a miracle. *Chest, 135*(6), 1643–1647. https://doi.org/10.1378/chest.08-2805.PMID:19497899;PMCID:PMC2821292

Feudtner, C. (2014). Responses from palliative care: Hope is like water. *Perspectives in Biological Medicine, 57*(4), 555–557. https://doi.org/10.1353/pbm.2014.0039 PMID: 26497242.

Garran, A. M., & Rasmussen, B. M. (2019). How should organizations respond to racism against health care workers? *AMA Journal of Ethics., 21*(6), E499-504. https://doi.org/10.1001/amajethics.2019.499 PMID: 31204990.

Hastings Center Report. (2004). A fifteen-year-old translator. With commentaries. *Hastings Center Report, 34*(3), 10–13.

International Association of Medical Interpreters. (2006). *Code of ethics*. Accessed February 19, 2021 from: https://www.imiaweb.org/code/default.asp

International Council of Nurses. (2012). *Code of ethics for nurses. Author*. https://www.icn.ch/sites/default/files/inline-files/2012_ICN_Codeofethicsfornurses_%20eng.pdf

Kleinman, A. (1988). *The illness narratives: Suffering, healing and the human condition*. Basic Books.

Kon, A. A., Davidson, J. E., Morrison, W., Danis, M., & White, D. B. (2016). Shared decision making in intensive care units: An American College of Critical Care Medicine and American Thoracic Society policy statement. *Critical Care Medicine, 44*(1), 188. https://doi.org/10.1097/CCM.0000000000001396.PMID:26509317;PMCID:PMC4788386

Lachman, V. D. (2014). Conscientious objection in nursing: definition and criteria for acceptance. *Medsurg Nurs, 23*(3) (May–JunE), 196–198. PMID: 25137800.

Lee, S., Robinson, E., Grace, P. J., Jurchak, M., & Zollfrank, A. (Published Online ahead of print April, 28, 2019). Developing a moral compass: Themes from the clinical ethics residency for nurses (CERN) final essays. *Nursing Ethics*. https://doi.org/10.1177/0969733019833125

Ng, Q. X., De Deyn, M., Lim, D. Y., Chan, H. W., & Yeo, W. S. (2020). The wounded healer: A narrative review of the mental health effects of the COVID-19 pandemic on healthcare workers. *Asian journal of psychiatry, 54*, 102258. https://doi.org/10.1016/j.ajp.2020.102258

Sue, D. W. (2010). *Microaggressions in everyday life: Race, gender, and sexual orientation*. John Wiley & Sons.

Tosone, C. (2012). Shared trauma. In C. R. Figley (Ed.), *Encyclopedia of Trauma: An interdisciplinary guide*. Sage.

Walker, M. U. (1993). Keeping moral space open: New images of ethics consulting. *The Hastings Center Report, 23*(2), 33–40.

Walters, K. L., Mohammed, S. A., Evans-Campbell, T., Beltran, R. E., Chae, D. H., & Duran, B. (2011). Bodies don't just tell stories, they tell histories. *Du Bois Review, 8*(1), 179–189.

Werner, E. A., Aloisio, C. E., Butler, A. D., D'Antonio, K. M., Kenny, J. M., Mitchell, A., Ona, S., & Monk, C. (2020). Addressing mental health in patients and providers during the COVID-19 pandemic. *Seminars in Perinatology, 44*(7), 151279. https://doi.org/10.1016/j.semperi.2020.151279

Weston, A. (2011). *A practical companion to ethics* (4th ed.). Oxford University.

Wicclair, M. R. (2011). *Conscientious objection in health care: An ethical analysis*. Cambridge University Press.

Willlis, D. G., Grace, P. J., & Roy, C. (2008). A central unifying focus for the discipline: Facilitating humanization, meaning, choice, quality of life, and healing in living and dying. *Advances in Nursing Science, 31*(1), E28–E40.

Part III
Ethical Issues Associated with Practice and Research

Chapter 7
Neonatal and Pediatric Acute and Palliative Care

Pamela J. Grace, Aimee Milliken, and Melissa Uveges

Abstract In this chapter we provide an overview of ethical issues arising in the context of neonatal and pediatric settings. Examples from acute, critical and palliative care environments are explored and nurses' roles as members of the healthcare team explicated. The chapter is organized from birth to adolescence, although there are areas where particular ethical considerations cross age groups. Specific emphasis is given to the role and limits of family decision-making.

7.1 Introduction

In this chapter we explore a range of ethical issues associated with caring for very early born babies to adolescents. A special emphasis is placed on examining nurses' roles and responsibilities in supporting decision making for children and their families. We use the term family broadly to include those who are formally or informally charged with making decisions for an infant, child, or adolescent. However, we recognize that sometimes a temporary caretaker, such as a foster family, may not have medical decision-making authority, and this will differ from country to country and depend on context and circumstances. A recent study conducted in the US revealed several possible scenarios related to decision making for a child in a temporary care situation that depends on context and circumstances (Seltzer et al., 2020). The decision may be: legally prescribed, determined by a team, or undertaken by approved foster parents. The study also found that sometimes decisions were made by a legally appointed guardian who might not know much about the infant or child

---

P. J. Grace (✉) · M. Uveges
William F. Connell School of Nursing, Boston College, Chestnut Hill, MA 02467, USA
e-mail: Gracepa@bc.edu

M. Uveges
e-mail: uveges@bc.edu

A. Milliken
William F. Connell School of Nursing, Boston College, Chestnut Hill, MA, USA
e-mail: aimee.milliken@bc.edu

© The Author(s), under exclusive license to Springer Nature B.V. 2022
P. Grace and A. Milliken (eds.), *Clinical Ethics Handbook for Nurses*, The International Library of Bioethics 93,
https://doi.org/10.1007/978-94-024-2155-2_7

(Seltzer et al., 2020). A problem exists when not much is known about the infant or child for whatever reason and a serious decision affecting their lives has to be made. In the last few decades a relatively new issue has surfaced concerning certain young adults who have a genetic or congenital disease and who are best treated by the pediatric specialists most familiar with them as they emerge into adulthood. Contrasting perspectives and attitudes from disparate countries and cultures, along with the state of the science, are used to provide insights for ethical decision making that serves the interests of infants, children, and adolescents. We use the term infants for age 0–2 in line with the American Academy of Pediatrics (2017). Where there is the possibility of ambiguity about what age group we are discussing we clarify. Finally, the issue of moral distress in nurses and others whose work necessitates close contact with children and their families is discussed and strategies for remedy suggested.

7.2 The Historical Development of Neonatal Intensive Care Units and Seminal Cases

The existence of specialized units designed to care for the needs of prematurely born infants or those who are born with serious physical problems is relatively recent. Their development coincides with the rapid evolution of biotechnological life-supporting and sustaining interventions as discussed in Chapter 3. Additionally, advances made in assisted reproductive technologies (ARTs) increasingly used in the developed world have as a negative sequelae an increase in the numbers of newborns born prematurely. Among the several reasons for this are an increased incidence of multiples, a trend to delay childbearing leading to decreased fertility and the desire to use ARTs, and there is emerging research to suggest that underlying pathophysiological reasons for infertility leading to the use of ARTs also increase the likelihood of prematurity (Institute of Medicine, 2007).

There is evidence that experimental technological advances such as incubators and naso-gastric feeding were used to try and support premature infants as far back as the turn of the century (National Institutes of Health [NIH], 1992). In the late 1800s Tarnier, a French obstetrician, recognized that premature infants could not maintain their body heat "and developed a crude isolette - a wooden box with a glass lid and a hot water bottle inside" (Payne, 2016) ... His work "contributed to a 28% decrease in infant mortality over three years at the French maternity hospital" (para, 2). From such beginnings, and with increased understanding of the special needs of preterm and extremely preterm infants, important interventions could be developed. These interventions were for the most part aimed at supporting their immature and developing organs, and ultimately survival. Roughly, in the 1950s mechanical ventilation, phototherapy for hyperbilirubinemia, and ventricular shunts to relieve cranial pressure became available. In the 1960s and 1970s more sophisticated feeding modes such as total parenteral nutrition became available and specialized neonatal intensive care started to be delivered in regional centers allowing concentrated high technology care, expertise, and treatment; however, these care settings also brought new problems for families living far from such centers who could not easily visit or access this type of care. Contemporarily, many more interventions have been, and continue to be, developed and are available usually in high level neonatal care units (NICUs) in academic medical centers in the US and elsewhere. In the US, neonatology was established as a specialty in 1960 with the inception of a neonatal intensive care unit at Yale, New Haven Hospital spearheaded by Louis Gluck (Gartner et al., 1992). Many countries now have the equivalent of neonatal intensive care units (NICUs) and the ethical issues associated with these units are diverse and complex. One of the biggest issues is the lack of degree of certainty about prognosis. That is, the ability to predict which infants requiring NICU care will go on to develop normally with little sequelae and which will not, is still relatively poorly understood, complicating both parental and clinical team ethical decision making. Moreover, questions of how to balance suffering with potential for life, quality of life, and the interests of the family unit are prevalent in NICUs, and it is often the nurses who are at the front lines of navigating the consequences of these decisions. Thus, it is critical that nurses are able to communicate their concerns in an articulate and informative way as discussed in detail in Chapter 4. When nurses are asked to carry out decisions with which they do not agree they can suffer moral distress which, as discussed in Chapters 1 and 2, can lead to them distancing from patients or leaving the profession which is problematic for patients, families, and the nurses themselves (Epstein & Hamric, 2009; Settle, 2014).

7.3 Principles of Parental and Team Decision-Making for Premature and Critically Ill Neonates

Another tricky issue for all involved with the care of seriously ill newborns is the problem of when continued treatment might be clinically ineffective or negatively impact the quality of life for the infant, though quality of life judgments are inherently subjective and deeply personal. Partly because of the uncertainty related to prognosis for many infants who are very premature or who are born with or develop other serious conditions, the question of when to opt for comfort measures versus continuing attempts at curative or life-sustaining treatments can be difficult. Additionally, there are sometimes uncertainties about who the decision-makers should be, how to share the decision-making and in the case of intractable conflicts who will have ultimate decision-making authority. Ethically, how should the final decision be made when a conflict exists? The healthcare team may have a more realistic understanding of the baby or infant's likely survival or potential for suffering. Yet in some countries, parental engagement in decision making is seen as important, given that the healthcare team may have biases about treatment options and overestimate the burdens of long-term outcomes, like disability, which may not reflect the values of parents (Garret et al., 2017; Penticuff & Arheart, 2005; Saigal & Doyle, 2008; Saigal et al., 2000).

A Norwegian study asking nurses and physicians, among other team members, their perspective on decision-making concluded that although parents should have a voice and should be well-informed and their circumstances understood, ultimately the healthcare team should be the decision-makers in life or death matters (Ursin & Syltern, 2018). Ursin and Syltern (2018) as a result of their study also concluded that healthcare team decision-making was most likely to "promote the best interest of both parents and the child" (p. S 572). Thus, parents would be relieved of some of the decision-making burden including the possibility of regret and the best interests of the child safeguarded from decisions that perhaps unconsciously reflect parental interests rather than the infant's. However, the family will be responsible for the complex care of a premature child who survives but has severe morbidities that require ongoing care and attention. Moreover, there are economic costs, social costs and costs to other children in the family whose interests may be side-tracked in favor of the one whose needs are the greatest (Anderson et al., 2007; Marquis et al., 2019). But individualized, case-based decision-making means that in some cases infants with similar physical conditions and sequelae might be treated differently than each other, which could constitute discrimination based on the infant's contextual circumstances.

In the US, the predominant clinical decision-making model used in pediatrics is shared decision-making, where ideally providers offer input on potential treatments and parents offer input on values and preferences that help shape which treatment option is in the best interests of the child. Indeed, the first 'Baby Doe' rules (1983) in the US. were initiated by the Reagan Government because of publicity about an infant born with Down syndrome and tracheoesophageal atresia. In consultation with the pediatrician, the family decided not to surgically repair the atresia, but to withhold fluids and let the infant die. This would not have been considered ethically permissible for another infant born without the cognitive challenges associated with Down' syndrome in the absence of other severe physical challenges. There were negative reactions to this situation, especially from the clinicians and nurses who were charged with caring for the infant. As a result, an amendment was added to the US Rehabilitation Act which established that not treating such infants was a breach of civil rights (Kopelman, 2005; White, 2011). Although this law was eventually negated by the US Supreme Court, a later law amended the existing Child Abuse, Protection and Treatment Act to forbid withholding an indicated treatment which would constitute neglect under the law. This law is still in place but has not resulted in prosecutions to-date. Nevertheless, its implications do hover in the background of decision-making in NICU's in the US, thus adding to decision-making complexity. An older review of the literature detailing practices in a variety of countries (Levin, 1990) revealed that differences among countries were generally based on "(1) the resources available; (2) social attitudes about the use of medical interventions and about disability; (3) the roles, experiences and values of decision-makers; and (4) the law" (p. 901). A more recent large-scale study (Helenius et al., 2020) related to determining redirection of care based on perceptions of 'futility' for premature births suggests continued differences based on these factors. This was concluded to be partly responsible for the differences in outcomes among countries.

7.3.1 Moral Status

Another issue that accompanies decision-making in NICU's concerns the moral status or standing of a neonate. One philosophical description of moral status asserts, "an entity has (full) moral status if and only if it or its interests morally matter to some degree for the entity's own sake" (Jaworski & Tannebaum, 2018). The implications of this are that moral status depends on some level of cognitive capacity and ability to experience life in some form. However, for certain religions the fact that an infant is a product of human beings, regardless of cognitive potential, means that infant should be assigned moral status and in having moral status should have his or her life protected, regardless of the child's ability to experience that life. Thus, a problem that often arises in making difficult decisions about the ongoing care of seriously ill infants is that of varying beliefs about whether, and under what conditions, quality of life trumps 'bare physical' life. Concerning a newborn, the idea of quality of life is different from that of an adult who has experienced life and has projects values and preferences. For adults what constitutes quality-of-life (QOL) inevitably has subjective aspects. That is, the adult has a perspective on what constitutes an acceptable level of QOL. For newborns and infants who have not developed preferences, beliefs, and values, QOL considerations focus on **potential** to live a minimally meaningful life (Powers & Faden, 2006). By that we mean that the child has the future capacity to engage cognitively with the world surrounding them and can experience such things as relationships, emotions such as joy etc. In the absence of such potential, especially in the presence of likely suffering the issue of potentially medically ineffective interventions may be raised.

7.3.2 Medically Ineffective Treatments and Care Redirection

The term medical futility is often used to describe interventions that cannot achieve their intended goal. The trouble, of course, with this idea is that it can be difficult to differentiate what interventions are futile in an absolute sense from those that offer a sliver of hope either for physical continuance or some eventual quality of life, especially due to the prognostic uncertainty inherent in pediatrics. Despite many attempts at defining "futility" (Schneiderman et al., 1990), the term remains subjective and a working definition elusive. More recently, the Society of Critical Care Medicine has recommended using the phrase "potentially inappropriate treatment" referring to treatments for which there is "no reasonable expectation that the patient will improve sufficiently to survive outside the acute care setting" or when there is "no reasonable expectation that the patient's neurologic function will improve sufficiently to allow the patient to perceive the benefits of treatment" (Kon et al., 2016, p. 1769).

For parents, sometimes a miniscule amount of hope from an intervention can be something they cling to and this is not surprising. The birth of their infant has been anticipated for several months and to be faced with decision-making for a young infant is an incredibly difficult task. It can be an especially burdensome responsibility for first-time parents of a newborn. Parents, generally, do not understand the future implications of their child's clinical problem, even if they can understand the current meaning. But developing understanding takes time and is a process. We also know that experiencing decisional conflict is common in the context of uncertainty and takes time to resolve (LeBlanc et al., 2009). Thus, our ethical responsibilities as nurses and other healthcare providers caring for this population are to understand the issues and provide support and resources. Transparency in providing information is key but so is an understanding of the psychological effects of learning that a hoped-for joyous occasion has been impacted by illness.

There are three (or more) possible religious and/or philosophical perspectives on when a living human entity—regardless of whether they are considered to have **full** moral status—should have their lives prolonged with life sustaining treatments (LST). The presence of these differing perspectives adds to decision making complexity and can give rise to conflict. As described above, one philosophical perspective is that maintaining a 'bare (physical) life' when there is no potential for experience is not reasonable per se., because human life is most importantly experiential. This perspective can nevertheless be challenged when families have strong reasons for maintaining, or maintaining for a period of time, a life that is unlikely to be experienced in some meaningful way. Families or others involved in decision making may believe the value of human life is absolute and cessation of efforts to prolong life are medically and morally unconscionable. Additionally, a family may need time to process the information and feel more confident that the course of action is best for the infant. Moreover, it may not be possible to accurately judge potential because of difficulties in prognostication. A second perspective is that it is an injustice to sustain the intractably painful life of an infant whose condition is itself life limiting, essentially abrogating the duty of non-maleficence (doing no harm). It is unjust because it serves some purpose other than the best interests of the child. The best interest of the child is best defined as that which "will benefit the infant, produce the least amount of harm, and include the cultural traditions of the parents" (Settle, 2018, p. 218). A third perspective is that a human child is to be treated as having human rights regardless of ability to claim or make use of those rights, just because that infant or child is born of human parents. This latter perspective relies on ideas about the existence of a supreme being or higher power that confers moral status on all human beings, whose lives have value in any form. It should be noted, though, that this perspective does not entail a prohibition against stopping interventions that are determined to be medically ineffective.

7.3.3 Providing Parental Support

Contemporarily, in many countries it is recognized that parents should be involved in decision-making for their newborns because they are the experts on their family and its resources. They, for the most part, have developed a strong emotional investment in their child over the prenatal period. However, they need adequate information and in a way that allows them to process its meaning in terms of their and their child's life. They may also need psychological support to make a decision that is the best possible for the infant, one that maximizes benefits and minimizes harms, including inadvertent harms. Parental judgment can also be skewed by denial of the seriousness of the situation. As noted by Jerud and Knowlton (2018), while

> the collaborative approach has many benefits ... appropriate participation in decision making necessitates that parents have accurate beliefs about the probable outcomes for their child (who is dependent) on their decisions...denial precludes authentic parental participation in collaborative decision making and thus warrants intervention. It is therefore the duty of the neonatologist to ensure that denial is not inappropriately resulting in decisions that are not in a child's best interest, that oppose goals the parents might hold if not in a state of denial, or that breach the harm threshold. (pp. 34–35)

While Jerud and Knowlton (2018) have a point, in situations like this that are inevitably complex, care must be taken not to put too much power in the hands of a singular clinician. Such cases are usually best reviewed by an ethics committee as discussed in Chapter 6.

Another source of ambiguity that can complicate parental decision-making for a critically ill infant is receiving inconsistent messages from various members of the healthcare team. Such conflicts add to the burden of parents who then become even more unsure about the best course of action. The following example highlights this problem.

Baby A is born at 29 weeks with known hydrops fetalis. The family lost a prior infant due to the same condition. Hydrops fetalis is a condition that causes fluid build-up in the fetus' tissues and organs, leading to severe, life-threatening swelling. Many different immune and non-immune diseases and medical complications can cause hydrops fetalis. There are several underlying causes for this condition and the survival rate to term is very low. While rarely infants will survive and live a normal life with aggressive interventions, most do not (Santos et al., 2011). Seven days of intensive rescue treatments have failed to improve Baby A's prognosis. The NICU physicians and the pediatric cardiologist think that a few more days might permit some improvement in physical condition, while the NICU nurses are concerned that the extent of Baby A's suffering is too much given the likely prognosis. Baby A's parents sense the tensions and are losing confidence in the medical team. While they desperately hope that Baby A will survive with a reasonable quality of life, if this is not a likely outcome then they would like more time with him as long as this would not cause him additional suffering. However, they are not sure that continuing aggressive treatment is the right course to pursue. They are confused about what the best course of action would be.

Besides the importance of the healthcare team all conveying the same message to parents, research reveals that: it is easier for families to understand the situation and be engaged in decision-making under the following conditions:

- Information is provided clearly and in everyday language and the families understanding is solicited

- Families are treated as contextually situated and their individual concerns are accounted for
- Supports based on their individual needs are provided
- An interdisciplinary team who can fill out the perspectives and provide a variety of resources outside of pure information needs is involved.

(Boss et al., 2016, p. 223)

However, the scant research on how information is actually provided to families reveals that up to 80% of conversations in family meetings is provided by the physician, the individual needs and concerns of the family were often left out and other perspectives not sought (Boss et al., 2016). A brief informal review of the status of family involvement in decision-making in Europe, Scandinavia, The Netherlands and Australia found that involvement of families in decision-making for critically ill neonates varies both across and within countries. However, the question is less about how it is done and more about how it ought to be done. Certainly, families have a big stake in what sort of interventions are being provided to their infants and, as the proxy-decision makers charged with making decisions that are in the best interests of their infant, should be involved. This points to an urgent need for nurses to be involved and to advocate that the individual concerns of family be addressed. Similarly, nurses play an important role in ensuring the ethical care of young children and adolescents. This next section provides a discussion of common problems that arise in the care of children and adolescents.

7.4 Issues in the Care of Children and Adolescents

Recurrent ethical themes that arise in the care of children and adolescents include: the developmental ability of the child to appreciate information and its meaning for them and for their future; parental worries about providing diagnostic information to children that may be harmful; parents (conscious or subconscious) focus on their own interests instead of that of the child; genetic testing issues (as discussed in Chapter 11); transitioning of care from pediatric to adult healthcare services; reproductive issues; exposure to abuse, neglect, and even human trafficking; end-of-life issues; and guardianship problems. Some of these themes are addressed in other chapters in this book. For example, the issue of medical futility is discussed in Chapter 4.

Much of a child's ability to determine his or her best interests depends on the level of emotional and cognitive development achieved as well as their past experiences. Additionally, the presence of supportive adults is critical to decisions that are in the best interests of the child (Gaylord, 2018). The parents and guardians of children are necessarily part of discussions about best courses of actions. For ease of discussion we use the term parents to stand for anyone who assumes primary responsibility for a child.

7.4.1 Balancing Autonomy and Beneficence

In Chapter 3 the concept of autonomy was defined in two ways. The first, derived from Immanuel Kant's (1724–1804) treatise on morality, asserts each mature human being is to be respected as having the same moral worth as everyone else because they have an in-built or 'a priori' structure for moral reasoning. The implication is that a higher power or creator is responsible for this inbuilt mechanism that only human beings possess. Kant provides a complex argument in support of this idea. But his conclusion is that it is immoral for people to use other people as mere objects that satisfy someone else's needs (extreme examples of this are slavery and contemporary problems such as the trafficking of human beings). This is also called the principle of respect for persons. Others have argued from a secular (non-religious basis) perspective that it is in each of our interests to be treated as morally important simply because any one of us could fall into the category of those who are not considered fully human. Chapter 12 provides a more detailed justification for this argument. From the past we know what terrible things can happen when groups of people are not seen as being of moral concern. Contemporarily, groups of displaced persons who have fled violence are often dehumanized, thus, subjected to inhumane treatment. The second sense of autonomy is related to the first but essentially means that because people (all things being equal) are rational beings they should be allowed to make their own decisions and might be expected to know themselves best. It follows logically that in healthcare settings this principle affirms a responsibility for clinicians to ensure the person has the information needed to make an informed and reasoned decision, which in turn requires understanding important particularities about the person in question. This second sense of autonomy is most pertinent to the care of children. When children lack the developmental capacity to make informed decisions for themselves, the adults around them are ethically charged with making good decisions on their behalf. This could be called 'autonomy by proxy' but is not autonomy in the usual sense of 'self-determination'. Exercising autonomy by proxy is, of course, tricky. Even when parents 'know' their children, they may not have adequate knowledge of the physical, psychological or developmental nuances of a health problem and its implications. Also, the emotional attachment most parents have to their children can distort decision-making and conflate parental needs with those of the child. Thus, when decision-making occurs in a hospital or clinic setting the best interest standard, as discussed earlier, is most often relied upon. As a reminder, the best interest standard focuses on enhancing benefits, controlling or diminishing possible harms and accounts for the cultural context of the parents (Settle, 2018). Thus, at times where especially difficult decisions have to be made, parents need the support of nurses and perhaps access to other supportive resources such as pastoral care, social work or counseling professionals.

Recently, the American Medical Association (AMA, 2019) recognized parental responsibilities in the Code of Medical Ethics Opinion 2.2.1. as also being to empower their children.

As the persons best positioned to understand their child's unique needs and interests, parents (or guardians) are asked to fill the dual responsibility of protecting their children and, at the same time, empowering them and promoting development of children's capacity to become independent decision makers. In giving or withholding permission for medical treatment for their children, parents/guardians are expected to safeguard their children's physical health and well-being and to nurture their children's developing personhood and autonomy. (AMA, 2019)

In turn, this implies that clinicians need to help parents fulfill this responsibility as discussed next.

7.4.2 Children's Involvement in Decision-Making

Major issues for nurses at the bedside tend to revolve around three themes: (1) The child should be involved in the decision-making but is not being included; (2) Parents are making decisions for their child that seem to the healthcare team or the nurses not to be in the child's best interests; (3) The child has strong ideas about what he or she wants but is being pressured either to accept or reject treatment.

7.4.2.1 Including or Excluding the Child from Decision-Making

A child's ability to appreciate the nuances and meanings of a proposed decision related to a course of treatment varies greatly depending on age, past experiences, and cognitive abilities (Alderson et al., 2006). It does not follow a straight line based on age, although developmental markers do play a role. In general, a four-year-old will not have developed as mature a sense of appreciation of consequences as a teenager. Determining the extent that a child should be involved in decision-making is difficult and is complicated by the number of other possible stakeholders. A critical factor in the determination is an evaluation of the benefits over risks (short and long-term) to the child of participation or non-participation and how necessary risks will be anticipated and minimized. A general principle is that a child is not given a choice of assenting or declining if a proposed treatment will be given anyway because it is necessary for that child's well-being. For example, a child would not be permitted to decline needed surgery for appendicitis. The risks of not performing surgery obviously outweigh the benefits. However, as much control as possible over the situation should be given to the child. One way to do this is to provide information in a sensitive and age-appropriate way, attending to the child's concerns. Where available, Child Life specialists, or similar support personnel, may be additional helpful resources to such children.

The European Charter for Children in Hospital (EACH, 2016) established children's rights in hospital settings in 1986 and has revised this several times since. Currently they include advice on how to talk to children about COVID-19. Article 4 lays out the child's right to information as follows:

- Information given to children should be based on the child's age and understanding and take into account their level of development;
- be informed by what the child already knows or imagines;
- include honest and simple explanations about their condition and treatment outcomes;
- explain the course of events to come, including what the child may see, smell, hear and feel include appropriately prepared verbal, audiovisual and written information, supported by illustrative models, play or other media presentations.
- Staff giving information should appreciate the child's capacity to comprehend information and express his or her views. Staff should encourage and answer questions, offering comfort when concern or fear is expressed (pp. 11–12)

When children have circumstances explained to them in a way that is tailored to their age and capacity to understand, and their concerns are heard, their sense of trust and control is enhanced as research undertaken in Spain (Noreña Peña & Rojas, 2014) with children 8–14 years highlights. Findings include the importance of "nursing staff behaviour as a key aspect in the exchange of information and communication of news as well as children's experience" (p. 245). However, some children in the study said they did not want to know details and that their parents could decide, so this possibility also has to be taken into account.

7.4.2.2 Parental Requests to Withhold Information

A problem encountered by pediatric nurses, especially in acute care settings, is that of being asked by parents to withhold information from their child because it would be too upsetting for them. For example, Lindsey is 11 years old. She has been admitted for treatment of a new diagnosis of acute myeloid leukemia. Her parents have not told her of her diagnosis, just that she has a 'virus' that needs to be treated in hospital. They are concerned that she is "an anxious child" and if she were told that she had leukemia it would diminish her body's ability to benefit from the chemotherapy. They want to be sure that the doctors and nurses do not reveal her diagnosis. There are several reasons why this is not good practice and might actually be harmful to Lindsey. Given that we need to respect parental wishes but remain focused on what is best for the child, one must navigate this situation carefully. The approach to this issue will differ depending on context and nuance. However, a good way to start is to explore with the parents what assumptions that they are making. Possible assumptions may be related to the family's cultural practices and beliefs. Is it usual in their culture to withhold information? Parents may assume that the child will not suspect or find out accidently, which would undermine trust both in them and in the healthcare team. They may assume there is no way to tell the child that preserves hope. Cole and Kodish (2013), provide some good strategies to assist families in considering what is in their child's best interests both short and long term. First it is important to validate the parents' right to protect their child, while helping them to see that what they are asking may actually do the opposite. Especially in those cases where a child's death is imminent (not the case with Lindsey at this point) parents have to live with the results of their decision-making and should be able to feel like they have done the right thing (Kreicbergs et al., 2005).

In this case, preserving Lindsey's trust in both her parents and the healthcare team is paramount. Studies suggest some themes for parents to understand:

1. The child may have an idea that something is not right, and they are not being told, thus imagining the worst.
2. The child may overhear, or accidently be told the truth by someone who is not party to the parents' wishes—undermining trust.
3. When evasive answers are given to the child's questions, the child may wonder what is going on.
4. Healthcare personnel may feel moral distress and a loss of sense of integrity when asked to do something they have strong reasons to know is not ethical.

Effective strategies are to discuss with parents the potential sequelae to their request and offer to either (1) help the parents talk to their child; or (2) give the parents some strategies for having the conversation with their child. It is also possible to give the parents some time to think about how they want to proceed without providers ceding their right to veracity should Lindsey ask questions.

7.4.2.3 Parental Decisions and Child's Best Interest

Occasionally parents seem determined to make decisions that either are not in the child's best interests or seem to work against the child's expressed wishes. Sometimes, the decision is based on religious grounds. Extreme examples include refusal of treatment based on religious doctrine. For example, in the US, the Christian Science parents of a child refused to allow treatment for lymphoma which had a predicted 40% chance of cure (Black, 2006). In other cases, Jehovah's Witness (JV) parents refuse blood for the child who is in danger from loss of blood. This causes great concern for nurses, physicians and other providers. It can give rise to moral distress especially when the risks of suffering and/or death are high. In the US, the courts typically support interventions necessary to save a child's life even against parental wishes and arguments that parents have a right to follow the dictates of their religion. Thus, freedom to practice their religion does not extend to exercising this right on behalf of a child. Parents are not permitted to exercise that right when it puts their child at high risk for death or other harms. In an often-cited case that was actually about labor laws, *Prince vs. Massachusetts* (1944), the US Supreme Court affirmed that parental rights of decision making for their children is not an absolute right. Moreover, similar arguments have been offered in Europe and Australia, among other countries (Woolley, 2005). So the question is, under which conditions is it permissible to override parental decision-making? This is an ethical issue of determining rights, risks, and benefits. Such cases sometimes end up in the courts. In another case, of a child with seizure disorder and developmental delays who had a major seizure, parents stopped treating the child. In this case, which ended up in the courts as a case of neglect, the chance of benefit from the treatments was high and the risks of not treating also high. Thus, courts overrode the parents decision-making rights (Black, 2006).

Alternatively, parents may not be psychologically or emotionally able to make good decisions for their child. An example of this is parents who refuse to allow their dying child to stop treatments and have comfort care or parents who do not want their child adequately treated for pain due to extreme grief or misconceptions about what this treatment may entail. At the extreme end of this continuum is the unnecessary death of a child due to parental decisions—for example from unreplaced blood loss—which would rob the child of later autonomous decision-making opportunities. What is at stake in this case is what has been called 'a child's right to an open future' (Millum, 2014). "The right protects the child against having important life choices determined by others before she has the ability to make them for herself" (p. 1). Basically the argument is that parents and or others should not infringe on the child's right to decide for themselves upon reaching maturity. However, there are countless other ways that a parent could rob the child of 'an open future'. For example, a parent could request genetic testing for their child to assess the child's risk of developing an adult-onset disease such as hereditary breast and/or ovarian cancer (BRCA1 or 2). If a child is tested and found to have a pathogenic variant in either gene, this will affect how that child looks at the future. Once one knows the results of a genetic test one cannot 'unknow'. Since this is an adult-onset disease, one prevailing view is that the child should be allowed to make a genetic testing decision for him or herself upon reaching the age of maturity. Chapter 11 outlines other views on this topic.

In another scenario where a child's future was endangered, Macauley and Fritzler (2014) describe, the case of a young boy with Guillain–Barre Syndrome (GBS), whose mother delayed treatment based on valuing the "natural healing processes" (p. 1). She eventually agreed to life saving treatments such as a ventilator because of threats to report her for child abuse. But while her son was ventilator-dependent she then tried to refuse the standard opioid addition to his medication routine citing fears of addiction. In this case while the mother ostensibly was working to help her son, her lack of understanding of consequences meant that she was not acting in her son's best interest. Knotty problems like this may not be resolvable by individual nurses but require a multi-disciplinary team such as an ethics committee to address. However, nurses can engage in preventive ethics, as discussed in Chapter 5. They can anticipate what is needed for the good care of a child and recognize emerging problems and barriers to that care. One way to do this is to listen to parental explanations of their beliefs and values and explore the meaning of these for the child in question. For the most part, listening to and building trust with the parents, along with evidence-informed explanations about such things as pain and healing, parental regret, children's needs can help the family make a good decision. However, when a parent persists in acting against the child's interests, we have responsibilities to place the child's needs at the forefront of decisions.

After-the-fact, a good strategy is to arrange a meeting with the staff involved to think about what was learned from the situation and what might be done differently in the future. Certainly, nurses need to be educated about the rights of children and how to articulate these in light of a situation where a child's interests are not being promoted whether intentionally or unintentionally.

7.5 Engaging in Self-Reflection, and Reflection on Practice

In Chapter 2 the importance of self-reflection and reflection on practice was discussed in relation to the development of nurse-patient interactions that are as non-judgmental as possible and elicit trust. Self-reflection allows the unearthing of biases and presuppositions so that they can be brought to the surface of consciousness and accounted for in the nurse-patient nurse-family interaction and in ethical decision-making. Reflection on practice concerns a willingness and ability to explore prior practice situations that did not have expected or intended results. It is necessary for the purpose of anticipating what is needed for improving future practice.

Both reflection and self-reflection require an acceptance that we are human and as such are influenced by our emotions and all of our prior acculturations such as upbringing, prevailing cultural values, education, and the extent of our exposure to different points-of-view. Developing the habit of self-reflection, is not easy but is improved with practice. Self-reflection can be uncomfortable as we realize that we have not always made the best or most well-considered decisions or that we hold conflicting values that need to be reconciled (Weston, 2011). Effective self-reflection—self-reflection that leads to well-considered decisions—is in an Aristotelian sense a virtue. For Aristotle, a virtue is developed over time and with practice. It is the result of cultivating habitual actions. It results in a balance between two excesses and is the practiced use of human reason to tame emotional reactions. For example, courage is a virtue that strikes a balance between reckless action (risky behavior) and timidity (not acting out of fear) in order to achieve a good end (Haggerty & Grace, 2008). At the end of Chapter 2 there is an exercise that can be used to develop self-reflection.

Associated with self-reflection is reflection-on-practice (Haggerty & Grace, 2008). Reflection-on-practice enhances clinical judgment and is needed for clinically wise actions. It can be enhanced in a team setting where various perspectives are considered, and the nuances of a case explored. Nursing ethics education where there is opportunity to discuss good practice and how to overcome obstacles to good practice is one route to enhance reflection. A consistent comment on post course evaluations from one of the Chapter author's (Grace) graduate nursing ethics classes is about how interactions with colleagues from disparate practice settings broadened the perspectives of these mostly seasoned nurses about practice issues. This finding is supported elsewhere in the literature and by the end-of-program essays from a yearlong Clinical Ethics Residency for Nurses (CERN) (Lee et al., 2020). Strategies for developing ethics discussion and ethics rounds are provided later. The need for such discussions is perhaps especially acute for nurses in pediatric settings because of the additional interests and concerns of family members that can inadvertently distract from an emphasis on the good of the child, especially when the child's perspective is not or cannot be known as in the setting of neonatal intensive care units.

7.6 Summary

Caring for newborns, infants and children is complicated by their extreme vulnerability in terms of cognitive development and dependence on the adults around them to make good decisions on their behalf. For neonates, what constitutes a good decision may not be clear as it is complicated by prognostic uncertainty. Moreover, the family—where this is available—will ultimately be responsible for providing long term care for seriously physically or psychologically compromised children and this in turn will have ripple effects on other family members. In some countries, families will be supported by societal resources; in others they may not. When they are not adequately supported, this responsibility may become an unsustainable burden on families, and this constitutes one of the injustices with which the nursing profession needs to concern itself. For children at varying levels of cognitive abilities, nurses and the healthcare team are ethically responsible for evaluating what the child needs. This may include assessing what the child knows and/or wants to know and how involved the child wants to be in the decision-making. We are also responsible for helping the child to talk to their parents about what they want and for helping parents to talk to their children about why they are deciding on a particular course of action.

References

Alderson, P., Sutcliffe, K., & Curtis, K. (2006). Children as partners with adults in their medical care. *Archives of Disease in Childhood, 91*(4), 300–303.

American Association of Pediatrics. (2017). Age limit of pediatrics. Accessed December 7, 2020 from https://pediatrics.aappublications.org/content/140/3/e20172151#:~:text=In%20the%20guidelines%20for%20choosing,12%20years%20of%20age%3B%20and%20(

American Medical Association. (2019). Opinion 2.2.1. Pediatric decision-making. Accessed October 6, 2020 from https://www.ama-assn.org/delivering-care/ethics/pediatric-decision-making

Anderson, D., Dumont, S., Jacobs, P., & Azzaria, L. (2007). The personal costs of caring for a child with a disability: A review of the literature. *Public Health Reports, 122*(1), 3–16.

Black, L. (2006). Limiting parents' rights in medical decision making. *AMA Journal of Ethics, 8*(10), 676–680.

Boss, R. D., Donohue, P. K., Larson, S. M., Arnold, R. M., & Roter, D. L. (2016). Family conferences in the neonatal intensive care unit: Observation of communication dynamics and contributions. *PediAtric Critical Care Medicine: A Journal of the Society of Critical Care Medicine and the World Federation of Pediatric Intensive and Critical Care Societies, 17*(3), 223.

Cole, C. M., & Kodish, E. (2013). Minors' right to know and therapeutic privilege. *AMA Journal of Ethics, 15*(8), 638–644.

EACH. (2016). European Association for Children in Hospital. Charter. https://www.each-for-sick-children.org/images/stories/2016/Charter_AUG2016_oSz.pdf

Epstein, E. G., & Hamric, A. B. (2009). Moral distress, moral residue, and the crescendo effect. *The Journal of Clinical Ethics, 20*(4), 330–342.

Garret, J. R., Carter, B. S., & Lantos, J. R. (2017). What we do when we resuscitate extremely preterm infants. *The American Journal of Bioethics, 17*(8), 1–3. https://doi.org/10.1080/15265161.2017.1341249

Gartner, L. M., Gartner, C. B., Gluck, L., & Butterfield, L. J. (1992). The care of premature infants: Historical perspective. *Health, 92*, 2786.

Gaylord, N. M. (2018). Nursing ethics and advanced practice: Children and adolescents. In P. J. Grace (Ed.), *Nursing ethics and professional responsibility in advanced practice* (pp. 237–258). Jones & Bartlett Learning.

Haggerty, L. A., & Grace, P. (2008). Clinical wisdom: The essential foundation of "good" nursing care. *Journal of Professional Nursing, 24*(4), 235–240.

Helenius, K., Morisaki, N., Kusuda, S., Shah, P.S., Norman, M., Lehtonen, L., Reichman, B., Darlow, B.A., Noguchi, A., Adams, M., & Bassler, D. (2020). Survey shows marked variations in approaches to redirection of care for critically ill very preterm infants in 11 countries. *Acta Paediatrica, 109*(7), 1338–1345.

Institute of Medicine (US). (2007). Preterm birth: Causes, consequences, and prevention. In R. E. Behrman, & A. S. Butler (Eds.), *Committee on understanding premature birth and assuring healthy outcomes*. National Academies Press. https://www.ncbi.nlm.nih.gov/books/NBK11363/

Jaworska, A., & Tannenbaum, J. (2018).The grounds of moral status. In E. N. Zalta (Ed.), *The Stanford encyclopedia of philosophy*. https://plato.stanford.edu/archives/spr2018/entries/grounds-moral-status/

Jerud, I., & Knowlton, S. (2018). When denial hurts the children: An argument for accountability of denial in parental decision making. *The American Journal of Bioethics: AJOB, 18*(9), 33–35. https://doi.org/10.1080/15265161.2018.1498950

Kon, A. A., Shepard, E. K., Sederstrom, N. O., Swoboda, S. M., Marshall, M. F., Birriel, B., & Rincon, F. (2016). Defining futile and potentially inappropriate interventions: A policy statement from the society of critical care medicine ethics committee. *Critical Care Medicine, 44*(9), 1769–1774. https://doi.org/10.1097/CCM.0000000000001965

Kopelman, L. (2005). Are the 21-year-old Baby Doe rules misunderstood or mistaken? *Pediatrics, 115*, 797–902.

Kreicbergs, U., Valdimarsdóttir, U., Onelöv, E., Björk, O., Steineck, G., & Henter, J. I. (2005). Care-related distress: A nationwide study of parents who lost their child to cancer. *Journal of Clinical Oncology: Official Journal of the American Society of Clinical Oncology, 23*(36), 9162–9171. https://doi.org/10.1200/JCO.2005.08.557

LeBlanc, A., Kenny, D. A., O'Connor, A. M., & Légaré, F. (2009). Decisional conflict in patients and their physicians: A dyadic approach to shared decision making. *Medical Decision Making, 29*(1), 61–68.

Lee, S., Robinson, E. M., Grace, P. J., Zollfrank, A., & Jurchak, M. (2020). Developing a moral compass: Themes from the Clinical Ethics Residency for Nurses' final essays. *Nursing Ethics, 27*(1), 28–39.

Levin, B. (1990). International perspectives on treatment choice in neonatal intensive care units. *Social Science & Medicine, 30*(8), 901–912.

Macauley, R. C., & Fritzler, L. J. (2014). Parental refusal of pain management: A potentially unrecognized form of medical neglect. *Palliative Medical Care, 1*(2), 5.

Marquis, S., Hayes, M. V., & McGrail, K. (2019). Factors that may affect the health of siblings of children who have an intellectual/developmental disability. *Journal of Policy and Practice in Intellectual Disabilities, 16*(4), 273–286.

Millum, J. (2014). The foundation of the child's right to an open future. *Journal of Social Philosophy, 45*(4), 522.

National Institutes of Health. (1992). *Neonatal intensive care: A history of excellence* (No. 92–2786). NIH Publication.

Payne, E. (2016). A brief history of advances in neonatal care. Accessed November 5, 2020 from https://www.nicuawareness.org/blog/a-brief-history-of-advances-in-neonatal-care

Peña, A. L., & Rojas, J. G. (2014). Ethical aspects of children's perceptions of information-giving in care. *Nursing Ethics, 21*(2), 245–256. https://doi.org/10.1177/0969733013484483 [Epub 2013 May 23 PMID: 23702897].

Penticuff, J. H., & Arheart, K. L. (2005). Effectiveness of an intervention to improve parent-professional collaboration in neonatal intensive care. *The Journal of Perinatal & Neonatal Nursing, 19*(2), 187–202.

Powers, M., & Faden, R. R. (2006). *Social justice: The moral foundations of public health and health policy.* Oxford University Press.

Prince v. Massachusetts (1944). 321 US. 158. Accessed December 7, 2020 from https://www.courtlistener.com/opinion/103933/prince-v-massachusetts/

Saigal, S., & Doyle, L. W. (2008). An overview of mortality and sequelae of preterm birth from infancy to adulthood. *The Lancet, 371*(9608), 261–269.

Saigal, S., Hoult, L. A., Streiner, D. L., Stoskopf, B. L., & Rosenbaum, P. L. (2000). School difficulties at adolescence in a regional cohort of children who were extremely low birth weight. *Pediatrics, 105*(2), 325–331.

Santo, S., Mansour, S., Thilaganathan, B., Homfray, T., Papageorghiou, A., Calvert, S., & Bhide, A. (2011). Prenatal diagnosis of non-immune hydrops fetalis: What do we tell the parents? *Prenatal Diagnosis, 31*(2), 186–195.

Schneiderman, L. J., Jecker, N. S., & Jonsen, A. R. (1990). Medical futility: Its meaning and ethical implications. *Annals of Internal Medicine, 112*(12), 949–954. https://doi.org/10.7326/0003-4819-112-12-949

Seltzer, R. R., Raisanen, T. S., Donohue, P. K., da Silva, T., Williams, E. P., Shepard, J., & Boss, R. D. (2020). Medical decision-making in foster care: Considerations for the care of children with medical complexity. *Academic Pediatrics, 20*(3), 333–340.

Settle, P. D. (2014). Nurse activism in the newborn intensive care unit: Actions in response to an ethical dilemma. *Nursing Ethics, 21*(2), 198–209. https://doi.org/10.1177/0969733012475254

Settle, M. D. (2018). Nursing ethics and advanced practice: Neonatal issues. In P. J. Grace (Ed.), *Nursing ethics and professional responsibility in advanced practice* (pp. 209–235). Jones and Bartlett Learning.

Ursin, L., & Syltern, J. (2018). In the best interest of the parents: Norwegian health personnel on the proper role of parents in neonatal decision-making. *Pediatrics, 142*(Supplement 1), S567–S573.

Weston, A. (2011). *A practical companion to ethics* (4th ed.). Oxford University Press.

White, M. (2011). The end at the beginning. *The Ochsner Journal, 11*(4), 309–316.

Woolley, S. (2005). Children of Jehovah's Witnesses and adolescent Jehovah's Witnesses: What are their rights? *Archive of Disease in Childhood, 90*, 715–719. https://doi.org/10.1136/adc.2004.067843

Resources

European Standard for Neonatal care: https://newborn-health-standards.org/
https://www.google.com/search?q=a+case+of+mixed+messages+in+the+nicu&rlz=1C1CHBF_e
nUS907US907&biw=1366&bih=663&tbm=isch&source=iu&ictx=1&fir=7RWyliKZX
wQjHM%252CvD9LxHZo0n1S7M%252C_&vet=1&usg=AI4_-kQnjDehcmYrR9nAMty
5wGjT7zYNOA&sa=X&ved=2ahUKEwiVrpvWypTsAhVdhXIEHdakDQgQ9QF6BAgEEAg#
imgrc=7RWyliKZXwQjHM

Chapter 8
Genetics: Nurses Roles and Responsibilities

Melissa K. Uveges and Andrew A. Dwyer

Abstract This chapter provides an overview of genetics and genomics and their importance in contemporary nursing practice. The fundamentals of what nurses need to know about the ethical aspects of genetic testing from deciding whether testing is important and for whom to helping persons with their decision-making, are provided. The use of genetic testing from preconception to disease monitoring are described. Additionally, the state of the science, the role of genetic counselors, problems of privacy and confidentiality and the complexity of informed consent are explored. The common thread throughout the chapter is an emphasis on how nurses can advocate for patients and families and help them navigate genetic/genomic healthcare.

8.1 Introduction

The Human Genome Project was an international research effort aimed at determining the sequence of the entire human genome and the genes that it contains (NHGRI, 2018, October 28). Since its completion in 2003, genetic and genomic technologies have grown exponentially and are increasingly being incorporated into healthcare (Hood & Rowen, 2013). As defined by the National Institutes of Health in the U.S, genetics is "the study of genes and their roles in inheritance," specifically the study of how certain traits or conditions are passed from one generation to the next (NHGRI, 2018, September 7). Genomics is a newer term and is defined as "the study of all of a person's genes (the genome), and the interaction of those genes with each other and the person's environment" (NHGRI, 2018, September 7). Nurses have been cited as critical personnel for the implementation of genetic and genomic technologies into clinical care (Williams et al., 2017). However, nurses worldwide lack genetics and genomics competencies, and therefore are challenged to provide

M. K. Uveges (✉) · A. A. Dwyer
Boston College William F. Connell School of Nursing, 140 Commonwealth Avenue, Maloney Hall 375, Chestnut Hill, MA 02467, USA
e-mail: uveges@bc.edu

A. A. Dwyer
e-mail: andrew.dwyer@bc.edu

© The Author(s), under exclusive license to Springer Nature B.V. 2022
P. Grace and A. Milliken (Eds.), *Clinical Ethics Handbook for Nurses*, The International Library of Bioethics 93,
https://doi.org/10.1007/978-94-024-2155-2_8

patients with the appropriate education and support related to these technologies (Calzone et al., 2014; Skirton et al., 2012; Williams et al., 2017). Nursing genetics and genomics competencies include understanding the ethical issues that arise with implementing genetics & genomics into care (Monsen, 2000). As described in depth in Chapter 2, ethical awareness and sensitivity are necessary for ensuring that nurses recognize the nature and extent of their professional obligations in specific settings, including settings where genetic and genomic technologies are prevalent (Milliken, 2018). In this chapter, we provide an overview of the major applications of genetics and genomics, discuss ethical issues prompted by the use of these applications, and implications for nursing practice as well as the disciplinary branch of the profession which is charged with developing knowledge for effective practice in dynamic world.

8.2 Genetic Screening and Testing: U.S. and International Perspectives

To begin, it is important to distinguish between genetic screening and genetic testing, as the indications and implications of each of these can be unique. Genetic screening does not diagnose a genetic condition per se. Rather, screening detects whether an individual is genetically predisposed to (or at risk of) developing a genetic condition, or if an individual may be a carrier of a genetic condition (American College of Obstetricians and Gynecologists [ACOG], 2019, September). Alternatively, genetic tests can be used for diagnostic purposes—to identify changes in chromosomes, genes, or gene products, such as protein levels—to confirm or rule-out a genetic condition. Both genetic screening and genetic testing can have important implications for health and/or family planning (Genetics Home Reference, 2020a, March 3). Moreover, genetic and genomic competencies may be considered "lifespan competencies" for nurses, as genomic information is relevant for preconception and prenatal testing, newborn screening, identifying disease susceptibility, screening and diagnosis, as well as for determining prognosis, informing therapeutic decision-making and monitoring disease burden and recurrence (Calzone et al., 2013). Nurses may well be the first persons encountered by individuals or families who seek information to aid their decision making.

8.2.1 Prenatal Genetic Screening and Testing

8.2.1.1 Prenatal Genetic Screening Tests

In the prenatal context, genetic screening is used to identify the risk of having a baby with a genetic condition. Carrier screening is one type of prenatal genetic screening used to identify whether a pregnant woman or her partner carry variants in one copy of a gene associated with an autosomal recessive condition (e.g. cystic fibrosis) (NICHD, 2017, January 31). In autosomal recessive conditions, only individuals harboring two copies of a mutation (i.e. one from each parent) will manifest the disease. Thus, a pregnant woman or her partner who undergo carrier screening do not themselves have the genetic disease. Rather the screening is to determine if they carry one copy of a genetic variant. If both the pregnant woman and her partner carry a variant in the same gene, their offspring could inherit the disease. As such, carrier screening is particularly important for couples engaged in reproductive planning. Carrier screening can be conducted pre-conception or after pregnancy is confirmed. Ideally, pre-conception counseling and testing occurs early so that couples can make informed reproductive decisions and can account for possible risks to future offspring (ACOG, 2017; ACOG, 2019, September). The exploration of beliefs, values, and risk tolerance are all important factors in making informed decisions. Partners who are both carriers for a specific condition may opt for assisted fertility using egg/sperm donation or pre-implantation genetic testing, discussed below, to avoid having an affected child. However, for some with strong religious beliefs, the possibility that an embryo that tests positive for the genetic defect might be destroyed is an important consideration.

Across countries, certain prenatal genetic screening tests are recommended during the first or second trimester for pregnant women (NICHD, 2017, January 31). Screening results are evaluated alongside other diagnostic tests to determine potential risk for the fetus being born with a certain genetic condition. One of the most well-known prenatal screenings conducted during the second trimester (at approximately 16–18 weeks gestation) is called the "quadruple" or "quad" screening, as it tests the levels of four different substances in the pregnant woman's blood (alpha fetoprotein, human chorionic gonadotropin, estriol, inhibin A) to identify potential neural tube defects and chromosomal abnormalities (American Pregnancy Association, 2019).

A newer prenatal screening test is called non-invasive prenatal testing (NIPT). This test screens the cell-free fetal DNA (from the placenta) in the pregnant woman's plasma at 9–10 weeks gestation (Pos et al., 2019). NIPT is considered a screening test because placental or maternal mosaicism (i.e. DNA alteration in some, but not all cells) can contribute to inaccurate screening results (Mardy & Wapner, 2016). As such, confirmatory or diagnostic testing is recommended following abnormal NIPT findings. NIPT is increasingly becoming routine care for pregnant women globally (Minear et al., 2015) because the testing window is early, and risk of miscarriage is lower compared to more invasive prenatal tests (see amniocentesis and chorionic villus sampling below). Still, ethical concerns remain. The low-risk nature of this test could potentially undermine the free and voluntary decision making of women who may wish to decline testing. For example, not testing could be viewed as irresponsible and/or unacceptable by healthcare providers, since NIPT requires a simple blood draw from the pregnant woman. However, opting for NIPT requires women to accept potential risks: the risk of carrying an affected fetus, the risk of inaccurate or inconclusive test results, and/or the risk of increased stress or anxiety related to screening results (Vanstone et al., 2015). Some women may find these risks unacceptable, posing challenges to universal NIPT policies. Another consideration is that as NIPT becomes increasingly routine, robust pre-test counseling and an appropriate informed consent process may be undermined, thus eroding informed decision making. Nurses can play a central role in promoting women's autonomy by ensuring access to informed choice materials or resources that explain NIPT, assessing whether information provided is sufficient for women's decision making, and supporting individualized values, beliefs and preferences, such that NIPT testing is voluntary. An important question to explore with the woman and her family (as desired), is what will be done given a positive finding (i.e. a result that shows a genetic variant).

Importantly, prenatal screening is not diagnostic. If prenatal genetic screening results are abnormal, suggesting risk for a genetic condition/birth defect, further screening or testing is recommended (ACOG, 2019, September). When deciding whether to obtain further genetic screening or testing, the American College of Obstetrics and Gynecology recommends that a pregnant woman and her partner consider their personal beliefs and values and reflect on how receiving additional screening/testing information might impact their decision making regarding a pregnancy (ACOG, 2019, September). International organizations, including the Society for Maternal–Fetal Medicine, also highlight the importance of informed decision making and women's autonomy in making decisions about prenatal screening tests (SMFM, 2015).

8.2.1.2 Prenatal Diagnostic Tests

Amniocentesis and chorionic villus sampling (CVS) are two prenatal diagnostic tests that may be indicated following a positive prenatal screening result. Alternatively, amniocentesis and CVS may be performed instead of prenatal screening, (i.e. NIPT). Amniocentesis is typically performed between weeks 15–20 of pregnancy and involves ultrasound-guided, fine needle aspiration of amniotic fluid for testing. Amniocentesis is highly accurate for detecting chromosomal abnormalities (e.g. Down syndrome/trisomy 21), neural tube defects (e.g. spina bifida) and genetic disorders (e.g. cystic fibrosis). However, amniocentesis cannot detect the severity of these conditions (American Pregnancy Association, n.d.-a) so a pregnant woman and her partner may feel uncertain about how to factor results into their pregnancy decision making. Additionally, risks associated with amniocentesis include bleeding, amniotic fluid leakage and possible miscarriage, (ACOG, 2019, January). CVS involves obtaining a placental tissue sample between weeks 10–13 of gestation. This test can detect chromosomal abnormalities as well as genetic disorders but does not identify neural tube defects (American Pregnancy Association, n.d.-b). The risk of miscarriage with CVS is slightly higher compared to amniocentesis (ACOG, 2019, January).

Prenatal diagnostic tests have broadened reproductive choice. At the same time, their use has raised concerns within the disability rights community. A chief concern centers around selective abortion of fetuses found to have what might be considered disabling genetic traits. Notably, the disability rights community does not hold monolithic, consensus views on what constitutes a "disabling trait." Rather, individuals within this community may hold disparate views on traits such as cleft lip and palate, hereditary deafness, cystic fibrosis, or sickle cell anemia. Regardless of how disabling traits are defined, the disability rights community is committed to ending discrimination and improving life for people living with disabilities. As such, the disability rights community supports the expressivist argument. This view posits that selective abortions express negative or discriminatory attitudes about the disabling trait as well as the individuals exhibiting the traits (Parens & Asch, 2003). A second major argument from disability rights advocates is that aborting fetuses with disabling traits demonstrates intolerance of diversity within the respective family and the broader society (Parens & Asch, 2003). If the pregnant woman and her partner decide to terminate the pregnancy, based on screening results, fewer individuals living with impactful genetic conditions will be born. A society without individuals with disabilities may not be attuned to the needs of diverse individuals. As a result, society could become less accommodating of differences (Ravitsky, 2017). Opponents of this view argue that prenatal diagnostic tests offer an opportunity for a pregnant woman and her partner to make informed choices. Specifically, testing enables the pregnant woman and her partner to prepare for the birth of a child with special needs. Interestingly, even when persons are aware and prepared for the delivery of an affected newborn, they still may face challenges accessing specialized services after their child is born (Ravitsky, 2017).

8.2.2 Newborn Screening

Newborn screening (NBS) is an example of population-level screening. In the U.S., NBS is performed on all babies shortly after birth to assess for infant hearing loss, heart disease, and a set of conditions that can impact normal development (March of Dimes, 2020). Similar screening programs are carried out in other countries. Globally, newborn screening is available in all 48 European jurisdictions, all Canadian provinces and some countries in the Middle East, North Africa, Latin America, and Asia Pacific (Therrell et al., 2015). The purpose of newborn screening is to detect potentially disabling or fatal conditions before signs or symptoms appear. After a newborn screening diagnosis, early intervention such as dietary changes to mitigate inborn errors of metabolism, can prevent nervous system damage; intellectual, developmental or physical disability; or even death (NICHD, 2017, September 1).

Newborn screening involves a blood test to detect genetic, metabolic, or endocrine conditions that develop in infancy or early childhood. The blood test is not a genetic test per se because it does not directly examine DNA. The test examines gene products (e.g. proteins) in an infant's blood. Such biomarkers are a proxy for DNA changes and suggest the presence of a genetic condition. In the U.S., state public health departments screen approximately 4 million babies annually in the U.S. Approximately 12,500 infants each year (roughly 1 in 300) are identified as having a NBS condition (NICHD, 2017, January 1).

Advances in genomics, like next-generation sequencing (NGS) technologies, are likely to change newborn screening practices. For example, in the U.S., the Eunice Kennedy Shriver National Institute of Child Health and Human Development (NICHD) and the National Human Genome Research Institute (NHGRI) have funded research to explore how genomic sequencing technologies could be integrated into NBS and how genomics could facilitate diagnosing metabolic disorders (Berg et al., 2017). Such NGS technologies include whole exome sequencing (WES)—a technique involving sequencing all the protein coding regions of the genome (i.e. exons). Whole genome sequencing (WGS) involves sequencing the entire DNA sequence of an individual—not just the protein coding exons (Genetics Home Reference, 2020b, March 3). Advantages of NGS include more sensitive and specific results, thereby decreasing false positives; expanding the list of rare conditions tested for; and informing/confirming a diagnosis, which can guide treatment for a child and identify disease risk in family members (Khan et al., 2016; Powell, 2018). At the same time, drawbacks include uncertainty interpreting some genetic findings (termed variants of uncertain significance, VUS), cost to public health programs and long turnaround times for results and interpretation (Powell, 2018).

One of the main ethical issues in newborn screening relates to parental consent for the long-term sample storage and use of dried blood spots leftover from newborn screening in secondary research. Secondary research on dried blood spots has been conducted in the U.S. and other countries (i.e. United Kingdom, Denmark, Italy, Australia, Germany, Sweden) (Rothwell et al., 2019). Prior to 2014, some states in the U.S. allowed dried newborn blood spots to be stored and used for research without parental consent. This practice may be permissible if samples are deidentified or the responsible Institutional Review Board (IRB) grants a waiver of consent. However, use outside of these parameters is a breach of the infant's privacy (Rothwell et al., 2019). In 2014, the Newborn Screening Saves Lives Reauthorization Act was passed requiring parental consent for secondary use of newborn blood spots collected after March 18, 2015 (Newborn screening saves lives reauthorization act, 2019). However, recent updates to the Common Rule (rules governing ethical conduct of research with human subjects in the U.S.) supersede the Reauthorization Act. Thus, parental consent for the use of de-identified specimens, including dried blood spots from newborn screening, is no longer required (Rothwell et al., 2019). This means, for example among other possibilities, that an infant's genetic data could be used in ways that are not aligned with parental values and preferences. In the aftermath of the legal controversy surrounding dried blood spots and the 2014 Reauthorization Act, several states have implemented an informed consent process for retaining and using dried blood spots for research (Rothwell et al., 2019).

8.2.3 Genetic Testing for Children and Adults

Diagnostic genetic tests, used to confirm or rule out a genetic condition, may be ordered by multiple types of healthcare providers, including advanced practice nurses, and are often collected by point of care nurses. Thus, it is important that these clinicians can respond to questions and access resources that facilitate informed decisions that are congruent with a patient or family's understanding, values and preferences. Clinicians consider a variety of factors when choosing the appropriate genetic test, including family history, patient age, physical exam findings, and specimen availability (Katsanis & Katsanis, 2013). In general, three types of genetic testing may be selected: chromosomal, molecular or biochemical testing. Table 8.1 summarizes types of genetic tests and offers an example(s) of each.

In cases where providers feel genetic testing is indicated, there is an ethical responsibility based on the goals of healthcare to prioritize the consent process, so patients have enough information to make an informed decision about the benefits, drawbacks and limitations to testing. Pre-test genetic counseling provides patients with information to help individuals and families understand the respective genetic test and the potential implications of test results. Informed by the history of the eugenics movement, as discussed in more detail later, genetic counseling is intentionally non-directive meaning a genetic counselor does not give advice about what the person should do. Rather, the counseling process includes value reflection to encourage individuals to make informed decisions that are aligned with their values and preferences. Providing appropriate informed consent for genetic testing can be challenging, especially given the limited availability of providers with genetic/genomic competencies or specialized genetic training. Nurses who do not specialize in genetics/genomics

Table 8.1 Types of genetic tests

Type of genetic test	Definition	Example(s)
Chromosomal	Analyzes whole chromosomes or longer strands of DNA to identify genetic changes (GHR, 2020a, March 3)	1. Karyotype- Identifies abnormal numbers (i.e. aneuploidies such as trisomy 21) or structures of chromosomes (NHGRI, n.d.) 2. Chromosomal microarray (CMA)- Identifies missing (deletion) or extra (duplication) chromosomal material (Baylor Genetics, 2021)
Biochemical	Does not involve direct examination of DNA, but rather, quantifies gene products, such as the amount or level of proteins in the patient's blood. Abnormalities detected through biochemical tests can indicate DNA changes and an underlying genetic condition (GHR, 2020a, March 3)	Newborn screening- screens for gene proteins, which can help detect genetic, metabolic, or endocrine conditions that would develop in infancy or early childhood without intervention
Molecular	Examines the DNA of a single gene(s) for changes, called variants or mutations (GHR, 2020a, March 3)	1. Single gene test- used to identify a variant in a specific gene 2. Multi-gene panel test- used to identify variants in multiple genes in parallel (Constantin et al., 2005)

still play an important role in supporting and advocating for patients and families weighing genetic testing decisions. Indeed, a key competency for professional nursing practice is to consider genetic and genomic information when taking health histories, conducting health and physical assessments, as well as when analyzing findings (Greco et al., 2012). After patients and families are identified as potentially benefiting from genetic/genomic services, nurses can be critical in supporting high quality decisions. First, registered and advanced practice nurses should provide current and credible information and technologies (e.g., patient decision aids) that facilitate informed decision making appropriate to the patient. Second, nurses can invite clients to reflect on their preferences and values by encouraging them to consider how they might use the test results to promote, maintain and restore health (see Table 8.2) (Greco et al., 2012) as exemplified in the following case.

Case: Returning Genetic Test Results
An advance practice nurse (APN) is seeing Allison in the clinic for a second appointment following genetic testing for hereditary breast and ovarian (*BRCA 1/2*). During Allison's first clinic visit, the APRN completed a thorough 3-generation family history, which revealed a significant risk of breast cancer for Allison. The APRN discussed the pros and cons of undergoing *BRCA 1/2* testing, what a positive result might mean, in terms of follow up for Allison and other relatives, as well as exploring Allison's values and preferences around testing. Allison decided to undergo testing. The APRN reviewed Allison's genetic test results, which revealed a variant in *BRCA 1* and plans to discuss test findings with Allison during today's visit. Several topics will be covered, including specific risk-reducing interventions for Allison based on the *BRCA 1* variant findings; how Allison might communicate her results to yet untested at-risk blood relatives; and what coping resources (i.e., patient support groups) are available for Allison and her family.

Genetic nursing competencies remain pertinent but may be more complex to implement when moving beyond single gene or panel testing. If single gene or gene panel testing (i.e. molecular testing) does not confirm a diagnosis, or if the diagnosis remains unclear, providers may consider whole exome sequencing (WES) or whole

Table 8.2 Supporting patients' decision making for genetic testing: questions to explore	Questions
	1. What do you understand to be the goals of this genetic test?
	2. What more would you like in the way of information?
	3. How would you describe a "positive" or "negative" genetic test result in this case? a. What steps might you take if you receive a positive vs. negative result?
	4. How do you see the results of the test impacting your life?
	5. Who besides you might be impacted by these results?
	6. What sorts of supports do you have/would you like to help you think this through?

genome sequencing (WGS). An important consideration for WES and WGS is how to handle the abundance of data produced from testing. In a diagnostic context, WES or WGS may be used to identify primary genomic findings. However, results may also include incidental, or secondary findings because testing examines all genes in the exome or genome. The American College of Medical Genetics and Genomics (ACMG) recommends that all clinical genomic sequencing tests include a report of incidental findings for 59 disease genes underlying 27 conditions that are considered 'medically actionable.' Actionable means there are effective preventive measures and treatments available. However, patients are not obliged to receive an incidental finding report and have the option of not receiving these results, and discussion of such decisions should be part of the informed consent process prior to WGS (Green et al., 2013; Kalia et al., 2017). Importantly, patients may not always be aware of this option, highlighting another area where involved nurses can support decision making. Reporting incidental findings for children who undergo whole exome (WES) or whole genome sequencing (WGS) has been hotly debated because three of the 27 conditions on the ACMG list are adult-onset only, meaning there is no action to be taken in childhood (Holm et al., 2019; Kalia et al., 2017; Ross & Clayton, 2019). Some argue that return of findings for adult-onset conditions could be in the child's best interest if results would benefit parents by informing them of a disease risk, enabling them to opt to receive testing, treatment, and remain capable of caring for their child (Holm et al., 2019). Others argue that best interests should remain focused on the child and that if parents' risk is to be known, parents themselves should be tested to determine their risk (Ross & Clayton, 2019). Another concern is that returning a child's results for an adult-onset condition violates the child's "right to an open future." The right to an open future preserves the child's right to make their own decision about receiving these results once they are an adult (Holm et al., 2019; Ross & Clayton, 2019). The following example depicts a case where adult-onset genetic testing was requested for a newborn.

Case: Genetic Testing for Adult-Onset Conditions in a Newborn
A young couple is expecting a baby and would like the baby to undergo genetic testing after birth for an adult-onset condition that is present in the family of the pregnant woman. The Genetics team is uncertain whether the request for testing should be honored. Testing an infant for an adult-onset disease is not common clinical practice, although testing occurs in research studies. Research protocols are subject to rigorous ethical scrutiny by institutional review boards/ethics committees to weigh the risks and benefits of testing and implications of possible results. Even if the infant's test results indicate increased risk for the respective genetic condition, findings are not diagnostic, and risk is not the same as a definitive diagnosis. Further, because the genetic condition in this scenario involves an adult onset of disease, there are no medical actions during childhood/adolescence that would prevent or ameliorate the condition. Thus, it is crucial to carefully explore the reasoning behind the testing request and discuss the implications for both the parents and their child. Non-maleficence, the obligation to do no harm, is an important principle for the team

to consider. In situations when some harm is unavoidable, the goal is to minimize potential harms.

8.2.4 Direct to Consumer Testing

Increasingly in the United States, and to a lesser extent internationally, individuals are seeking genetic information through direct-to-consumer (DTC) genetic testing (Hogarth et al., 2008). Historically, genetic testing was performed in the context of a face-to-face, detailed individual and family risk assessment by a healthcare provider. In such encounters, healthcare providers utilize professional practice guidelines to determine which genetic test(s) might be most appropriate for an individual. Prior to testing, the provider would offer education, genetic counseling, and obtain informed consent. Once results were obtained, the provider would meet with the patient, in person or by phone, to discuss the results, debrief and provide individualized recommendations. In contrast, DTC genetic testing is advertised directly to individuals though various media platforms (print, television, internet) and test kits are available for purchase directly from a company or pharmacy. Individuals who utilize DTC testing complete sample collection at home, mail the sample and receive results by phone, mail, or email. A healthcare provider may or may not be involved in ordering the test or interpreting the results (Loud, 2010).

Notably, the availability of DTC testing holds potential benefits, such as allowing for earlier detection of disease or disease management through increased access to testing without provider involvement. At the same time, DTC testing raises ethical concerns (Loud, 2010). Currently, there is little regulation of DTC testing and tests may not be valid, meaning they may not measure what they intend to measure. Further, an individual may access a DTC test without adequate context or counseling (Hudson et al., 2007). Thus, there is a danger that individuals may be harmed, physically or emotionally, by making important health decisions based on inaccurate, incomplete, or misunderstood information—particularly if a healthcare provider is not involved to help interpret or contextualize the results (Loud, 2010). For example, clinically unwarranted DTC tests might prompt unnecessary, invasive follow up testing/procedures. Negative DTC findings may create a false sense of assurance or alternatively, results may create unnecessary anxiety (Lippi, et al., 2011). Another consideration is that individuals may be harmed after learning unexpected information about family, such as non-relatedness (Genetics Home Reference, 2020a, July 7).

DTC testing removes the healthcare provider as gatekeeper to genetic testing and theoretically, allows greater access to testing. However, the limited role of healthcare providers in the process increases the likelihood that consumers will neither receive pre-test nor post-test counseling. Accordingly, DTC testing has important implications for the informed consent process. A central requisite of informed consent is the disclosure of information necessary for making a voluntary decision. For DTC companies who offer counseling, guidance may be limited to counselors reading

8 Genetics: Nurses Roles and Responsibilities

directly from test reports and not providing consumers with individualized implications (Udesky, 2010). Nurses are often asked for advice about whether someone should have DTC testing and relevant anticipated concerns. It is therefore important to ask the individual about their goals for seeking testing and assess how they will handle and cope with the test results. Nurses should appreciate the pros and cons of DTC testing, as well as concerns regarding unintended consequences.

One important consideration is that DTC genetic testing services follow a for-profit business model. Some DTC genetic testing businesses profit by selling access to consumer genomic data to third parties (i.e. researchers, insurers, law enforcement). Consequently, nurses should be aware of such practices and the threats to patient privacy and data protection (Hendricks-Sturrup & Lu, 2019). An additional threat to patient privacy is the lack of a chain of custody for DTC testing. Samples are submitted via mail and companies cannot verify the source of samples. Therefore, individuals may send a sample with their name, or another individual's sample without this other individual's full consent (Lippi et al., 2011). The following example involves a case of a patient requesting input from her primary care provider after receiving DTC results. While this case involves an advanced practice nurse in the U.S., nurses in other countries might well be asked to help their patients think through the meaning of, and their options related to, unexpected test results from DTC testing companies.

Case: An Advanced Practice Registered Nurses Interpretation of Findings from Direct-to-Consumer Testing
The APRN is a Family Nurse Practitioner in a busy primary care clinic. Today she is seeing a 37-year-old patient, Karen, for her annual physical examination. At the beginning of the clinical encounter, Karen mentions that she received the DTC testing kit from her boyfriend for her birthday, after discussing with him that it could be "fun" to see what it shows. Karen mentions she has brought her DTC test results to her appointment, as she would like help interpreting the findings. This scenario presents a challenging dilemma for the APRN, as far as determining her professional obligation. Indeed, ethical challenges around the nurse's obligations to help interpret genetic findings are increasingly common with the growth of DTC testing by the lay public. Since many in the lay public may lack genetic literacy and numeracy skills to accurately interpret DTC results, the APRN may feel a duty to help Karen interpret and understand her findings. However, the interpretation of findings is challenging as many findings are "variants of unknown significance" and it may not be clear how to advise Karen, in terms of the potential impact of variants on health. Moreover, the APRN may not have deep understanding of the specific disease(s) implicated in Karen's DTC test results. This is particularly salient as techniques vary across DTC companies and the sensitivity and specificity (i.e. markers employed and number of reads) may not accurately depict the individual's true risk. In addition, while a detailed 3-generation family history may be helpful in interpreting test results, some genetic variants may be de novo (i.e. spontaneous and not carried by other family members). If the APRN feels unqualified to counsel Karen, an alternative approach would be to provide her with information and a referral to meet

with a genetic counselor who has more in-depth knowledge and abilities in interpreting findings. With any scenario, the APRN's professional obligation is to be cognizant of a key genetic nursing competency—i.e., to provide credible, accurate, appropriate and current information, resources and services/technologies that facilitate patient decision-making—either by the APRN, or through referral to another qualified clinician.

8.3 Impact of Genetic Information

8.3.1 Informed Consent

Clinical genetics, or genetic research can have important social, economic, and/or psychological implications for patients/participants (Jamal, 2016). For this reason, informed consent is an important process that implicates nurses. Informed consent is not merely a signed document. It is the process of discussing risks, benefits, and potential alternatives of the relevant genetic/genomic application. Informed consent for genetic/genomic studies must clearly identify the purpose, limitations, possible outcomes following testing, as well as how results will be used and shared. Genetic counseling involves not only providing information but asking focused questions to elicit patient values and preferences. When testing is not urgent, individuals should be given ample time to reflect on their values and beliefs in relation to testing implications. In some cases, genetic or genomic testing may yield imprecise, uncertain or unactionable results. Helping a patient or research participant understand the possible outcomes is an essential part of managing patient/participant responses and future actions (Jamal, 2016). It also means that the nurse must understand something about the patient, their context, and life goals. This appreciation facilitates providing tailored information that is relevant to the individual and their family.

8.3.2 Privacy and Confidentiality

In addition to informed consent, patients and research participants ought to be informed about the steps that will be taken to protect their privacy, once genetic results are available. In the clinical context, genetic tests are selected based on the individual patient's history and presentation. In such settings return of results is routine and expected. In the research context, return of individualized results may or may not be part of the research protocol. For example, an individual may provide a DNA sample for genetic research on asthma—yet it is possible that using WES or WGS, researchers could find an actionable finding unrelated to asthma. In such cases, the lines between clinical genetics and research can become blurry. To manage such ethical, legal and social implications, research is required to undergo ethics review by an institutional review board (IRB). However, IRB policies regarding genetic research may vary regionally. Additionally, laws governing the return of results specific to genome sequencing currently vary by country (Thorogood et al., 2019). Regardless of setting, nurses can play a pivotal role in helping patients understand which results, if any, will be returned and inviting patients to reflect on the potential impact of results on health and wellbeing.

For example, disclosing genetic results could lead to certain types of discrimination. A key aspect of genetic privacy has to do with the heritability of genetic variants. If a patient receives genetic results that can be traced to other relatives, providers or researchers are then faced with the challenge of how to balance the individual patient's genetic privacy in light of the potential benefit of warning other family members about genetic risk. Like other providers, nurses are obligated to maintain confidentiality, yet there might be situations when a provider is warranted in overriding this duty. In the U.S., The President's Commission for the Study of Ethical Problems in Medicine and Biomedical and Behavioral Research (1983) identified several conditions that, if satisfied, could warrant disclosure of results to relatives. These include qualifications such as: reasonable efforts have failed to elicit the patient's voluntary consent to disclose results to family members; there is a high probability that harm will occur if information is withheld and the disclosed information could avert harm; the harm suffered would be serious; and appropriate precautions are taken to ensure that only the genetic information needed for diagnosis and/or treatment of the disease in question is disclosed (Jamal, 2016). From an ethical standpoint, identifying a concrete situation that clearly warrants disclosure to a family member remains up for debate. Recent legal cases involving autosomal dominant conditions (i.e. offspring have a 50% chance of inheriting the variant and getting the condition) have received attention and highlight when providers might consider non-consensually notifying family members of a genetic risk. In *ABC v. St. George's Healthcare NHS trust and others*, a plaintiff identified as "ABC" sued the UK National Health Service (NHS) because her father's physicians failed to reveal his diagnosis of Huntington's disease (an incurable, neurodegenerative disease). The plaintiff, pregnant at the time of her father's diagnosis, claimed she would have terminated the pregnancy if she knew of the Huntington's diagnosis, given that she had a 50% chance of inheriting the disease and then passing it onto her child. Ultimately, the court sided with the NHS, yet the case highlights situations that may legally challenge providers' duty to maintain patient confidentiality (Sokol, 2020). Organizational-based clinical or research ethics committees (IRBs) can be helpful resources for nurses and nurse researchers who feel it may be their duty to override patient privacy and inform relatives. Alternatively, nurses could seek out the advice of an external ethics expert or committee if these resources are not available within the organization/clinical environment.

8.3.3 Eugenics

Ethical concerns have been raised around specific applications of genetics; in particular, eugenics, or the manipulation of genes in an effort to improve the human species. Eugenics has traditionally been subdivided into positive eugenics and negative eugenics. Positive eugenics seeks to increase what a given society or political group considers desirable human traits through selective mating and use of reproductive technologies. In contrast, negative eugenics seeks to decrease what the group or society considers undesirable traits by preventing those who possess such traits from reproducing, or by utilizing assisted reproductive technologies (Jamal, 2016).

Formal human eugenics programs began in the late nineteenth century in parallel to increasing understanding of inheritance patterns discovered through Mendelian genetics (Jamal, 2016). Although the eugenics movement expanded across the globe, eugenic research programs were especially prevalent in the United States, Britain, and Germany. Infamous eugenics practices were used to justify the subjugation of certain races/populations including Jews, Blacks, and the Irish. Sterilization campaigns were organized to prevent propagation of alcoholics, orphans, epileptics, those with intellectual disabilities, as well as diseased or 'degenerate' persons. Such programs were extended to include African Americans and the poor. By the 1930's, the human rights violations evident in Nazi Germany propelled a de-escalation of eugenics in the United States. However, the history of eugenics continues to permeate genetics in the research context (Jamal, 2016). Understanding the history of eugenics is important for nurses interacting with patients whose care involves genetic testing, since some patients may raise concerns based on historical genetic abuses. Indeed, members of historically marginalized groups may be suspicious or distrustful of genetic healthcare. In addition, some consider modern-day assisted reproductive technologies (ART) to be facilitators of a "new eugenics" movement. Specifically, concerns include the possibility that a pregnant woman and her partner may use ART to select desirable traits in their offspring or decide whether to keep or terminate certain embryos (Sparrow, 2011).

8.3.4 Discrimination

Genetic discrimination is the act of treating individuals differently based on a gene variant or increased risk of an inherited condition (Genetics Home Reference, 2020b, July 7). Individuals considering genetic testing often cite concerns related to genetic discrimination by insurers or employers (Genetics Home Reference, 2020b, July 7). Nurses are likely to encounter patients who express such concerns, particularly in settings where genetic testing is embedded in clinical practice. In 2008, the U.S. federal government passed legislation to address such concerns regarding discrimination. The Genetic Information Nondiscrimination Act (GINA) protects individuals from genetic discrimination by health insurers and employers. However, GINA does not apply to other types of insurance, such as life, long-term care, or disability insurance (NHGRI, 2020; Zacharias et al., 2018). Further, GINA does not apply to certain groups of individuals, including those participating in the U.S. military Tricare coverage, veterans receiving care from the Veterans Health Administration, individuals receiving care from the Indian Health Service, or federal employees enrolled in the Federal Employee Health Benefits Plan (Jamal, 2016). Individuals may have concerns about future insurance eligibility based on genetic findings. It is important that nurses and other healthcare providers understand patient concerns regarding financial, social, or psychological discrimination in their country or territory of practice. In the U.S., sharing an individual's genetic health information is restricted under the Health Insurance Portability and Accountability Act (HIPAA) (NHGRI, 2020). However, HIPAA only applies to 'covered entities,' such as health plans, healthcare clearinghouses, and most healthcare providers. The law does not apply to other private businesses or public agencies in the same way (U.S. Department of Health and Human Services, 2013).

8.3.5 Access: Genetic Workforce Issues

Genetic screening and testing carry benefits as well as potential risks that are specific to the individual. Therefore, deciding whether or not to undergo genetic screening or testing can be complex. In addition to developing genetic competencies as part of their educational curriculum, nurses can benefit from an interprofessional approach. Nurses can consult and collaborate with genetic specialists with specialized training in genetics and genomics including genetic counselors and medical geneticists.

Genetic counseling is a field that began in the United States in 1969 to help address personalized decision-making needs of patients and families regarding their genetic health (National Society of Genetic Counselors, 2020; Ormond et al., 2018). Certified genetic counselors (CGCs) receive advanced training in medical genetics as well as counseling. Their role is to provide personalized education for individuals to help them understand genetic risk based on personal and family medical history. CGCs provide information on relevant genetic tests that may be ordered by providers (including advanced practice registered nurses) (National Society of Genetic Counselors, 2020). Genetic counselors also help patients interpret genetic test results and to make informed health decisions for themselves and their family. Genetic counseling has a discipline-specific code of ethics enumerating the profession's goals and values that guide practice (National Society of Genetic Counselors, 2017). Based on historical abuses in the genetic realm, a key tenet of genetic counseling practice is a non-directive approach when communicating with patients and families.

The number of genetic counselors in the U.S. has risen dramatically as genomic healthcare has grown. Growth of 27% annually is projected to continue over the next decade, yet the demand for CGCs continues to outpace the supply (Bureau of Labor Statistics, 2020; Hoskovec et al., 2018). The shortfall of CGCs is due to several factors, including the falling cost of genetic tests, increased access to testing, and the expansion of genetics and genomics from specialty clinics to primary care (Hoskovec et al., 2018). Internationally, the genetic counseling profession is in various stages of development (Ormond et al., 2018). In 2018, there was an estimated 7,000 trained genetic counselors in 28 countries, meaning not all countries have genetic counselors (Abacan et al., 2019). In many countries, the estimated number of per-capita genetic counselors ranges widely, and most countries lack either national or regional regulation (Abacan et al., 2019). A recent landscape review shows that in many countries, nurses work as genetic counselors (i.e. United Kingdom and several Scandinavian countries) (Calzone et al., 2018).

Medical geneticists are another group of genetic specialist provider who are in short supply. Shortages of CGCs and medical geneticists mean the healthcare workforce is not adequate to meet the growing demand for genetic services (Campion, 2019; Maiese et al., 2019). Lack of access to trained genetic healthcare providers, both in the U.S. and globally, contributes to disparities in accessing and using genetic technologies (IOM, 2009; NASEM, 2018b). Other contributing factors to disparities include: fragmented health care systems with poor linkages to specialty care; limited patient genetic literacy/numeracy skills; varied cultural perceptions of genetic testing; inadequate insurance coverage, prior insurance approval requirements and expensive copayments; geographic variation; and implicit bias around use of genetic technology for certain populations (IOM, 2009; Tuckson et al., 2013). In some contexts, nurses may help fill gaps where there are limited numbers of genetic specialists. The International Society for Nurses in Genetics (ISONG) is one professional organization committed to nurses specializing in genetics and to developing genetic nursing competencies. Indeed, as nurses are the most numerous group of trained healthcare professionals, there is a push to enhance genetic and genomic nursing competencies to meet the need for trained genetic/genomic health professionals (Greco et al., 2012). Working with ISONG and other nursing stakeholders, the Global Genomic Nursing Alliance (G2NA) has recently launched a roadmap for accelerating genomics into nursing globally (Tonkin et al., 2020).

8.4 Genetic Research and Biobanks

As technology has advanced, there has been a tremendous growth in genetic and genomic research. Much of this research requires the storage of biospecimens (i.e. human blood, tissue, cells, DNA, RNA, or protein). Biospecimens contain genetic information, which, when analyzed, can identify genetic variants associated with disease (Mashke, 2008). Biobanks are repositories that accept, process, store, and distribute biospecimens and data for use in research. Recently, virtual biobanks have been established. Virtual biobanks are electronic databases that store biological specimen information and make data available without the need to access the physical sample(s) (DeSouza & Greenspan, 2013).

Nurse scientists, research nurse coordinators, and clinical research and practice nurses need to be aware of the potential ethical issues associated with biobanking to facilitate biobanking practices (Sanner et al., 2015). For example, nurses involved in collecting biospecimens for genetic research ought to be aware of issues involving informed consent. Informed consent for biospecimen donation to a biobank necessitates the research team ensure participants are able to balance the risks and benefits of the way their specimen might be used in research and make a decision based on these risks and benefits (Grady et al., 2013). The informed consent process should include how the participant's identity will be protected, and the safeguards used to protect participant data (Sanner et al., 2015). Individuals who donate samples to biobanks do so at a specific point in time, perhaps during a routine clinical or surgical procedure or sometimes in relation to a specific research study. Informed consent can become an issue if researchers wish to use these biospecimens for reasons other than the original study purpose. Ensuring biobank participants are properly informed about the ways their biospecimen(s) might be utilized has been a topic of much discussion. Indeed, ISONG has developed a position statement for nurses regarding biobanks that highlights best practices and ethical concerns specific to nursing practice (ISONG, 2013).

One suggestion for dealing with the issue of informed consent for biospecimens in biobanks is to obtain broad consent from participants. Broad consent means that biospecimens will be used for an unspecified range of future research, with a few restrictions (Grady et al., 2013). While broad consent is not as specific as study-specific consent, it offers more restrictions than "blanket consent," which allows unlimited use (Grady et al., 2013). Some bioethicists have suggested a tiered or tailored consent process as an alternative approach. Under a tiered consent model, individuals are given choices about which types of research their biospecimen may be used for. Tiered consent may involve the use of a checklist, where the participant indicates which types of research for which they would approve the use of their biospecimen. Each type of consent has a different level of control for the participant. Additionally, there is a potential participant burden as well as cost and administrative burden for the researcher (Grady et al., 2013).

Another biobank consideration relates to the question of returning individual results to participants. The majority of U.S. and international research guidelines support the ethical mandate of returning research results, especially if they are medically actionable. Currently, there are no policies governing when or if biobank research results may benefit the participant (Cardigan et al., 2017). A 2018 consensus study report, titled *Returning Individual Research Results to Participants: Guidance for a New Research Paradigm*, advocates for more collaborative and transparent research practices involving human biospecimen use. The report makes recommendations regarding the return of results on a study-by-study basis. One proposed approach for improving the return of results process is to engage community groups and advocacy organizations to ensure that participant values are elicited and incorporated into practices (NASEM, 2018a). Many nurse researchers are familiar with community-participatory-based research methods. As such, we envision that nurses could play a key role in influencing future biobank return of results guidelines.

8.5 Summary

In this chapter we explored the major applications of genetics and genomics in healthcare. Our purpose was to raise awareness about the ethical issues that nurses may face in the course of their practice and to provide resources and strategies for them to use. A clearer understanding of the relevant implications of genetic tests will assist nurses in meeting their goals of supporting patients' decision making and wellbeing. We began the chapter by describing the landscape of prenatal genetic screening and diagnostic genetic testing. Context was provided about the reasons for newborn screening efforts globally. Our review of the main types of genetic tests for children and adults—chromosomal, molecular or biochemical –clarified the conditions under which the test might be selected and suggested. It is also important for nurses to understand the range of effects that increased access to genetic testing provided by direct-to-consumer companies can have on those accessing them. It is, of course, best if people can be advised of those implications ahead of accessing them and this may well be a role of a nurse who is asked for advice, but the nature of DTC renders this less likely. Thus, nurses may need to provide assistance and access to resources when a person receives unexpected results and does not know what to do next. We underscored the ethical importance of the informed consent process for genetic/genomic applications as well as privacy and confidentiality concerns resulting from genetic/genomic findings. Our discussion uses the history of eugenics and its implications for the potential abuses of genomic information as a lens to highlight the potential for discrimination of various sorts based on genetic test findings. We note growing concern around access to genetic/genomic services in light of the shortage of genomic specialists to meet burgeoning demand. The role of nurses with training in genomic competencies is discussed as a means to fill existing gaps in access and use of genomic healthcare. Last, we describe ethical, legal and social implications related to genetics/genomic research. The common thread throughout the chapter is an emphasis on how nurses can advocate for patients and families and help them navigate genetic/genomic healthcare.

References

Abacan, M., Alsubaie, L., Barlow-Stewart, K., Caanen, B., Cordier, C., Courtney, E., Davoine, E., Edwards, J., Elackatt, N. J., Gardiner, K., Guan, Y., Huang, L., Malmgren, C.L., Kejriwal, S., Kim, H. J., Lambert, D., Lantigua-Cruz, P. A., Lee, J. M. H., Lodahl, M., …Wicklund, C. (2019). The global state of the genetic counseling profession. *European Journal of Human Genetics, 27*(2), 183–197. https://doi.org/10.1038/s41431-018-0252-x

American College of Obstetricians and Gynecologists [ACOG]. (2019, September). *Prenatal genetic screening tests*. Retrieved March 17, 2020, from https://www.acog.org/Patients/FAQs/Prenatal-Genetic-Screening-Tests?IsMobileSet=false

American College of Obstetricians and Gynecologists [ACOG]. (2017). Carrier screening for genetic conditions: Committee Opinion No. 691. *Obstetrics and Gynecology, 129*, e41–55.

American College of Obstetrics and Gynecologists [ACOG]. (2019, January). *Prenatal genetic diagnostic tests*. Retrieved March 24, 2020, from https://www.acog.org/patient-resources/faqs/pregnancy/prenatal-genetic-diagnostic-tests

American Pregnancy Association. (2019, October 25). *Quad screen test*. Retrieved March 17, 2020, from https://americanpregnancy.org/prenatal-testing/quad-screen/

American Pregnancy Association. (n.d.-a). *Amniocentesis*. https://americanpregnancy.org/prenatal-testing/amniocentesis/

American Pregnancy Association. (n.d.-b). *Chorionic villus sampling*. https://americanpregnancy.org/prenatal-testing/chorionic-villus-sampling/

Baylor Genetics. (2021). *Postnatal CMA*. Retrieved February 9, 2021, from https://baylorgenetics.com/cma/

Berg, J. S., Agrawal, P. B., Bailey, D. B., Jr, Beggs, A. H., Brenner, S. E., Brower, A. M., Cakici, J. A., Ceyhan-Birsoy, O., Chan, K., Chen, F., Currier, R. J., Dukhovny, D., Green, R. C., Harris-Wai, J., Holm, I. A., Iglesias, B., Joseph, G., Kingsmore, S. F., Koenig, B. A., Kwok, P. Y., ... Wise, A. L. (2017). Newborn sequencing in genomic medicine and public health. *Pediatrics, 139*(2), e20162252. https://doi.org/10.1542/peds.2016-2252

Bureau of Labor Statistics, U.S. Department of Labor, *Occupational Outlook Handbook*. (2020, April 10). Genetic counselors. Retrieved January 23, 2021, from https://www.bls.gov/ooh/health care/genetic-counselors.htm

Calzone, K., Jenkins, J., Culp, S., Caskey, S., & Badzek, L. (2014). Introducing a new competency into nursing practice. *Journal of Nursing Regulation, 5*(1), 40–47 [PubMed: 25343056].

Calzone, K. A., Jenkins, J., Nicol, N., Skirton, H., Feero, W. G., Green, E. D. (2013). Relevance of genomics to healthcare and nursing practice. *Journal of Nursing Scholarship, 45*(1), 1–2 [PubMed 23368676].

Calzone, K. A., Kirk, M., Tonkin, E., Badzek, L., Benjamin, C., & Middleton, A. (2018). The global landscape of nursing and genomics. *Journal of Nursing Scholarship, 50*(3), 249–256.

Campion, M., Goldgar, C., Hopkin, R. J., Prows, C. A., & Dasgupta, S. (2019). Genomic education for the next generation of healthcare providers. *Genetics in Medicine, 21*(11), 2422–2430.

Cardigan, R. J., Edwards, T. P., Lassiter, D., Davis, A. M., & Henderson, G. E. (2017). "Forward-thinking" in U.S. biobanking. *Genetic Testing and Molecular Biomarkers, 21*(3), 148–154.

Constantin, C. M., Faucett, A., & Lubin, I. M. (2005). A primer on genetic testing. *Journal of Midwifery & Women's Health, 50*(3), 197–204.

DeSouza, Y. G., & Greenspan, J. S. (2013). Biobanking past, present, and future: Responsibilities and benefits. *AIDS, 27*(3), 303–312.

Genetics Home Reference [GHR]. (2020a, March 3). Genetic testing. Retrieved March 7, 2020 from https://ghr.nlm.nih.gov/primer/testing/genetictesting

Genetics Home Reference [GHR]. (2020a, July 7). *What are the benefits and risks of direct-to-consumer genetic testing?* Retrieved July 13, 2020, from https://ghr.nlm.nih.gov/primer/dtcgen etictesting/dtcrisksbenefits

Genetics Home Reference [GHR]. (2020b, March 3). *What are whole exome sequencing and whole genome sequencing?* Retrieved March 10, 2020, from https://ghr.nlm.nih.gov/primer/testing/seq uencing

Genetics Home Reference [GHR]. (2020b, July 7). *What is genetic discrimination?* Retrieved July 13, 2020, from https://ghr.nlm.nih.gov/primer/testing/discrimination

Grady, C., Eckstein, L., Berkman, B., et al. (2013). Broad consent for research with biological samples: Workshop conclusions. *American Journal of Bioethics, 15*(9), 34–42.

Greco, K.E., Tinley, S., & Seibert, D. (2012). *Essential genetic and genomic competencies for nurses with graduate degrees*. American Nurses Association and International Society of Nurses in Genetics.

Green, R. C., Berg, J. S., Grody, W. W., et al. (2013). ACMG recommendations for reporting of incidental findings in clinical exome and genome sequencing. *Genetics in Medicine, 15*(7), 565–574.

Hendricks-Sturrup, R. M., & Lu, C. Y. (2019). Direct-to-consumer genetic testing data privacy: Key concerns and recommendations based on consumer perspectives. *Journal of Personalized Medicine, 9*(2), 25.

Hogarth, S., Javitt, G., & Melzer, D. (2008). The current landscape for direct-to-consumer genetic testing: Legal, ethical, and policy issues. *Annual Review of Genomics and Human Genetics, 9,* 161–182. https://doi.org/10.1146/annurev.genom.9.081307.164319

Holm, I. A., McGuire, A., Pereira, S., Rehm, H., Green, R. C., Beggs, A. H., & The BabySeq Project Team. (2019). Returning a genomic result for an adult-onset condition to the parents of a newborn: Insights from the BabySeq project. *Pediatrics, 143*(s1), s37–s43.https://doi.org/10.1542/peds.2018-1099H

Hood, L., & Rowen, L. (2013). The human genome project: Big science transforms biology and medicine. *Genome Medicine, 5,* 79. https://doi.org/10.1186/gm483

Hoskovec, J. M., Bennett, R. L., Caery, M. E., DaVanzo, J. E., Dougherty, M., Hahn, S. E., LeRoy, B. S., O'Neal, S., Richardson, J. G., & Wicklund, C. A. (2018). Projecting the supply and demand for certified genetic counselors: A workforce study. *Journal of Genetic Counseling, 27*(1), 16–20.

Hudson, K., Javitt, G., Burke, W., Byers, P., & American Society of Human Genetics Social Issues Committee. (2007). ASHG statement* on direct-to-consumer genetic testing in the United States. *Obstetrics and Gynecology, 110*(6), 1392–1395. https://doi.org/10.1097/01.AOG.0000292086.98514.8b

Institute of Medicine [IOM]. (2009). *Genetic service delivery: The current system and its strengths and challenges.* In Innovations in service delivery in the age of genomics: Workshop summary. Institute of Medicine (US) Roundtable on Translating Genomic-based research for health. National Academies Press.

International Society of Nurses in Genomics [ISONG]. (2013). *Position statement: Genetic biobanking for research.* Retrieved June 5, 2020, from https://www.isong.org/resources/Documents/PS_Genetic%20Biobanking%20for%20Research%20Position%20Statement_February%202013.pdf

Jamal, L. (2016). Ethical and policy issues in clinical genetics and genomics. In C. E. Kasper, T. A. Schneidereith, & F. R. Lashley (Eds.), *Lashley's essentials of clinical genetics in nursing practice* (pp. 443–453). Springer.

Kalia, S. S., Adelman, K., Bale, S. J., et al. (2017). Recommendations for reporting of secondary findings in clinical exome and genome sequencing, 2016 update (ACMG v2.0): A policy statement of the American College of Medical Genetics and Genomics. *Genetics in Medicine, 19*(2), 249–255.

Katsanis, S. H., & Katsanis, N. (2013). Molecular genetic testing and the future of clinical genomics. *Nature Reviews Genetics, 14*(6), 415–426.

Khan, C. M., Moore, E. G., Leos, C., & Rini, C. (2016). Patient hopes for diagnostic genomic sequencing: Roles of uncertainty and social status. *European Journal of Human Genetics, 24,* 803–808.

Lippi, G., Favaloro, E. J., & Plebani, M. (2011). Direct-to-consumer testing: More risks than opportunities. *The International Journal of Clinical Practice, 65*(12), 1221–1229.

Loud, J. T. (2010). Direct-to-consumer genetic and genomic testing: Preparing nurse practitioners for genomic healthcare. *The Journal of Nurse Practitioners, 6*(8), 585–594.

Maiese, D. R., Keehn, A., Lyon, M., Flannery, D., Watson, M., & Working groups of the National Coordinating Center for seven regional genetics service collaboratives. (2019). Current conditions in medical genetics practice. *Genetics in Medicine, 21*(8), 1874–1877.

March of Dimes. (2020, July). *Newborn screening tests for your baby.* Retrieved February 9, 2021, from https://www.marchofdimes.org/baby/newborn-screening-tests-for-your-baby.aspx

Mardy, A. & Wapner, R. J. (2016) Confined placental mosaicism and its impact on confirmation of NIPT results. *American Journal of Medical Genetics Part C* (Seminars in Medical Genetics). 172C, 118–122.

Mashke, K. J. (2008). Biobanks: DNA and research. In M. Crowley (Ed.), *From birth to death and bench to clinic: The hastings center bioethics briefing book for journalists, policymakers, and campaigns* (11–14). The Hastings Center.

Milliken, A. (2018). Nurse ethical sensitivity: An integrative review. *Nursing Ethics, 25*(3), 278–303.

Minear, M. A., Lewis, C., Pradhan, S., & Chandrasekharan, S. (2015). Global perspectives on clinical adoption of NIPT. *Prenatal Diagnosis, 35*(10), 959–967. https://doi.org/10.1002/pd.4637. Epub 2015 September 25. PMID: 26085345; PMCID: PMC5065727.

Monsen, R. B. (2000). An international agenda for ethics in nursing and genetics. *Journal of Pediatric Nursing, 15*(4), 212–216.

National Academies of Sciences, Engineering, and Medicine [NASEM]; Health and Medicine Division; Board on Health Sciences Policy. (2018a). Downey, A. S., Busta, E. R., Mancher, M., et al., eds. *Returning individual research results to participants: Guidance for a new research paradigm.* National Academies Press.

National Academies of Sciences, Engineering, and Medicine [NASEM]. (2018b). *Understanding disparities in access to genomic medicine: Proceedings of a workshop.* The National Academies Press. https://doi.org/10.17226/25277

National Human Genome Research Institute [NHGRI]. (2018, September 7). *Genetics vs. genomics fact sheet.* Retrieved March 7, 2020, from https://www.genome.gov/about-genomics/fact-sheets/Genetics-vs-Genomics

National Human Genome Research Institute [NHGRI]. (2018, October 28). *What is the Human Genome Project?* Retrieved March 20, 2020, from https://www.genome.gov/human-genome-project/What

National Human Genome Research Institute [NHGRI]. (2020, February 24). *Privacy in genomics.* Retrieve March 20, 2020, from https://www.genome.gov/about-genomics/policy-issues/Privacy

National Human Genome Research Institute [NHGRI]. (n.d.) *Karyotype.* https://www.genome.gov/genetics-glossary/Karyotype

National Institute of Child Health and Human Development [NICHD]. (2017, January 1). *How many newborns are screened in the United States?* Retrieved May 6, 2020, from https://www.nichd.nih.gov/health/topics/newborn/conditioninfo/infants-screened

National Institute of Child Health and Human Development [NICHD]. (2017, January 31). *What tests might I need during pregnancy?* Retrieved May 5, 2020, from https://www.nichd.nih.gov/health/topics/preconceptioncare/conditioninfo/tests-needed

National Institute of Child Health and Human Development [NICHD]. (2017, September 1). *What is the purpose of newborn screening?* Retrieved January 13, 2021, from https://www.nichd.nih.gov/health/topics/newborn/conditioninfo/purpose#:~:text=The%20purpose%20of%20newborn%20screening%20is%20to%20detect%20potentially%20fatal,of%20a%20disease%20or%20condition

National Society of Genetic Counselors. (2017). *NSGC code of ethics.* Retrieved July 13, 2020, from https://www.nsgc.org/p/cm/ld/fid=12

National Society of Genetic Counselors. (2020). *Who are genetic counselors?* Retrieved July 13, 2020, from https://www.nsgc.org/page/whoaregeneticcounselors-473

Newborn screening saves lives reauthorization act of 2019, H.R. 2507, 116th Cong. (2019). https://www.congress.gov/bill/116th-congress/house-bill/2507/text?q=%7B%22search%22%3A%5B%22newborn+screening+saves+lives%22%5D%7D&r=1&s=1

Ormond, K. E., Laurino, M. Y., Barlow-Stewart, K., Wessels, T., Macaulay, S., Austin, J., & Middleton, A. (2018). Genetic counseling globally: Where are we now? *American Journal of Medical Genetics Part C, Seminars in Medical Genetics, 178*(1), 98–107.

Parens, E., & Asch, A. (2003). Disability rights critique of prenatal genetic testing: Reflections and recommendations. *Mental Retardation and Developmental Disabilities Research Reviews, 9*, 40–47.

Pos, O., Budis, J., & Szemes, T. (2019, May 31). Recent trends in prenatal genetic screening and testing. *F1000 Research* (F1000 Faculty Rev), 764. https://doi.org/10.12688/f1000research.16837.1 [PubMed 31214330].

Powell, C. M. (2018). What genome sequencing can offer universal newborn screening programs. *Hastings Center Report, 48*(2), S18-19.

Ravitsky, V. (2017). The shifting landscape of prenatal testing: Between reproductive autonomy and public health. *Hastings Center Report, 47*(6), S34-40.

Ross, L. F., & Clayton, E. W. (2019). Ethical issues in newborn sequencing research: The case study of BabySeq. *Pediatrics, 144*(6), e20191031.

Rothwell, E., Johnson, E., Riches, N., & Botkin, J. R. (2019). Secondary research uses of residual newborn screening dried bloodspots: A scoping review. *Genetics in Medicine: Official Journal of the American College of Medical Genetics, 21*(7), 1469–1475. https://doi.org/10.1038/s41436-018-0387-8

Sanner, J., Yu, E., & Nomie, K. (2015). Nursing and biobanking. *Advances in Experimental Medicine and Biology, 864*, 157–163.

Skirton, H., O'Connor, A., & Humphreys, A. (2012). Nurses' competence in genetics: A mixed method systematic review. *Journal of Advanced Nursing, 68*(11), 2387–2398. https://doi.org/10.1111/j.1365-2648.2012.06034.x. Epub 2012 May 20. PMID: 22607038.

Sokol, D. (2020). ABC of medical confidentiality. *BMJ (Clinical Research ed.), 368*, m857. https://doi.org/10.1136/bmj.m857

Sparrow, R. (2011). A not-so-new eugenics: Harris and Savulescu on human enhancement. *Hastings Center Report, 41*(1), 32–42.

The Society for Maternal-Fetal Medicine Publications Committee. Society for Maternal-Fetal Medicine [SMFM] special report: SMFM statement: Clarification of recommendations regarding cell-free DNA aneuploidy screening. *American Journal of Obstetrics and Gynecology* (2015). Retrieved December 8, 2020, from https://www.ajog.org/article/S0002-9378(15)01191-6/pdf

Therrell, B. L., Padilla, C. D., Loeber, J. G., Kneisser, I., Saadallah, A., Borrajo, G. J. C., & Adams, J. (2015). Current status of newborn screening worldwide: 2015. *Seminars in Perinatology, 39*, 171–187.

Thorogood, A., Dalpé, G., & Knoppers, B. M. (2019). Return of individual genomic research results: Are laws and policies keeping step? *European Journal of Human Genetics: EJHG, 27*(4), 535–546. https://doi.org/10.1038/s41431-018-0311-3

Tonkin, E., Calzone, K. A., Badzek, L., Benjamin, C., Middleton, A., Patch, C., & Kirk, M. (2020). A roadmap for global acceleration of genomics integration across nursing. *Journal of Nursing Scholarship, 52*(2), 329–338.

Tuckson, R. V., Newcomer, L., & De Sa, J. M. (2013, April 10). Accessing genomic medicine: Affordability, diffusion, and disparities. *JAMA, 309*(14), 1469–1470.

Udesky, L. (2010). The ethics of direct-to-consumer testing. *The Lancet, 376*(9750), 1377–1378. https://doi.org/10.1016/S0140-6736(10)61939-3

U.S. Department of Health and Human Services. (2013, July 26). *Who must comply with HIPAA privacy standards?* https://www.hhs.gov/hipaa/for-professionals/faq/190/who-must-comply-with-hipaa-privacy-standards/index.html

Vanstone, M., Yacoub, K., Giacomini, M., Hulan, D., & McDonald, S. (2015). Women's experiences of publicly funded non-Invasive prenatal testing in Ontario, Canada: Considerations for health technology policy-making. *Qualitative Health Research, 25*(8), 1069–1084. https://doi.org/10.1177/1049732315589745

Williams, J. K., Feero, W. G., Leonard, D. G. B., & Coleman, B. (2017). Implementation science, genomic precision medicine, and improved health: A new path forward? *Nursing Outlook, 65*, 36–40.

Zacharias, R. L., Smith, M. E., & King, J. S. (2018). The legal dimensions of genomic sequencing in newborn screening. *Hastings Center Report, 48*(2), S39-41.

Chapter 9
Ethical Issues in Psychiatric and Mental Health Care

Julie P. Dunne, Emma K. Blackwell, Emily Ursini, and Aimee Milliken

Abstract Persons with mental health concerns are encountered in all areas of nursing practice. While this chapter specifically addresses ethical issues in psychiatric and mental health nursing, the information is pertinent for nurses across settings. A major issue in psychiatric and mental health settings is the problem that cognitive difficulties can interfere with making reasoned choices and processing information. We discuss ways to mitigate the harm such difficulties can cause to a person's sense of dignity and even physical safety. We also discuss the limits that have to be placed on a person's freedom when others are at risk of harm from their actions. The roles of stigma and bias and their compounding influences on mental health are explored along with mindfulness strategies to facilitate recognition and control of implicit and explicit biases. Additionally, the evolving role of telehealth and personal data storage are examined related to how sensitive information is protected. An important responsibility of nurses related to individuals with unmet mental health needs is addressing problems with access to mental health care. Various approaches to influencing problematic policies are suggested.

9.1 Stigma and Implicit Bias

Mental health is defined by the World Health Organization (WHO) as "a state of well-being in which the individual realizes his or her own abilities, can cope with life's normal stresses, can work productively and fruitfully, and can make a contribution to society" (WHO, 2020). The importance of mental wellness is not only essential

---

J. P. Dunne · E. K. Blackwell · E. Ursini
William F. Connell School of Nursing, Boston College, Chestnut Hill, Newton, MA 02467, USA
e-mail: julie.dunne@bc.edu

E. Ursini
e-mail: ursinie@bc.edu

A. Milliken (✉)
William F. Connell School of Nursing, Boston College, Chestnut Hill, MA, USA
e-mail: aimee.milliken@bc.edu

© The Author(s), under exclusive license to Springer Nature B.V. 2022
P. Grace and A. Milliken (eds.), *Clinical Ethics Handbook for Nurses*, The International Library of Bioethics 93,
https://doi.org/10.1007/978-94-024-2155-2_9

in psychiatric settings, but across healthcare. Nurses care for the whole person, which includes addressing mental health needs that also influence physical wellbeing. Nurses in all fields will encounter ethical issues related to the mental health of patients. Further, nurses in all fields need to consider personal mental health including as it relates to therapeutic use of self and the risk for secondary trauma in professional settings. Recognizing the widespread impact of stigma and bias in mental health is a first step to providing ethical psychiatric nursing care.

Stigma has impacted those with mental illness and the care that they receive throughout history. For example, during medieval times and the Renaissance, beliefs around demonic possession in mental health conditions were common. In the eighteenth and nineteenth centuries, individuals with mental illness were often considered unintelligent or dangerous and kept separate from society (Corrigan et al., 2005). Systematic efforts to reduce stigma around mental illness began in Canada, the United Kingdom, the United States and globally with the World Psychiatric Association in the 1990s (Corrigan et al., 2012; Stuart, 2008). However, notions that mental health conditions are shameful or that individuals with psychiatric illnesses are dangerous are still pervasive today (Seeman et al., 2016). These beliefs place blame on the individual with mental illness and create barriers to accessing healthcare.

Misconceptions about the etiology of mental illness are reinforced by a variety of factors. For example, popular media generally depicts individuals with eating disorders as privileged (e.g. white, upper-class) women carelessly choosing to engage in behaviors such as restriction or purging (Mitchison et al., 2014) and the news often stereotypes individuals with schizophrenia as violent (Bevilacqua Guarniero et al., 2017; Yang & Parrott, 2018). Language and communication, or lack thereof, also play a role in stigmatization of mental illness. Terminology like "addict" or "insane" have historically negative connotations and are used in insulting or prejudiced ways (Hayward & Bright, 1997). Further, objective discussion around mental illness is often limited in professional settings, but also among families and friend-groups, perpetuating the belief that it is something to be ashamed of or to hide.

These stigmas and stereotypes about mental health result in implicit bias, or unconscious judgments about the world and others based on perceptions, attitudes or memories (Narayan, 2019). Specifically, in order to understand and respond to the environment, humans rely on past experience and information to categorize events and people. When this categorization or judgment is shaped by stereotypical beliefs around mental health, it results in worse patient outcomes, insufficient care including inadequate assessments, inappropriate diagnoses and treatment, less time spent addressing patient's need and a lack of follow up (FitzGerald & Hurst, 2017; Narayan, 2019). This is compounded by implicit bias around race, gender, sexuality, weight stigma and other factors (Bailey et al., 2017; FitzGerald & Hurst, 2017; Fuss et al., 2018).

Examples of implicit bias in psychiatric nursing are as follows:

- A nurse has seen multiple news clips about violent crimes involving persons with schizophrenia. Based on these memories, the nurse unconsciously responds by

spending less time with patients who have this diagnosis even though only a minority of persons with schizophrenia are violent (Varshney et al., 2016).
- A nurse is raised in a family where mental illness is not discussed. The nurse has unconsciously internalized the belief that mental illness is "bad" or "scary" and fears working with patients with psychiatric disorders. This results in inadequate treatment planning and follow up because the nurse fails to ask the patient for input.

Due to its unconscious and hidden nature, implicit bias can help explain the disconnection that sometimes occurs between the intention to treat all patients equally and behaviors that differ from this, such as spending less time with a patient due to internalized stigma around mental health or, as an example, overlooking a diagnosis of bulimia nervosa in an African-American male patient due to bias around mental health, race and gender (FitzGerald & Hurst, 2017). As described earlier in this textbook (e.g. Chapter 1), when individuals or groups of individuals are treated differently from others, all persons in a society are at greater risk of dehumanization. As professionals, nurses are responsible for promoting social justice (Berwick, 2020; Grace & Willis, 2012). In order to do this, nurses, who are responsible for providing optimal care for any patient, must become aware of personal implicit biases in order to reduce injustices in healthcare and in society.

9.1.1 Mindfulness

Mindfulness is one means of addressing implicit bias in healthcare settings. Mindfulness is paying attention, with openness, to the present moment (Kabat-Zinn & Hanh, 2009). Mindfulness promotes emotion regulation and understanding, self-related processes including self-monitoring and attentional control including cognitive flexibility (Schuman-Olivier et al., 2020). In healthcare settings, nurses can take time to mindfully notice thoughts or emotions as they arise, including awareness of implicit biases. Nurses can also notice body sensations which may signal discomfort or anxiety in particular situations. This awareness through increased mindfulness will help nurses to understand and monitor their thoughts, emotions and body sensations and to act more compassionately towards patients (Burgess et al., 2017; Narayan, 2019). One specific practice that nurses can use comes from Mindfulness Based Cognitive Therapy (MBCT) and is called the "Three Minute Breathing Space" (Segal et al., 2018).

Instructions for the "Three Minute Breathing Space"

Step 1: Take one minute to become aware of thoughts, feelings and body sensations occurring in the present moment

Step 2: Take one minute to redirect attention to focus on the physical sensations of breathing

Step 3: Take one minute to expand awareness to the body including posture and facial expression and bring this "expanded awareness" to the next moments of your day. (Segal et al., 2018)

Mindfulness practices, such as the "Three Minute Breathing Space" also promote extinction learning and behavior change (Schuman-Olivier et al., 2020). Through mindfulness, nurses may be able to address biases and act in a less-biased and more equitable way when caring for patients. For example, following a "Three Minute Breathing Space" nurses can then choose how to skillfully and morally respond to a given situation from a place of expanded awareness. Treating patients as equally morally worthy is required by nursing codes of ethics. It facilitates trust in nurses and in exchange the elicitation of information necessary to provide good care. Specifically, mindfulness promotes quality care resulting in more safe and patient-centered practices, as well as the quality of caring leading to increased empathy and responsiveness (Epstein, 2017).

Skillfully responding to implicit bias may include increased opportunities for contact with stigmatized groups, such as those with mental illness (Corrigan et al., 2012; Narayan, 2019) and increased education about addressing stigma (Corrigan et al., 2012). Individuation and perspective taking in which nurses work to see each person as unique and consider the patient's thoughts and feelings (Narayan, 2019) and actions such as counter stereotyping and stereotype replacing in which nurses replace automatic biased thoughts with positive images and examples or intentionally act with compassion after self-reflection on biases (Institute for Healthcare Improvement, 2017) are also useful ways to address implicit bias. Implicit bias, and the related issues of structural racism, inequity, and social determinants of health, can create issues with access to care.

Additional resources are:

- Continuing Education "Addressing Implicit Bias in Nursing: A Review" https://doi.org/10.1097/01.NAJ.0000569340.27659.5a
- The Institute for Healthcare Improvement: http://www.ihi.org

9.2 Access to Care

9.2.1 Social Determinants of Mental Health

Many factors, including genetic, biological, and environmental factors, impact the trajectory of one's health. Over time, these factors and determinants of health (e.g. income, food and housing insecurity, early childhood development, etc.) have been placed at the forefront of research on important influences on health outcomes as they often mediate access to healthcare services. Between 2008 and 2018, scientific literature focused on understanding more about the social determinants of health increased by nearly 2000% (Shim & Compton, 2018), as time and time again, research emphasized the permeating reach of social determinants on health. The Centers for

Disease Control and Prevention (CDC) define social determinants of health as the conditions of the places in which an individual lives, learns, works and plays (CDC, 2021). These conditions impact an individual's access to health care and health outcomes throughout the entire lifespan, from infancy to older adulthood. As such, the United Nations has emphasized eliminating poverty, reducing inequality, developing sustainable cities and communities, and peace, justice, and strong institutions as four of the items on the 2030 Agenda for Sustainable Development (United Nations, 2015). Chapter 11 discusses issues of structural disadvantage and injustice in greater detail.

The advantages, disadvantages and experiences of individuals are not uniform across the world, or even within a given country or city. Opportunities, wealth, education and health care are not distributed equally. These inequities result in divergent patterns of health across different populations, subpopulations and individuals. They create health disparities, as certain populations are allocated resources and goods that others are not (Shim & Compton, 2019). These disparities benefit those who are born into and encounter more advantages throughout the lifespan, while those without the same sorts of advantages suffer. As people experience stress related to a consistent lack of resources and goods, the prolonged anxiety response physically alters brains and bodies making these individuals more susceptible to a variety of conditions (Yaribeygi et al., 2017). For instance, the experience of a greater number of adverse childhood experiences (ACEs) is correlated with increased risk for various cancers, heart disease, sexually transmitted diseases, lung and liver diseases, and skeletal fractures (Sederer, 2016). The CDC defines ACEs as potentially traumatic events occurring between ages of 0–17, including things like the experience of violence and neglect, or witnessing violence (CDC, 2020b). These experiences induce the stress response that is tied to poor health outcomes.

Social determinants of health also impact mental health. There are disparities between access to and specialization of mental health services, outcomes and quality of care for different populations (Shim & Compton, 2019). An understanding of these experiences and outcomes points to the need to combat disparities. For example, children who've survived multiple ACEs are not only at risk for the aforementioned physical health risks, but are also at a higher risk for mood, anxiety and substance use disorders, and suicidal ideation (Mersky et al., 2013). Physical abuse has been associated with lifelong attention deficit hyperactivity disorder (ADHD), post-traumatic stress disorder (PTSD) and bipolar disorder (Sugaya et al., 2012). Lower levels of education, related to various other social determinants such as poverty resulting in underfunded schools, is associated with a greater risk of late-life depression (Chang-Quan et al., 2010). Poverty in childhood has been associated with the experiences of PTSD, major depressive disorder and arrests in adulthood (Nikulina et al., 2011). Beyond childhood, adults and older adults experience the effects of social determinants of mental health. Specifically, those with the lowest incomes in a location are 1.5–3 times more likely to experience depression or anxiety (Ridley et al., 2020). In industrialized countries, unemployment and job insecurity can severely impact mental health. In the United States, there is a link between suicide rates and unemployment rates (Reeves et al., 2012).

Further, studies have found that experiences of discrimination and prejudices are highly correlated with poor mental health outcomes, including depression and PTSD. In New York City, individuals identifying as Black or Latinx reported higher posttraumatic stress following Hurricane Sandy than others. Across the United States, LGBTQ+ (lesbian, gay, bisexual or transgender) and racial/ethnic minorities more often report poor mental health (Alegría et al., 2019). This bias, stigmatization, and racism, compounded with factors such as income and housing inequality which often stems from systemic and historical marginalization, may result in further lack of access to mental health care. In response to these factors and their potential to negatively impact the world, the US Department of Health and Human Services designated a 10-year goal of improving social and physical environments to promote health (Office of Disease Prevention & Health Promotion, 2020). While the United States is used here as an example, these issues occur on a global scale.

On a nurse-patient level, there are several steps that can be taken to address and prevent negative health outcomes through screening individuals based on age cohort. Awareness of such interventions may help reduce nurse moral distress and burnout when working with individuals from disadvantaged backgrounds. This lessens the feelings of helplessness that lead to moral distress. For children, adolescents, and young adults, assessing and addressing issues related to trauma, education and poverty is important (Shim & Compton, 2019). Early-interventions such as community-sponsored after-school care programs, increased food bank access and education mentorship programs can serve as a protective factor against the poor mental health outcomes. One successfully implemented program offered a high-quality preschool program for those living in poverty in Ypsilanti, Michigan, resulting in students achieving both higher incomes in the workplace and increased education levels in adulthood (Schweinhart, 2007). For adults, screening for issues related to income, housing, employment, legal status and other personal areas and referring for additional support prevented worsening mental health outcomes (Kenyon et al., 2007).

9.2.2 Health Insurance and Mental Health Parity

The role of public or private insurance and other means of accessing affordable healthcare varies across the globe. In low-income and middle-income countries, the monetary equivalent of less than $2 dollars per person is spent yearly on mental health. This creates a huge treatment gap, and manifests in economic losses resulting from things such as sick days, decreased productivity and work. In 2010, worldwide, the equivalent of an estimated 2.5–8.5 trillion dollars was lost as a result of mental and neurological disorders. An additional 12 billion days in the 36 largest countries in the world are lost yearly, attributed to anxiety and depression disorders (Chisholm et al., 2016). Even in developed countries, limited funds are allocated to addressing mental health needs and health insurance often does not cover preventive mental health treatment. In 2013, 2.4 trillion dollars were spent on healthcare in the United

States. However, of this, only 187.8 billion was spent on mental health and substance use disorders (Winerman, 2017) even though about one in five adults live with mental illness (NIMH, 2021). Limited funding raises ethical issues related to distributive justice. Despite evidence that mental health challenges can lead to the aforementioned losses in productivity and related health issues, mental-health related supports and services are not funded on the same scale as interventions targeted at many other diseases, including cardiac disease and cancer.

In the United States, some measures have been enacted to try to improve access to mental healthcare. The Paul Wellstone and Pete Domenici Mental Health Parity and Addiction Equity Act of 2008 mandated that private health insurances not restrict what they will pay toward mental health related costs more than they would toward medical and surgical costs (Centers for Medicare & Medicaid Services, n.d.). With this Act, restrictions on the number of visits or other costs to treat someone's mental health condition must not be different from those imposed on treating someone's physical health condition. While a step in the right direction, the Act does not address the ratio of mental health providers to physical health providers within one's network, meaning that a patient may have access to only a few mental health providers and a great number of physical health providers. This forces individuals to search for out of network treatment (e.g. clinicians that do not participate in the health plan), resulting in high costs for mental healthcare. There is a large disparity in costs for out of network care resulting in those with behavioral conditions spending much more than those with physical conditions (Xu et al., 2019).

Even with insurance, behavioral health clinicians who treat disorders such as substance use disorder and major depressive disorder have very little participation in private health plans. For instance, in one study, only 62% of psychiatrists listed accepted new, privately insured patients (Xu et al., 2019). This means that even when health care plans include behavioral health clinicians, many do not accept new patients, as they are in high demand, and there are often long wait times for those seeking care. Access is a challenge even for physicians. Between 2004 and 2005, two-thirds of primary care physicians reported that they were unable to get outpatient mental health services for patients (Cunningham, 2009). These limitations again represent issues of justice and highlight the need for more accessible mental healthcare.

Due to the difficulty in accessing mental health care even with insurance, nurses in psychiatric and other settings may face ethical dilemmas related to weighing the risks of long wait times for low-cost care versus referring patients to expensive out-of-network providers. Nurses can work to support lobby efforts to expand access to care, especially since effective mental healthcare has been shown to have great economic advantages worldwide (e.g. In 2016, Chisholm and colleagues determined that returns for increased, effective depression and anxiety treatment between the years of 2016 and 2030 would result in 147 billion dollar return worldwide, and 43 million extra years of healthy life over this period).

9.2.3 Open Notes and Cures Act

In 2012, Sweden launched an Open Notes Service through which all citizens, besides adolescents, could read notes from non-psychiatric settings. This practice was hoped to enhance patient involvement in their care. The decision to include psychiatric notes in this practice varied county by county. In the month prior to implementation, many psychiatric health care practitioners did not expect Open Notes to be beneficial (Petersson & Erlingsdottir, 2018a, 2018b). Indeed, after a year and a half, many clinicians reported that the benefits to Open Notes were not realized (e.g. only 5.7% of clinicians believed that their patients reading Open Notes took better care of themselves, and only 8% of clinicians believed that patients reading Open Notes were taking their medication more regularly). Only 14.2% of clinicians believed that there was more patient-clinician trust. However, some of the major concerns expressed by commentators prior to implementation of this practice were found to be baseless. For example, only a few clinicians reported spending significantly more time with patients due to patient questions, writing less candidly in their notes, and spending more time writing notes. Ultimately, there was very little negative impact of Open Notes on practice (Petersson & Erlingsdottir, 2018a). More research is needed, however, to ascertain the benefits versus problems with this patient empowerment strategy.

The United States Federal Cures Act of 2021 ensures that patients have access to their own electronic health information. The act mandates open notes, including in psychiatric settings. The Office of the National Coordinator for Health Information Technology (ONC) defines that act's purpose as ease of access limited by complicated online software, and to prevent blocking of information. (ONC, n.d.; Petersson & Erlingsdottir, 2018b). As this act is implemented, more research will be required to determine whether the benefits of accessing one's own health information outweigh the potential ethical challenges. For example, some have worried that immediate access to clinical information in the medical record, without the assistance of a provider to explain or contextualize the data, may cause confusion, loss of trust, or undue stress.

While some research has been mixed, the induction of Open Notes and the Cures Act have been shown to increase patient autonomy, as patients are empowered to read and be more involved in their own healthcare, taking on a "partner" role with the clinical team (Blease et al., 2020). This more equal role can also foster a therapeutic alliance between the patient and clinician leading to more congruent and therapeutic care. Patients can refer back to their notes in times of crisis to remind themselves of coping strategies, grounding techniques and other important therapeutic activities (Blease et al., 2020). Moreover, the Cures Act may increase professionalism as clinicians are forced to think in a less biased manner about their patients because the documentation should be professional and impartial as it may be read by patients. This practice of less biased note taking might lead, albeit inadvertently, to more unprejudiced care.

9.3 Privacy and Confidentiality

9.3.1 Mandated Reporting

Due to their role in the healthcare setting, the way nurses interact with patients can intentionally or unintentionally reveal situations of potential or actual abuse and neglect. In some countries, such as the United States, nurses are among the persons designated as mandated reporters of abuse and neglect in particular populations. Which populations—children, adults, or the elderly—nurses are obligated to report when abuse or neglect is suspected varies from state to state. However, the obligation is legally enforced (Boyd, 2018). This includes suspected instances of both child and elder abuse, and in some states intimate partner violence, with failure to report resulting in fines. Many other countries also have mandatory reporting laws for child abuse (McTavish et al., 2017). Instances of abuse are unfortunately not uncommon, with one in seven children in the United States experiencing child abuse and neglect per year (CDC, 2020a) and one in ten people aged 60 and older living at home who experience elder abuse and neglect (CDC, 2020c) in the United States. While the responsibility of the nurse as a mandated reporter is critical in ensuring the safety and well-being of members of the society, it is important to delve into the impact this role may have on privacy, trust and on the therapeutic relationship nurses have with their patients. Perhaps especially where reporting of intimate partner violence is legally required (as it is in some US states) and there is extreme risk to the abused, the nurse may be forced to choose between the legal requirement of reporting and the ethical action of protecting the victim: a risk versus benefit decision. In settings where this might occur it is important to know what one's resources are and who might be consulted for assistance.

Nurses are placed in a role of "narrow surveillance" (Fraser et al., 2010) where they must identify potential instances of abuse and neglect within the time frame of their interaction with patients. In Fraser and colleagues' study (2010), it was noted there could be confusion about when and what to report, as reporting was seen as an important responsibility. Reporting erroneously could cause harm and there were many individual and contextual factors involved that had to be accounted for. For example, studies have shown that difficulties arise when identifying emotional abuse which can be subtle in its presentation (Fraser et al., 2010). In Fraser and colleagues (2010) study of nurses' experiences identifying child abuse and neglect, training was perceived as helpful in aiding nurses to feel equipped for the responsibility of identification and reporting. An important role of nursing education would be to emphasize how to recognize signs of emotional abuse and the role of individual perception in abuse and neglect to aid in increasing successful future identification. Ethical challenges may arise for nurses when one is uncertain regarding suspected abuse or neglect, as reporting potential abuse and neglect can be a lifesaving and protective step, yet an erroneous report can strain the family in question. Further, mandated reporting often requires infringement on confidentiality, a critical component of a successful therapeutic relationship, and this can erode trust. While the safety of those potentially abused outweighs the confidentiality of the therapeutic relationship, it is nonetheless ethically challenging not to honor the agreement of the relationship (Steinberg et al., 1997). When possible, the nurse's status as a mandated reporter should be disclosed at the outset of a therapeutic relationship. Keeping both the understanding that any suspicion should be reported and that this can impact the therapeutic relationship in mind, nurse who is faced with such challenges in their practice should seek appropriate training and know what their resources and supports are.

9.3.2 Stigma, Privacy and Data Sharing

The use of technology in healthcare has allowed rapid knowledge development and improvements in patient care delivery but have also augmented problems for protecting patient privacy. Researchers are encouraging the open use of patient data in order to guide scientific endeavors and promote new discoveries (Walsh et al., 2018). However, with these exciting and promising new developments arise questions regarding the ethical obligation of upholding patient privacy. Investigating the benefits and drawbacks of sharing data within the psychological community and its relationship to nursing ethics is a critical concern.

Open data sharing involves the use of unstructured and qualitative data reported by the clinician in the medical record, which includes sensitive patient information, relationship data, information about past trauma, and medical history (Walsh et al., 2018). While contributing important knowledge to the field of psychology and psychiatry, there are associated risks to the patient that have to be considered. Among the risks is that of stigma, as discussed earlier. Privacy breaches can occur inadvertently as a result of equipment upgrades, server violations, and issues with identity and attribute disclosure. Transparency in disclosing potential risks is critical for ensuring patient informed consent. More work is needed on protecting an individual's privacy including greater de-identification of data and a tiered approach for data sharing that considers the risks and consequences of data sharing at different levels and within different contexts (Walsh et al., 2018).

As new applications and other sources of sharing patient information become available, nurses need to ensure they understand the implications for patients and can adequately inform them of these. Especially for those applications that are publicly available, and these are increasing exponentially, nurses have an advisory role. Studies have determined that some of the privacy practices of prominent applications involve their ability to share information with third parties that include linkable identifiers, something that users are not aware of or able to anticipate (Huckvale et al., 2019). Nurses can educate patients who desire to use available applications for managing their mental health about the ways their data may be used, and help them balance the risks and benefits so that patients are enabled to make informed decisions.

9.3.3 Telepsychiatry

In addition to electronic healthcare data, as healthcare evolves, and especially in light of the COVID-19 pandemic, telepsychiatry has become a promising way to provide patient care. Telepsychiatry allows provider and patient interaction at a distance through the use of internet platforms and telephone calls (Hubley et al., 2016). Telepsychiatry allows for medical care that is relatively easy to access and decreases barriers to care such as travel time and transport coordination. Patients and providers report a general satisfaction with telepsychiatry, with those in rural areas rating it as even more successful in meeting their needs as compared to those in suburban areas.

With the growing popularity of this form of medical care, it is important to evaluate how telepsychiatry changes the way that healthcare is provided and received, as well as considerations around confidentiality. First, this form of healthcare inherently places a larger emphasis on listening to and relying upon patient self-report. Lacking the ability to sit face-to-face with patients places an even greater value on traits, or ethical "virtues" such as honesty, candor, and accountability in patient-provider interactions (Rutenberg & Oberle, 2008). Providers specifically report concerns regarding the therapeutic relationship, citing that this type of care presents its own unique challenges. From the perspective of patients, studies have indicated that they report experiencing the same level of comfort disclosing information via telehealth, but lower levels of satisfaction regarding feeling supported and encouraged by their providers (Hubley et al., 2016). With the widespread transition to telehealth during the COVID-19 pandemic, more research is needed to ascertain whether these trends remain accurate. Factors such as lack of access to a private space may impact confidentiality and nurses should be aware of these limitations. To address this limitation, nurses may encourage clients to ensure access to a quiet space prior to making an appointment. If this is not possible, patients may be advised to let their provider know, and increase privacy through strategies such as wearing headphones or utilizing white noise to make this experience as private as possible.

While some studies indicate that telehealth can help diminish healthcare disparities associated with in-person care, others find that telehealth may exacerbate existing disparities and the influence of systemic racism. As telehealth becomes more popular, it is essential to investigate its specific impact on existing disparities associated with in person visits (Chunara et al., 2020). For example, it is important to note that technological barriers to video calls reflect pre-existing healthcare disparities (Strowd et al., 2020). This is evident through a study on the rapid implementation of telehealth during the COVID-19 pandemic indicating that those who are older, Black, male, and receive Medicare or Medicaid support (which are types of US social services) are less likely to adopt video visits (Chunara et al., 2020). Indeed, although the proportion of Black patients accessing telemedicine services has increased, these levels are still lower compared to white patients (Chunara et al., 2020).

Ethical challenges arise throughout psychiatric care and some new challenges are specific to telepsychiatry. These telehealth-specific issues can lead to stress and burnout among nurses. Good clinical judgment and critical thinking skills specific to this environment are needed to overcome barriers to developing the nurse-patient relationship and thus gathering the data that enables the nurse to provide optimal care despite the virtual environment. These skills are especially important when there is a question of danger to the patient. An ability to navigate the balance between the competing principles of nonmaleficence and autonomy for their patients when the understanding of the severity of medical issues may differ between patient and provider (Rutenberg & Oberle, 2008). As discussed in earlier chapters, while promoting patient autonomy is extremely important, in a telepsychiatry setting when a patient's capacity for judging what is in his or her best interests may be in doubt, a risk versus benefit decision has to be made. As an example, consider a patient who reveals that he is very angry at a family member and having thoughts of violence but reports that he can control these thoughts and has never acted on them in the past. The nurse has to determine the likelihood of the patient acting on these feelings now. The nurse has to evaluate whether the patient's decision not to go to a facility (which would cost more money) is too risky to honor in light of the potential harm to the family member and what best action to take next. Nurses working in settings where such issues arise have responsibilities to develop their ethical decision-making capacities, have a grasp of the range of possible actions, and know what their resources for dealing with such emergencies are. Increased continuing education regarding ways in which to conceptualize and work through these sorts of ethically challenging situations may aid in reducing the risk of telehealth nurse burnout which in turn can be deleterious to good patient care.

9.3.4 Therapeutic Use of Self as a Nurse

Developing a therapeutic relationship between nurse and patient is an essential component involved in providing successful psychiatric nursing care. A therapeutic relationship is one that facilitates "meeting (the patient's) nursing needs, to the mutual satisfaction of the nurse and the patient" (McQueen, 2000, p. 274). Part of fostering this therapeutic relationship involves emotional work on the part of the nurse, along with the use of social skills and personal qualities (McQueen, 2000). The way in which therapeutic relationships develop may be unique to each nurse-patient relationship, but share three main fundamental qualities: empathetic understanding, genuineness, and unconditional positive regard (McQueen, 2000).

The therapeutic use of oneself is one way to foster therapeutic relationships and may manifest through the act of self-disclosure. Self-disclosure involves sharing information about oneself to one's patients. Its use can convey an understanding, and normalize patient experiences, along with promoting patient reciprocity (Ashmore & Banks, 2002). Each of these outcomes may be quite successful in the development and continuation of a therapeutic relationship. However, one must consider the effect of both under- and over-disclosing information. Nurses who under-disclose may have trouble encouraging patients to engage in therapeutic activities because the foundation of genuineness and trust has not been established. On the other hand, when nurses over-disclose information, this may interfere with the nurse's ability to help with the patients' well-being, thus undermining the goal of the relationship (Ashmore & Banks, 2002). It is essential for nurses to balance the content and quantity of self-disclosure in a way that is most therapeutic for the patient while also considering their own privacy and maintenance of professional boundaries. When deciphering what personal information to disclose to patients, it is valuable to encourage nurses to ask themselves how sharing specific pieces of information would benefit their patients. Additionally, it is important that the nurse's motive behind sharing this information is not based on the hope for secondary gain.

Other aspects of the nurse-patient relationship are transference and countertransference. Transference refers to an unconscious response of a patient towards a nurse, while countertransference refers to an unconscious response of a nurse towards a patient (O'Kelly, 1998). It is common for a nurse to experience countertransference as patients may unconsciously remind them of family members, loved ones, or even those in their lives that they dislike or have poor relationships with (O'Kelly, 1998). Countertransference can be recognized through a nurse's strong emotional reaction toward a patient that may cause them to act in ways that are different from how they normally would. This may manifest as either over-involvement or withdrawal from the relationship depending on the nature of the countertransference. In these instances, the role of the nurse is to work towards recognition of countertransference and the way that it influences thoughts, feelings, and behaviors toward patients (O'Kelly, 1998). A way to diminish the effect of countertransference once recognized is to verbalize this recognition of countertransference to colleagues or to step away from the relationship if it is no longer therapeutic. In instances where countertransference interferes with the care that the nurse is providing, the quality of care may be hindered. According to nursing theorist Hilgard Peplau, nurses must be able to understand themselves and their own needs before they can meet the needs of their patients (O'Kelly, 1998; Peplau, 1991). Thus, according to her perspective, the nurse-patient relationship is inherently ethical when the basis of this relationship is to promote patient well-being (Gastmans, 1998). Nurses must be able to recognize factors that promote and diminish from this goal in order to ensure that they are fostering a therapeutic relationship.

9.4 Restrictions on Autonomy

9.4.1 Involuntary and Voluntary Treatment

While receiving psychiatric care, it is the responsibility of healthcare providers to ensure that patients are afforded treatment options that allow them to maintain their personal freedom to the greatest possible extent (Saraceno et al., 2003). This is in an effort to promote their overall good by providing them the autonomy to facilitate their sense of control over their health. In the inpatient psychiatric setting, patients may be either admitted voluntarily or involuntarily. While this is so in the United States, many other countries have similar legal recourse when the safety of the person or others in their environment are at risk of harm. A voluntary admission is associated with obtaining informed consent from patients, reflecting an individual's acceptance of their physician's recommendation for their hospitalization. A voluntary admission nevertheless warrants transparency about under which conditions the person's voluntary admission might change to an involuntary one. For example, a patient is admitted voluntarily to the psychiatric ward of an institution. However, she then develops hallucinations and is delusional about a family member who she believes is trying to poison her. It is determined that although she now wishes to leave the institution, it is too risky for her to do so. A court order to continue hospitalization involuntarily may be obtained.

Involuntary hospitalization requires a legal order, in the United States and elsewhere. These can usually be obtained quickly and on an emergency basis. It enables an institution to legally prevent a patient from leaving. It may, or may not, also ensure the patient accepts the treatment needed to either restore to baseline or manage symptoms. Ultimately, the hope is for the person to function safely in society. Involuntary commitment to an institution is a serious move. There is a relatively long history worldwide of using psychiatry as a weapon to control dissidents, and to remove 'undesirables' from society (Van Voren, 2016). Thus, involuntary hospitalization should be used in rare circumstances wherein the patient in question is considered to be at risk of harming themselves or others if not in inpatient treatment (Saraceno et al., 2003). The underlying concept of involuntary admission is that in specific occasions this decision is made in the best interest of the patient and protects public safety. An example of an involuntary admission that is in the best interest of the patient is on that of suicidality. There is evidence that such hospitalization resulted in a reduction of suicidality over time and across countries related to treatment received (Giacco & Priebe, 2016). The ethical basis for such an admission hinges on the concept that, generally, suicidality is viewed as a manifestation of an underlying psychiatric issue that we have an obligation to treat in order to return the patient to their baseline. Involuntary admissions for dangerousness to self or others protects both patients and those that are at risk of harm from the person, however the goal in both cases is to facilitate a return to self-control. Involuntary admission remains controversial and not to be undertaken lightly. When a psychiatric condition interferes with a person's ability to judge reality and that person or others are a risk of harm it may be warranted in order to return the person to a state where they no longer pose a risk to themselves or others.

Involuntary admission has been noted to exacerbate feelings of alienation and dissatisfaction and may result in unwillingness to adhere to treatment recommendations (Monahan et al., 1995), or, alternatively, it may empower the patient. The temporary restriction of autonomy in order to promote a "good" for the patient is ethically justifiable, however it is important to try to limit associated harms. What underlies patient experience of their hospital admission lies in their individual perceptions of their hospitalization, which is influenced by the way in which they are treated (Monahan et al., 1995).

The psychiatric nurse is responsible for ensuring that human dignity is preserved (Monahan et al., 1995). Preserving human dignity and respect are especially important in psychiatric settings for providing a sense of security (Johnson & Delaney, 2007). Continued knowledge developments of the field of psychology offer promise for reducing the rate of involuntary psychiatric admissions including through the use of crisis resolution teams and outpatient programs (Schmitz-Buhl et al., 2019).

9.4.2 De-escalation

As a nurse in any setting, the utilization of de-escalation techniques is a necessary element of competent patient care. De-escalation is a term used to encapsulate the psychosocial interventions utilized to redirect patients to a calmer mental space (Berring et al., 2016). Using de-escalation techniques successfully benefits all patients and nurses on the unit, avoids the use of measures such as chemical and physical restraints, and keeps nurses and patients safe. There are four key elements of successful de-escalation: knowing yourself, knowing the patient, knowing the situation, and knowing how to communicate (Berring et al., 2016). Those who are successful at de-escalating situations build rapport with their patients and consider why they may be behaving the way they are. It is important to take the time and effort to understand each of these elements to successfully de-escalate a situation. Further, what may appear to be a suddenly erupting situation, or one that has no known precipitants, under close observation may be due to a myriad of smaller irritants (Johnson & Delaney, 2007). Regardless of how a situation escalates, noticing the beginning of escalation is a key component of successful intervention (Johnson & Delaney, 2007). Time is another key component of de-escalation, with those who successfully de-escalate a situation being able to identify the most impactful time in which to intervene, as stepping in too early or too late may escalate the situation further (Johnson & Delaney, 2007).

Successful de-escalation depends on a number of factors, often including techniques utilized that are highly individualized to each patient. While there is no uniform way in which de-escalation should occur, it is important to provide psychiatric nurses with the mindset, tools, and training to prepare them to aid patients in reaching a calmer mental space. Additionally, identifying nurses who are prepared and willing to patiently utilize de-escalation techniques with the main goal of avoiding measures such as chemical and physical restraints unless absolutely necessary is essential for quality patient care. Successful attributes for nurses to display when de-escalating a situation include empathy, care, humor, and calmness (Berring et al., 2016). For patients on a psychiatric unit, fear may surround the role of de-escalation, with the perception that restraints will ultimately be utilized. While it is the perception of nurses and patients that restraints are the "worst case," there is an opportunity within this setting to shift this culture to a mutual understanding that all involved wish for peaceful solutions (Berring et al., 2016). To propel this shift, psychiatric nurses should be educated in depth regarding ways to successfully de-escalate situations prior to being on the unit and practicing nurses will benefit from continuing education measures. Further, education should be centered around discouraging the use of coercive measures with patients, which are perceived as dehumanizing to patients and are often not ethically supportable (Berring et al., 2016). Including patient perspectives in these measures may additionally aid in fostering empathy and understanding on the part of the nurse.

9.4.3 Chemical and Physical Restraints

Although utilized as a last resort, restraints often hold a role in the practice of a psychiatric nurse. Both chemical and physical restraints may be used when a patient is determined to be at imminent risk of harming themselves or others. Chemical restraints involve the administration of medication to calm the patient and de-escalate the situation, and physical restraints involve limiting the patient's mobility in order to promote safety. At its core, the act of restraining someone diminishes a persons' autonomy, which the nurse is responsible for upholding under Codes of Ethics. Further, nurses must consider how restraining a patient plays into the balance between beneficence and nonmaleficence (Mohr, 2010). This may be ethically taxing, as the nurse must take the entirety of the situation into account to ultimately make the decision that restraint will most likely benefit the patient and at the same time poses little risk of harm. Further, in many cases these decisions have to be made relatively quickly.

Since the use of restraints is troubling to nurses, this element is often cited as a reason for stepping away from acute psychiatric care (Bigwood & Crowe, 2008). However, in certain instances the use of restraints is viewed as the only option to ensure the safety of the patient and staff members. While restraints may be deemed necessary, evidence has determined the presence of misuse and abuse of restraints within the nursing field (Mohr, 2010). The misuse of restraints must be addressed, as it results in patient harm and consequences as tragic and severe as death. This intervention meant to ultimately promote safety may instead result in a great deal of damage to patient well-being. The act of restraining someone chemically or physically is an ethically weighty decision (Mohr, 2010), especially given the particular vulnerability of the psychiatric patient population.

Increased education regarding the proper use of restraints is called for within the nursing community. Education will help ensure that nurses understand the relevant indications, use, and adherence to rules including guidelines such as time limitations. It is essential that nurses are informed of all other means of creating a safe environment in their units, including the utilization of de-escalation techniques prior to considering restraints of any kind.

Ethical challenges may arise when nurses disagree with their colleagues' decisions to restrain patients. The presence of such disagreements speak to the importance of fostering communication skills within the nursing community, along with the importance of fostering critical thinking skills and clinical judgement in relation to the ethical challenges that nurses in the psychiatric setting may face. This you-tube video clip demonstrating how de-escalation works with a one-on-one encounter may be helpful: https://www.youtube.com/watch?v=6B9Kqg6jFeI.

9.5 Collaborative Recovery

9.5.1 Trauma-Informed Care

Trauma-informed care is care based on the role that trauma and traumatic stress play in a patient's behavior and cognitions. The American Psychological Association (APA) defines trauma as the emotional response of an individual to their experiencing or witnessing of a situation that could, or seemed as though it could, cause death or injury (APA, 2013). Experiences of trauma are associated with emotional dysregulation, substance use disorder, self-harm, hyperarousal, sleep disturbances, excessive guilt, cognitive errors, flashbacks and triggers (SAMHSA, 2014a).

The concept of, and support for, trauma-informed care emerged in the 1970s as the awareness of domestic trauma and its aftermath increased and subsequent rape crisis centers and women's shelters emerged. It was further pushed forward as child-advocacy and child-abuse centered care emerged in the 1980s. By the 1990s, researchers looked at these past examples of trauma-informed care, and the post-traumatic stress experiences of soldiers returning from the Vietnam War to analyze how clinicians could aid those who experienced trauma; thus the title of trauma-informed care was born. However, some insightful and compassionate clinicians had been practicing this sort of care for years, informed by various movements such as feminism, without having a name for it (Wilson et al., 2013).

SAMHSA, the Substance Abuse and Mental Health Services Administration, defines trauma-informed approach as dependent on six principles: (1) safety (2) trustworthiness and transparency (3) peer support (4) collaboration and mutuality (5) empowerment, voice, and choice (6) cultural, historical and gender issues. First, the patient should feel physically and psychologically safe. The decisions made by the providers must be clear and encourage trust. Peer support suggests working with other trauma survivors to share stories, build trust and establish hope. The relationship between clinician and patient should be a partnership, without any hierarchies of power. Additionally, the organization providing care should foster an environment where staff and patients feel safe and empowered to make choices about their treatment and experiences. Lastly, cultural, historical and gender issues should inform care by ensuring the impact of historical and general trauma is recognized and addressed (SAMHSA, 2014b). SAMHSA also offers the 4 R's: key assumptions necessary to a trauma-informed approach. These include: providers have an understanding and **realization** about trauma's impact on patients, providers are able to **recognize** the signs of trauma within a patient, the provider **responds** by using the above six principles, the provider **resists re-traumatization** of the patient (SAMHSA, 2014b).

Leadership, including nursing leadership, is important in implementation of trauma-informed care. A visible and committed staff, united in the goal of trauma-informed care has been associated with better patient outcomes and the inclusion of nurses in not only collecting data but analyzing and working to suggest improvements in care has contributed to more effective and enhanced adoption of trauma-based care (Muskett, 2014). Additional strategies found to be helpful in addressing trauma include routine screening of clients for trauma histories and satisfaction surveys specific to trauma-informed care. The development of a staff culture committed to the value of trauma-informed care also necessitates effective training of staff in trauma-informed care (Muskett, 2014). Trauma-informed care can lead to a reduction in substance use and psychiatric symptoms, increased safety, self-esteem and relationships in children, and is correlated with increased housing stability. It is cost-effective as it does not cost more than other therapeutic interventions and may actually reduce the need for crisis-based services, such as hospitalizations (Hopper et al., 2010).

One concern for those analyzing trauma-informed care guidelines is the loose structure. When talking to clinicians, most are in favor of trauma-informed care, but few can define it, and those who can often have different definitions because of variations in training (Berliner & Kolko, 2016). This may result in moral distress. As such, there is a need for an increasingly unified approach to trauma informed care.

Trauma-informed care is not only important in the psychiatric setting but has benefits in the general practice setting, too. In medical settings, understanding the influence of a patient's trauma is important because these experiences can result in long term negative health outcomes, including issues such as cardiovascular disease, decreased immune function, and decreased attention to physical health and pain (Schnurr & Green, 2004). However, evidence suggests a minority of family practice doctors screen for childhood trauma, if ever (Weinreb et al., 2010). Asking patients about their past trauma can improve the therapeutic alliance (Tomaz & Castro-Vale, 2020). Nurses and other providers outside of psychiatry should receive training in trauma-informed care as this can also improve identification of trauma and referral to appropriate care, thereby improving outcomes.

9.5.2 Patient-Centered Care

Trauma-informed care is centered around the trauma experiences of a patient, and a patient's reactions to the trauma experience. *Patient-centered care* focuses on the patient as well, concerning itself with the specific needs and lived experience of the patient, which may or may not include trauma. Patient-centered care, rather than focusing on the specific needs of the provider or larger organization, is an obligation in all of nursing practice, not only in the psychiatric nursing setting. It shifts the decision-making role to the patient, allowing patients to speak for themselves and encouraging the provider to be an active listener. This structure empowers patients to take control of their healthcare. Patient-centered care has been associated with higher patient satisfaction, better outcomes and improved adherence to care regime (Hensley, 2012). Patient centered care is also associated with better recovery, better emotional health, reduced diagnostic tests and reduced need for referrals, improving cost and efficiency (Stewart et al., 2007).

The Picker Institute identifies 8 dimensions of patient-centered care. These are applicable in the psychiatric setting and include:

1. Respect for the patient's values, preferences and expressed needs: This allows the patient's treatment planning to shift into a partnership as the patient is able to assert their values and influence their treatment plan.
2. Information and education: This encourages open communication and mandates the full scope of information provided to the patient so that they can make informed decisions.
3. Improved access to care: Access to care means that patients can receive care in a setting that is easy, safe and comfortable for the patient.
4. Provision of emotional support to relieve fear and anxiety: This humanizes the person behind the disease, removing stigma associated with working with psychiatric patients.
5. Involvement of family and friends: This allows family/friends to advocate for the patient.
6. Continuity and secure transition between health care settings: This supports the patient as they transition between different aspects of their psychiatric care as well as their transition to their outside lives, ensuring stability.
7. Physical comfort: This allows patients to be comfortable in their environment, in safe and comfortable settings while in psychiatric care and while in their outside lives.
8. Coordination of care: This allows the patient to be effectively treated by all members of the team (Davis et al., 2005; Hensley, 2012).

Patient centered care is applicable even, and perhaps especially, in situations where a patient is admitted involuntarily or in forensic mental health settings. However, patient-centered care among these populations is considered more complicated. For example, the settings of forensic mental health must prioritize safety over calm and comfort, and treatment is not always elective. These factors may foster an environment where patients may not desire to participate in their own care (Livingston et al., 2012). In one forensic hospital located in British Columbia, researchers staged an intervention focused on patient-centered care, involving changes such as increased patient empowerment, engagement and altered therapeutic milieu and found that patients and clinicians viewed as satisfactory the level of recovery-oriented care and held positive views about the therapeutic milieu. Furthermore, a higher level of personal recovery in patients was correlated with greater empowerment and lower internalized stigma (Livingston et al., 2012). Studies such as these suggest that patient-centered care is applicable in many settings.

9.6 Psychological Impacts of COVID-19 on Nurses

Regardless of specialty, nurses have faced unprecedented stress across the globe as a result of the COVID-19 pandemic. Increased rates of depression (Ettman et al., 2020; Lai et al., 2020), anxiety (Cao et al., 2020; Lai et al., 2020), eating disorders (Phillipou et al., 2020) and substance use (Pollard et al., 2020) have been reported and nurses are no exception to these statistics. Being on the front lines of the pandemic puts nurses at increased risk for emotional and/or moral distress and burnout while attempting to cope with secondary trauma and navigate systemic issues.

Many nurses in areas hard-hit by the pandemic were re-deployed to areas in need of additional staff, creating stressors around working in an unfamiliar environment, and increased exposure to critical illness and death. Nurses and nurse leaders often worked beyond their normally scheduled hours, both by choice and out of necessity. Nurses and other clinicians, particularly in the early days of the pandemic, worried about the transmissibility of COVID-19 and whether they were putting themselves or their families at risk for death simply by showing up for work. The extent of the nurse's "duty to care" was often called into question: is there a "duty" to provide care even if it means risking one's own health? Is this morally obligatory, or supererogatory?

Early data have shown that the psychological impacts of the pandemic on nurses are far reaching. For example, nurses in China who were involved in the direct care of patients with COVID were more likely to experience depression, anxiety, insomnia, and emotional distress (Lai et al., 2020). Nurses too often become socialized to the idea that caring for others comes at the expense of caring for themselves and they may not be aware of resources to prevent or treat mental health concerns. Further, personal, and professional stigma towards nurses with psychiatric needs may present additional barriers to appropriate care.

Resources for promoting nurses' mental wellbeing:

- APNA Well-Being Initiative and Nurses Guide to Mental Health Support Services: https://www.apna.org
- American Nurses Association (ANA) Happy App: https://www.happythemovement.com/ana
- https://www.2020yearofthenurse.org/
- https://rcni.com/nursing-standard/features/how-covid-19-affecting-nurses-mental-health-and-what-to-do-about-it-159456
- https://www.nursingtimes.net/news/mental-health/global-nursing-body-issues-warning-on-nurse-mental-health-during-covid-19-crisis-30-04-2020/
- https://www.ispn-psych.org/mental-health-links
- https://www.nursingtimes.net/news/covid-19-are-you-ok/

9.6.1 Secondary Trauma

Secondary trauma, sometimes referred to as "vicarious trauma," occurs when nurses bear witness to the highly stressful events of other's lives. Secondary trauma is common in mental health nursing, but also in critical and emergency care, pediatrics, oncology and midwifery (Missouridou, 2017). During the COVID-19 pandemic, nurses working in hospitals have watched as patients faced uncertainty, physical isolation, invasive medical procedures and even death without the benefit of having loved ones present due to restrictions on visitation. On top of this, many patients, including some psychiatric patients and children, do not have the cognitive or developmental capacity to understand the rationale for various restrictions in place (though in certain areas, exceptions to visitation restrictions were made for these particularly vulnerable groups). Facing these traumas has put healthcare workers, including nurses, at risk for developing psychological symptoms (e.g. insomnia, emotional distress) or mental health conditions (e.g. depression, anxiety) (Lai et al., 2020). While the longitudinal effects of secondary trauma from COVID are yet to be seen, specialists are predicting an ongoing "secondary pandemic" of increased mental health concerns (Choi et al., 2020).

There are many consequences of exposure to trauma, including cognitive and mood changes, sleep disturbance and hyperarousal (American Psychiatric Association, 2013; Choi et al., 2020). Among nurses, emotions associated with trauma may be difficult to process and various patterns of behavior including disengagement, overinvolvement or maladaptive coping may occur (Missouridou, 2017). Specifically, these responses to trauma may result in worse patient care and lack of self-care by nurses, both of which present ethical concerns. Nurses, including those in nursing leadership roles, can reduce the impact of secondary trauma by fostering organizational awareness and promoting teamwork. Programs focused on building resilience may be particularly useful for healthcare workers (Choi et al., 2020). Other specific ways to reduce the burdens of secondary trauma include attending or encouraging staff to attend ongoing trainings, promoting self-care both in and outside of work and providing opportunities for or seeking out clinical supervision (Choi et al., 2020; Missouridou, 2017).

9.6.2 Mental Health Workforce

In addition to the consequences of the COVID pandemic on nurses' wellbeing, the "secondary pandemic" of increased mental illness (Choi et al., 2020) has implications for the mental health workforce. A paucity of mental health providers, including psychiatric nurses, existed before the pandemic (American Psychiatric Nurses Association [APNA], 2019; Substance Abuse and Mental Health Services Administration [SAMHSA], 2019) and the need for mental health treatment is now expanding. In the

United States, the current workforce of mental health nurses is aging and lacks diversity (Phoenix, 2019). Rural areas are especially struggling with too few psychiatric providers, including mental health nurses (Phoenix, 2019). To support the growing need for mental health treatment, all nurses should receive education on recognizing and treating common illnesses like anxiety, depression and substance use disorders. Increased availability of specialized educational opportunities will also be important to diversify the mental health nursing workforce. Finally, allowing nurses and psychiatric nurse practitioners to practice to the full extent of their education and training will increase access to mental healthcare (APNA, 2019).

In addition to supporting efforts to increase the number of nurses and other providers working in mental health, changes to insurance requirements and the use of new technology to expand access to mental healthcare will also be useful. For example, insurance companies can continue to reimburse for telepsychiatry which will allow for providers to reach rural and other underserved populations more easily. Funding can be allocated to mental health start-ups, including app-based therapy platforms, companies that help facilitate insurance reimbursement for providers and other tech-enabled mental health services, such as online screening or self-help tools.

9.7 Case Studies

9.7.1 Case 1: Implicit Bias

A nurse is working on a medical-surgical floor at a community hospital and is assigned to care for an incarcerated individual while they are on the unit. In addition to physical health needs, the patient has a history of major depression and opioid use disorder. Despite the patient reporting a high level of pain, the nurse notices that, according to the patient's chart, the patient has not been receiving pain medication.

1. What role might implicit bias have in this patient's care or lack of care?
2. How can the nurse work to recognize and reduce personal implicit bias that may arise?
3. How can the nurse practice patient centered care for this individual?

Case Resolution: The nurse recognizes the existence of bias and stigma towards individuals with mental illness, substance use disorders and who are incarcerated, including among nurses and other healthcare workers. Implicit bias results in subpar assessments, inappropriate diagnoses, treatment and follow up, and less time spent addressing patient's needs. Therefore, the nurse understands that inadequate pain management may be a result of implicit bias against this patient. The nurse uses mindfulness and stereotype replacing to reduce personal implicit bias that may arise. The nurse also considers the role that social determinants of health, like socioeconomic status, early childhood development and education play in access to healthcare and healthcare outcomes and the role that race/racism has on social determinants of health. Through this knowledge and self-reflection, the nurse works to adequately address the patient's pain. The nurse utilizes patient centered care by allowing the patient to speak for themselves and works to be an active listener.

9.7.2 Case 2: Therapeutic Use of Self

A nurse on an inpatient psychiatric unit is caring for a patient who is nearing discharge. The patient has been hospitalized for 3 weeks and many other patients on the unit turn to this individual for advice. The patient has some overlapping interests with the nurse and reminds the nurse of a close and supportive friend of theirs. The patient often asks the nurse, "how are you doing today?" The nurse feels a sense of closeness to and fondness for the patient and notices a tendency to want to respond by sharing frustration at hospital administration or worries about a particular family member who is struggling.

1. Awareness is an important part of the therapeutic use of self. What personal emotions or reactions should the nurse be aware of in this situation?
2. Consider the pros and cons of sharing personal feelings of frustration or worries with this patient?
3. What could the nurse do within their professional community to navigate the countertransference they are experiencing?
4. What could the nurse do outside of their professional community to navigate the countertransference they are experiencing?
5. How might the nurse's code of ethics inform their decisions in this case, and guide them regarding establishing professional boundaries?
6. What ethical implications might follow from blurred professional boundaries?

Case Resolution: The nurse acknowledges the feelings of closeness to and fondness for the patient and the positive countertransference that they are experiencing. The nurse recognizes that these types of reactions are normal but that an awareness that they are happening is important in maintaining professional boundaries and the nurse's privacy. The nurse recognizes that although sharing frustration or worry with the patient might foster a sense of rapport, it may shift the focus away from the patient's psychiatric needs or cause the patient to feel responsible for the nurse's mental health, which may impact the care the patient receives. The nurse attends bi-weekly peer-supervision with other nurses and consults with their manager to appropriately process this countertransference. The nurse also utilizes self-care strategies, like walking for 30 min three times weekly and limiting the number of extra shifts they sign up for in order to help manage the frustration and worry that they are feeling.

9.8 Summary

In the prior discussion several issues of ethical importance to nurses working in psychiatric and mental health settings were discussed and strategies for ethical practice with people suffering from mental illness or mental health disorders, provided. Additionally, these insights and strategies will be helpful for all of those encountering mental health issues in practice. While we could not cover all possible eventualities, the content of this chapter along with the tools for ethical decision making that are available in Chapters 1, 2 and 3 equip nurses for ethical decision making in settings where mental health issues present. The current COVID-19 pandemic has illuminated the fact that mental health issues can affect any one of us, thus inter- and intra-disciplinary collaborations may be needed to resolve problems and to provide support.

References

Alegría, M., NeMoyer, A., Bagué, I. F., Wang, Y., & Alvarez, K. (2018). Social determinants of mental health: Where we are and where we need to go. *Current Psychiatry Reports, 20*(11), 95.

American Psychiatric Association. (2013). *Diagnostic and statistical manual of mental disorders* (5th ed.). American Psychiatric Publishing.

American Psychiatric Nurses Association [APNA]. (2019). *Expanding mental health care services in America: The pivotal role of psychiatric-mental health nurses.* https://www.apna.org/files/public/Resources/Expanding_Mental_Health_Care_Services_in_America-The_Pivotal_Role_of_Psychiatric-Mental_Health_Nurses_04_19.pdf

Ashmore, R., & Banks, D. (2002). Self-disclosure in adult and mental health nursing students. *British Journal of Nursing, 11*(3), 172–177.

Bailey, Z. D., Krieger, N., Agénor, M., Graves, J., Linos, N., & Bassett, M. T. (2017). Structural racism and health inequities in the USA: Evidence and interventions. *The Lancet, 389*(10077), 1453–1463.

Berliner, L., & Kolko, D. J. (2016). Trauma informed care: A commentary and critique. *Child Maltreatment, 21*(2), 168–172.

Berring, L. L., Pedersen, L., & Buus, N. (2016). Coping with violence in mental health care settings: Patient and staff member perspectives on de-escalation practices. *Archives of Psychiatric Nursing, 30*(5), 499–507.

Berwick, D. M. (2020). The moral determinants of health. *JAMA, 324*(3), 225–226.

Bevilacqua Guarniero, F., Bellinghini, R. H., & Gattaz, W. F. (2017). The schizophrenia stigma and mass media: A search for news published by wide circulation media in Brazil. *International Review of Psychiatry, 29*(3), 241–247.

Bigwood, S., & Crowe, M. (2008). 'It's part of the job, but it spoils the job': A phenomenological study of physical restraint. *International Journal of Mental Health Nursing, 17*(3), 215–222.

Blease, C. R., Walker, J., Torous, J., & O'Neil, S. (2020). Sharing clinical notes in psychotherapy: A new tool to strengthen patient autonomy. *Frontiers in Psychiatry, 11*, 1–4.

Boyd, M. (2018). *Psychiatric nursing: Contemporary practice* (6th ed.). Wolters Kluwer Health/Lippincott Williams & Wilkins.

Burgess, D. J., Beach, M. C., & Saha, S. (2017). Mindfulness practice: A promising approach to reducing the effects of clinician implicit bias on patients. *Patient Education and Counseling, 100*(2), 372–376.

Cao, W., Fang, Z., Hou, G., Han, M., Xu, X., Dong, J., & Zheng, J. (2020). The psychological impact of the COVID-19 epidemic on college students in China. *Psychiatry Research, 287*, 112934.
Centers for Disease Control and Prevention. (2020a, May 13). *Elder abuse.* https://www.cdc.gov/violenceprevention/elderabuse/index.html
Centers for Disease Control and Prevention. (2020b, April 3). *Preventing adverse childhood experiences.* https://www.cdc.gov/violenceprevention/aces/fastfact.html?CDC_AA_ref Val=https%3A%2F%2Fwww.cdc.gov%2Fviolenceprevention%2Facestudy%2Ffastfact.htmll
Centers for Disease Control and Prevention. (2020c, April 7). *Preventing child abuse and neglect.* https://www.cdc.gov/violenceprevention/childabuseandneglect/fastfact.html
Centers for Disease Control and Prevention. (2021, January 26). *Social determinants of health: Know what affects health.* https://www.cdc.gov/socialdeterminants/index.htm
Centers for Medicare and Medicaid Services. (n.d.). *The Mental Health Parity and Addiction Equity Act (MHPAEA).* https://www.cms.gov/CCIIO/Programs-and-Initiatives/Other-Insurance-Protections/mhpaea_factsheet
Chang-Quan, H., Zheng-Rong, W., Yong-Hong, L., & Qing-Xiu, L. (2010). Education and risk for late life depression: A meta-analysis of published literature. *International Journal Psychiatry Medicine, 40*(1), 109–124.
Chisholm, D., Sweeny, K., Sheehan, P., Rasmussen, B., Smit, F., Cuijpers, P., & Saxena, S. (2016). Scaling-up treatment of depression and anxiety: A global return on investment analysis. *The Lancet Psychiatry, 3*(5), 415–424.
Choi, K. R., Heilemann, M. V., Fauer, A., & Mead, M. (2020). A second pandemic: Mental health spillover from the novel coronavirus (COVID-19). *Journal of the American Psychiatric Nurses Association, 26*(4), 340–343.
Chunara, R., Zhao, Y., Chen, J., Lawrence, K., Testa, P. A., Nov, O., & Mann, D. M. (2020). Telemedicine and healthcare disparities: A cohort study in a large healthcare system in New York City during COVID-19. *Journal of the American Medical Informatics Association, 28*(1), 33–41.
Corrigan, P. W., Morris, S. B., Michaels, P. J., Rafacz, J. D., & Rüsch, N. (2012). Challenging the public stigma of mental illness: A meta-analysis of outcome studies. *Psychiatric Services, 63*(10), 963–973.
Corrigan, P. W., Kerr, A., & Knudsen, L. (2005). The stigma of mental illness: Explanatory models and methods for change. *Applied and Preventive Psychology, 11*(3), 179–190.
Cunningham, P. J. (2009). Beyond parity: Primary care physicians' perspectives on access to mental health care: More PCPs have trouble obtaining mental health services for their patients than have problems getting other specialty services. *Health Affairs, 28*(Suppl. 1), w490–w501.
Davis, K., Schoenbaum, S. C., & Audet, A. M. (2005). A 2020 vision of patient-centered primary care. *Journal of General Internal Medicine, 20*(10), 953–957.
Epstein, R. (2017). *Attending: Medicine, mindfulness, and humanity.* Simon and Schuster.
Ettman, C. K., Abdalla, S. M., Cohen, G. H., Sampson, L., Vivier, P. M., & Galea, S. (2020). Prevalence of depression symptoms in US adults before and during the COVID-19 pandemic. *JAMA Network Open, 3*(9), e2019686–e2019686.
FitzGerald, C., & Hurst, S. (2017). Implicit bias in healthcare professionals: A systematic review. *BMC Medical Ethics, 18*(1), 19.
Fraser, J. A., Mathews, B., Walsh, K., Chen, L., & Dunne, M. (2010). Factors influencing child abuse and neglect recognition and reporting by nurses: A multivariate analysis. *International Journal of Nursing Studies, 47*(2), 146–153.
Fuss, J., Briken, P., & Klein, V. (2018). Gender bias in clinicians' pathologization of atypical sexuality: A randomized controlled trial with mental health professionals. *Scientific Reports, 8*(1), 1–9.
Gastmans, C. (1998). Interpersonal relations in nursing: A philosophical-ethical analysis of the work of Hildegard E. Peplau. *Journal of Advanced Nursing, 28*(6), 1312–1319.
Giacco, D., & Priebe, S. (2016). Suicidality and hostility following involuntary hospital treatment. *PloS One, 11*(5), e0154458.

Grace, P. J., & Willis, D. G. (2012). Nursing responsibilities and social justice: An analysis in support of disciplinary goals. *Nursing Outlook, 60*(4), 198–207.

Hayward, P., & Bright, J. (1997). Stigma and mental illness: A review and critique. *Journal of Mental Health, 6*(4), 345–354.

Hensley, M. A. (2012). Patient-centered care and psychiatric rehabilitation: What's the connection? *The International Journal of Psychosocial Rehabilitation, 17*(1), 135–141.

Hopper, E. K., Bassuk, E. L., & Olivet, J. (2010). Shelter from the storm: Trauma-informed care in homelessness services settings. *The Open Health Services and Policy Journal, 3*(1), 80–100.

Hubley, S., Lynch, S. B., Schneck, C., Thomas, M., & Shore, J. (2016). Review of key telepsychiatry outcomes. *World Journal of Psychiatry, 6*(2), 269–282.

Huckvale, K., Torous, J., & Larsen, M. E. (2019). Assessment of the data sharing and privacy practices of smartphone apps for depression and smoking cessation. *JAMA Network Open, 2*(4), e192542–e192542.

Institute for Healthcare Improvement, IHI Multimedia Team. (2017, September 28). *How to reduce implicit bias.* http://www.ihi.org/communities/blogs/how-to-reduce-implicit-bias

Johnson, M. E., & Delaney, K. R. (2007). Keeping the unit safe: The anatomy of escalation. *Journal of the American Psychiatric Nurses Association, 13*(1), 42–52.

Kabat-Zinn, J., & Hanh, T. N. (2009). *Full catastrophe living: Using the wisdom of your body and mind to face stress, pain, and illness.* Delta.

Kenyon, C., Sandel, M., Silverstein, M., Shakir, A., & Zuckerman, B. (2007). Revisiting the social history for child health. *Pediatrics, 120*(3), 734–738.

Lai, J., Ma, S., Wang, Y., Cai, Z., Hu, J., Wei, N., Wu, J., Du, H., Chen, T., Li, R., Tan, H., Kang, L., Yao, L., Huang, M., Wang, H., Wang, G., Liu, Z., & Hu, S. (2020). Factors associated with mental health outcomes among health care workers exposed to coronavirus disease 2019. *JAMA Network Open, 3*(3), e203976–e203976.

Livingston, J. D., Nijdam-Jones, A., & Brink, J. (2012). A tale of two cultures: Examining patient-centered care in a forensic mental health hospital. *The Journal of Forensic Psychiatry & Psychology, 23*(3), 345–360.

McQueen, A. (2000). Nurse–patient relationships and partnership in hospital care. *Journal of Clinical Nursing, 9*(5), 723–731.

McTavish, J. R., Kimber, M., Devries, K., Colombini, M., MacGregor, J., Wathen, C. N., Agarwal, A., & MacMillan, H. L. (2017). Mandated reporters' experiences with reporting child maltreatment: A meta-synthesis of qualitative studies. *BMJ Open, 7*(10), e013942.

Mersky, J. P., Topitzes, J., & Reynolds, A. J. (2013). The impact of adverse childhood experiences on health, mental health and substance use in early adulthood: A cohort study of an urban, minority sample in the U.S. *Child Abuse & Neglect, 37*(11), 917–925.

Missouridou, E. (2017). Secondary posttraumatic stress and nurses' emotional responses to patient's trauma. *Journal of Trauma Nursing, 24*(2), 110–115.

Mitchison, D., Hay, P., Slewa-Younan, S., & Mond, J. (2014). The changing demographic profile of eating disorder behaviors in the community. *BMC Public Health, 14*(1), 943.

Mohr, W. K. (2010). Restraints and the code of ethics: An uneasy fit. *Archives of Psychiatric Nursing, 24*(1), 3–14.

Monahan, J., Hoge, S. K., Lidz, C., Roth, L. H., Bennett, N., Gardner, W., & Mulvey, E. (1995). Coercion and commitment: Understanding involuntary mental hospital admission. *International Journal of Law and Psychiatry, 18*(3), 249–263.

Muskett, C. (2014). Trauma-informed care in inpatient mental health settings: A review of the literature. *International Journal of Mental Health Nursing, 23*(1), 51–59.

Narayan, M. C. (2019). CE: Addressing implicit bias in nursing: A review. *The American Journal of Nursing, 119*(7), 36–43.

National Institute of Mental Health. (2021). *Mental illness.* https://www.nimh.nih.gov/health/statistics/mental-illness.shtml#:~:text=Mental%20illnesses%20are%20common%20in,mild%20to%20moderate%20to%20severe

Nikulina, V., Widom, C. S., & Czaja, S. (2011). The role of childhood neglect and childhood poverty in predicting mental health, academic achievement and crime in adulthood. *American Journal of Community Psychology, 48*(3–4), 309–321.

Office of Disease Prevention and Health Promotion. (2020, October 8). *Social determinants of health*. https://www.healthypeople.gov/2020/topics-objectives/topic/social-determinants-of-health

Office of the National Coordinator for the Health Information Technology. (n.d.). *ONC's Cures Act Final Rule supports seamless and secure access, exchange and use of electronic health information*. https://www.healthit.gov/curesrule/

O'Kelly, G. (1998). Countertransference in the nurse-patient relationship: A review of the literature. *Journal of Advanced Nursing, 28*(2), 391–397.

Peplau, H. E. (1991). *Interpersonal relations in nursing: A conceptual frame of reference for psychodynamic nursing*. Springer.

Petersson, L., & Erlingsdottir, G. (2018a). Open notes in swedish psychiatric care (part 1): Survey among psychiatric care professionals. *JMIR Mental Health, 5*(1), e11

Petersson, L., & Erlingsdottir, G. (2018b). Open notes in Swedish psychiatric care (part 2): Survey among psychiatric care professionals. *JMIR Mental Health, 5*(2), e10521.

Phillipou, A., Meyer, D., Neill, E., Tan, E. J., Toh, W. L., Van Rheenen, T. E., & Rossell, S. L. (2020). Eating and exercise behaviors in eating disorders and the general population during the COVID-19 pandemic in Australia: Initial results from the COLLATE project. *International Journal of Eating Disorders, 53*(7), 1158–1165.

Phoenix, B. J. (2019). The current psychiatric mental health registered nurse workforce. *Journal of the American Psychiatric Nurses Association, 25*(1), 38–48.

Pollard, M. S., Tucker, J. S., & Green, H. D. (2020). Changes in adult alcohol use and consequences during the COVID-19 pandemic in the US. *JAMA Network Open, 3*(9), e2022942–e2022942.

Reeves, A., Stuckler, D., McKee, M., Gunnell, D., Chang, S., & Basu, S. (2012). Increase in state suicide rates in the USA during economic recession. *The Lancet, 380*(9856), 1813–1814.

Ridley, M., Rao, G., Schilbach, F., & Patel, V. (2020). Poverty, depression, and anxiety: Causal evidence and mechanisms. *Science, 370*(6522).

Rutenberg, C., & Oberle, K. (2008). Ethics in telehealth nursing practice. *Home Health Care Management & Practice, 20*(4), 342–348.

Saraceno, B., Funk, M., Pathare, S., & Minoletti, A. (2003). *Mental health legislation and human rights: Mental Health policy and service guidance package*. World Health Organization.

Schmitz-Buhl, M., Gairing, S. K., Rietz, C., et al. (2019). A retrospective analysis of determinants of involuntary psychiatric in-patient treatment. *BMC Psychiatry, 19*, 127.

Schnurr, P. P., & Green, B. L. (2004). Understanding relationships among trauma, posttraumatic stress disorder, and health outcomes. In P. P. Schnurr & B. L. Green (Eds.), *Trauma and health: Physical health consequences of exposure to extreme stress*. (Chapter 10, pp. 247–275). American Psychological Association.

Schuman-Olivier, Z., Trombka, M., Lovas, D. A., Brewer, J. A., Vago, D. R., Gawande, R., Dunne, J. P., Lazar, S. W., Loucks, E. B., & Fulwiler, C. (2020). Mindfulness and behavior change. *Harvard Review of Psychiatry, 28*(6), 371.

Schweinhart, L. J. (2007). Outcomes of the high/scope Perry preschool study and Michigan school readiness program. In *Early child development: From measurement to action* (pp. 87–102). World Bank.

Sederer, L. I. (2016). The social determinants of mental health. *Psychiatric Services, 67*(2), 234–235.

Seeman, N., Tang, S., Brown, A. D., & Ing, A. (2016). World survey of mental illness stigma. *Journal of Affective Disorders, 190*, 115–121.

Segal, Z. V., Williams, M., & Teasdale, J. (2018). *Mindfulness-based cognitive therapy for depression*. Guilford Publications.

Shim, R. S., & Compton, M. T. (2018). Addressing the social determinants of mental health: If not now, when? If not us, who? *Psychiatric Services, 69*(8), 844–846.

Shim, R. S. & Compton, M. T. (2019). The social determinants of mental health. In L. W. Roberts (Ed.), *The American Psychiatric Association publishing textbook of psychiatry* (7th ed., Chapter 6, pp. 163–175). American Psychiatric Association Publishing.

Steinberg, K. L., Levine, M., & Doueck, H. J. (1997). Effects of legally mandated child-abuse reports on the therapeutic relationship: A survey of psychotherapists. *American Journal of Orthopsychiatry, 67*(1), 112–122.

Stewart, M. A., Brown, J. B., Donner, A., & McWhinney, I. R. (2007). The impact of patient-centered care on outcomes. *The Journal of Family Practice, 49*(9), 796–804.

Strowd, R. E., Strauss, L., Graham, R., Dodenhoff, K., Schreiber, A., Thomson, S., Ambrosini, A., Thurman, A. M., Olszewski, C., Smith, L. D., Cartwright, M. S., Guzik, A., Wells, R. E., Munger Clary, H, Malone, J., Ezzeddine, M, Duncan, P. W., & Tegeler, C. (2020). Rapid implementation of outpatient teleneurology in rural Appalachia: Barriers and disparities. *Neurology: Clinical Practice, 11*, 232–241.

Stuart, H. (2008). Fighting the stigma caused by mental disorders: Past perspectives, present activities, and future directions. *World Psychiatry: Official Journal of the World Psychiatric Association (WPA), 7*(3), 185–188.

Substance Abuse and Mental Health Services Administration. (2014a). Understanding the impact of trauma. In *A treatment improvement protocol: Trauma-informed care in behavioral health services* (Chapter 3, pp. 59–90). US Department of Health and Human Services.

Substance Abuse and Mental Health Services Administration. (2014b). *SAMHSA's concept of trauma and guidance for a trauma-informed approach [Fact sheet]*. Department of Health and Human Services. https://ncsacw.samhsa.gov/userfiles/files/SAMHSA_Trauma.pdf

Substance Abuse and Mental Health Services Administration [SAMHSA]. (2019). *Behavioral health workforce report*. https://www.samhsa.gov/sites/default/files/behavioral-health-workforce-report.pdf

Sugaya, L., Hasin, D. S., Olfson, M., Lin, K., Grant, B. F., & Blanco, C. (2012). Child physical abuse and adult mental health: A national study. *Journal of Traumatic Stress, 25*(4), 384–392.

Tomaz, T., & Castro-Vale, I. (2020). Trauma-informed care in primary health settings-which is even more needed in times of Covid-19. *Healthcare (Basel, Switzerland), 8*(3), 340.

United Nations. (2015). Transforming our world: The 2030 agenda for sustainable development. https://sdgs.un.org/2030agenda

van Voren, R. (2016). Ending political abuse of psychiatry: Where we are at and what needs to be done. *BJPsych Bulletin, 40*(1), 30–33.

Varshney, M., Mahapatra, A., Krishnan, V., Gupta, R., & Deb, K. S. (2016). Violence and mental illness: What is the true story? *Journal of Epidemiology and Community Health, 70*(3), 223–225.

Walsh, C. G., Xia, W., Li, M., Denny, J. C., Harris, P. A., & Malin, B. A. (2018). Enabling open-science initiatives in clinical psychology and psychiatry without sacrificing patients' privacy: Current practices and future challenges. *Advances in Methods and Practices in Psychological Science, 1*(1), 104–114.

Weinreb, L., Savageau, J. A., Candib, L. M., Reed, G. W., & Fletcher, K. E. (2010). Screening for childhood trauma in adult primary care patients: A cross-sectional survey. *Primary Care Companion to the Journal of Clinical Psychiatry, 12*(6).

Wilson, C., Pence, D. M., & Conradi, L. (2013). Trauma-informed care. In *Encyclopedia of social work*. NASW Press and Oxford University Press.

Winerman, L. (2017). By the numbers: The cost of treatment. *Monitor on Psychology, 48*(3), 80.

World Health Organization. (2020). *Mental health*. https://www.who.int/mental_health/who_urges_investment/en/

Xu, W. Y., Song, C., Li, Y., & Retchin, S. M. (2019). Cost-sharing disparities for out-of-network care for adults with behavioral health conditions. *JAMA Network Open, 2*(11), e1914554–e1914554.

Yang, Y., & Parrott, S. (2018). Schizophrenia in Chinese and US online news media: Exploring cultural influence on the mediated portrayal of schizophrenia. *Health Communication, 33*(5), 553–561.

Yaribeygi, H., Panahi, Y., Sahraei, H., Johnston, T. P., & Sahebkar, A. (2017). The impact of stress on body function: A review. *EXCIL Journal: Experimental and Clinical Sciences, 16*, 1057–1072.

Chapter 10
Research on Human Subjects: Nurses Roles and Responsibilities

Pamela J. Grace and Aimee Milliken

Abstract Nurses encounter the human subjects of research in many different settings and their relationships with the person who is on a research protocol may take any of a number of different forms. They may: be asked for their advice about whether a person should participate in a study, care for someone who is on a research protocol, or serve as a research protocol coordinator or a member of the research team. Some nurses with advanced degrees may serve as principal investigators who design and implement research studies. Regardless of role, if they are enacting a role because they are nurses with nursing expertise, then nursing perspectives and values ought to predominate over research values when these seem to conflict. People who are trying to decide whether to take part in a study need good information in a form that permits them to grasp the implications for them and perhaps for their families. It is important for both the research subject and the integrity of the research protocol, that nurses understand the history of research ethics, the risks and benefits of human subjects' research and their ethical responsibilities to the subject. This chapter provides a brief history of the development of research using human beings, illustrating both benefits and pitfalls. Ethical principles associated with the protection of human beings are detailed. Throughout, different types of studies are discussed along with their special considerations. Finally, we provide some case discussions to serve as concrete examples of issues, along with strategies that nurses can use to resolve problems they encounter.

P. J. Grace (✉)
William F. Connell School of Nursing, Boston College, Chestnut Hill, Boston, MA 02467, USA
e-mail: Gracepa@bc.edu

A. Milliken
William F. Connell School of Nursing, Boston College, Chestnut Hill, MA, USA
e-mail: aimee.milliken@bc.edu

10.1 Introduction

10.1.1 Subject Versus Participant

In this chapter we refer to people who are enrolled in research studies of various sorts as subjects. This is the term that is used internationally. However, there is contemporary debate about whether it is more respectful to call them participants. The thought is that a participant is one who is voluntarily engaging in the research (Hurley, 2019). But as Hurley (2019) notes, "(B)eyond engagement, it suggests the individual has some ownership or investment in the research project in question, or in its outcomes or findings" (p. 2). However, there are compelling reasons not to abandon the term 'subjects'. For example, not all who are the subjects of research are willing participants. Research on groups, studies using big data, with those who are cognitively impaired or cognitively undeveloped are not able to voluntarily consent. Persons enrolled in research can rarely be said to be on an equal footing with the researcher. Hurley (2019) argues that the term "subject" remains important. It helps us overcome the problem of "real power and knowledge asymmetries between researchers and those upon whom research interventions or procedures are done, or about whom information is being collected" (p. 3).

10.1.2 Research Benefits, Burdens and Injustice

The results of research on human beings have greatly improved the human potential for living a good life and/or overcoming disease. However, it is also true that unethical research has caused immeasurable suffering with lasting impacts. While currently in most countries regulations and safeguards have been instituted to protect human subjects, risks remain. They do so for many reasons. Problems can occur after the start of an approved protocol and between periods of direct oversight by regulators. Study design may also be problematic and subject to bias and abuses, despite institutional oversight. Nurses may be the first or only ones to recognize problems occurring at the subject-intervention interface or when it is recognized that subject circumstances, preferences, or sense of the study's burdens have changed (DeBruin et al., 2011). Another major reason for risk is that research on human subjects is primarily aimed at developing knowledge that can benefit groups of people or even a society. Thus, there is a tendency to prioritize the common good over the good of the individual, even when this may result in burdensome or potentially harmful impacts for the individual. Yet to lose sight of the individual subject as important is and has been problematic for society. What is important about societies is they are made up of individuals who, ideally anyway, contribute in different ways to its functioning (Grace, 2018). This tension between individual and societal good illustrates the difficulty of relying on a particular moral theory for direction as discussed in earlier chapters. There is an obvious clash of values between consequentialist theoretical ideas about what it is good for human beings to pursue, and deontologic perspectives. Consequentialism theorizes that what it is good for humans to pursue is the greatest good for the greatest number and allows for the possibility that it is permissible to disadvantage some people in order to benefit the majority. Whereas deontologic (duty-based) theoretical ideas hold that above all human beings must be respected as individuals and not used solely as an object enabling others to reach their goals (as examples of treating people as objects, slavery and human trafficking are both practices that use human beings as mere objects to benefit others). Reconciling these tensions is a job for the field of inquiry that is research ethics.

There are a host of other issues associated with research that can put a subject at risk, perhaps inadvertently. For example, an oncology patient who is enrolled in a drug study, may be inclined to view the site principal investigator (PI) as they would their own physician or healthcare provider, yet the main goal of the PI is to maintain the study integrity so that the results are reliable. This is an example of the concept of therapeutic misconception. Lidz and Appelbaum (2002) note this occurs, "when a research subject fails to appreciate the distinction between the imperatives of clinical research and of ordinary treatment, and therefore inaccurately attributes therapeutic intent to research procedure" (V. 57). This line is often blurred for cancer patients as disease progresses and effective lines of standard therapy become exhausted, and enrollment in clinical trials is pursued as a "last ditch" effort.

Another example of potential risk to subjects involves the fact that researchers are rewarded, in various ways for completed and published studies. The rewards can include promotion, easier access to future grants, and even the possibility of profits if the researcher has interests in the company sponsoring the study. This was a major problem in the Jesse Gelsinger case described in more detail later. Jesse, a teenager, agreed to take part in this Phase I trial of a gene vector. He experienced an overwhelming immune response and died. Although there were many problems with the research process, a major issue was the economic incentive for the researcher. Subsequently it was discovered that, "the principal investigator held $13 million in equity in Genovo, the biotechnology firm supplying the viral vector used in the trial" (Kong, 2005, p. 205). Thus there may be incentives that distort a research team's perspective and cause them to disregard two of the principles that guide research on human subjects, respect for persons and beneficence. These warrants of these principles are described in detail later. Persons with terminal diseases may enroll in a study in the hopes they will be cured, even when the study is not aimed at cure. There is also a risk of subtle inducements to participate in terms of reimbursement. In the case of research on children, parents might be persuaded by the idea of financial help and override the child's unwillingness to be in the study. As the chapter progresses these issues are exemplified and the nurse's role in advocating is clarified. First, though, we trace the history of research ethics as it developed internationally. This foundation sets the context for discussing the various issues and describing strategies for moving toward their resolution. Insights from cognitive psychology studies are helpful in understanding how human motivations related to research can become distorted.

10.2 A Brief History of Biomedical Research Ethics and Associated Regulations

While there has been a long history of efforts to understand illness and health by observation and experimentation, before the early 1900s these studies were mostly small in scope and not subject to regulations of any sort. For reasons given shortly, research efforts expanded exponentially in the 1900s and with this expansion the risks for inadvertent or advertent abuse of research subjects were exacerbated.

10.2.1 Defining Human Subjects Research

A comprehensive definition of research on human subjects is provided by the World Health Organization Manual (WHO, 2011). It is defined as,

> any social science, biomedical, behavioural, or epidemiological activity that entails systematic collection or analysis of data with the intent to generate new knowledge, in which human beings: are exposed to manipulation, intervention, observation, or other interaction with investigators either directly or through alteration of their environment; or become individually identifiable through investigator's collection, preparation, or use of biological material or medical or other records. (p. 40)

Other available definitions are similar in scope. One can see from this definition that there is quite a variety in types of research and their procedures. Studies may be *qualitative* in nature, seeking a better understanding of the meaning of experienced phenomena such as post-partum depression, child abuse, moral distress so on. These studies, for the most part, rely on subject perceptions of their experiences, although there are observational aspects as the researcher or assistants note such things as change in affect, or in the case of ethnography, how a social unit interacts. Some studies are *observational.* In these studies an investigator simply documents observations and analyzes data, but there are no interventions or changes in the care that would have been given or in other contextual features. *Interventional* studies on the other hand, are those in which "the investigator manipulates the subject or the subject's environment for the purpose of modifying one or more health-related biomedical or behavioral processes and/or endpoints" (National Institutes of Health, 2018). Clinical trials, such as drug studies are interventional in nature whether or not they randomize either a placebo (a substance with no therapeutic effect) or standard of care and an active substance. Finally, already existing data or human material may be analyzed for various purposes. An important thing to keep in mind is that harms are possible in any of these types of studies and should be anticipated, guarded against or where necessary minimized within the bounds of reasonableness. Ethical oversight committees, known as Institutional Review Boards in the United States, are charged with ensuring harms for a proposed study are as minimal as is feasible. Additionally, people have a right to be as fully informed as possible so as to enable them to make a decision that is in line with their values, preferences and the way they have lived their lives. This right to informed consent whether by the potential participant or an appropriate surrogate is a human right as described next.

10.2.2 Human Rights

Moral theorizing from Ancient Greek times to the present has sought to understand the place of human beings in the world. As noted earlier, resulting theories have different answers, however almost all recognize the importance of individual human beings and the need to respect them. The theories of Immanuel Kant (1724–1804) and Jean-Jacques Rousseau (1712–1778) have been influential in modern thinking and are based on the human ability to reason. Kant's quest was to establish "the supreme principle of morality" (Kant, 1965/1785, p. 321), discussed in more detail in Chapter 3. While, due to the perspectives during that time, women and children were not considered as being fully rational, children developmentally and women because their'nature is caring and nurturing' nevertheless, for Kant, they could strive towards rationality (Varden, 2017) and the ability to decide right actions based on using the internal 'format' of the categorical imperative. As a reminder, the categorical imperative essentially asserts that those actions that fit the format "Act only according to that maxim by which you can at the same time will that it should become a universal law" (Kant, 1965/1785, p. 339). This ability for self-imposed moral rules gives human beings an inviolable status of being an 'end in themselves', not subject to the will of others and not to be used by others as purely a means to their ends. This idea of individual human moral importance underlies the UN Declaration of Human Rights (1948). There are 190 nations that have signed on to this declaration.

10.2.3 Barriers to Honoring Human Rights

However, advances in cognitive science tend to highlight the problem that human beings do not always act as rationally as they might suppose even when intentionally trying to reason through a problem (van Gaal et al., 2012). Additionally, while Kant's theory proposes every human being to be of equal importance from a moral perspective, this is an ideal that is often not honored because of the tension between it and human desires for power and advantage. This permits the dehumanization of individuals and groups (Vaes et al., 2021). A huge problem in research, as well as in life, is that if a group of persons is not considered 'fully human' for some reason, it may be seen as morally permissible to exploit them (as evidenced by slavery, human trafficking, the Tuskegee syphilis study and so on). Contemporarily, the concept of human rights addresses such flaws emphasizing the idea that because human beings have common interests in surviving and flourishing, they ought to respect other human beings as having the same interests (Weston, 2011). Moreover human rights hold across countries and borders. The importance of human rights was codified after

WWII in the United Nations (1948) as the *Universal Declaration of Human Rights* in response to the harms inflicted by Nazis on the Jewish people and other people considered undesirable. At that time It was signed by 48 countries.

10.2.4 Nursing and Human Rights

As a profession, nursing ascribes to the idea of the pre-eminent importance of each individual person regardless of prior circumstances and deeds. As noted in the preamble of the International Council of Nursing's Code of Ethics (2012)

> Inherent in nursing is a respect for human rights, including cultural rights, the right to life and choice, to dignity and to be treated with respect. Nursing care is respectful of and unrestricted by considerations of age, colour, creed, culture, disability or illness, gender, sexual orientation, nationality, politics, race or social status.

The American Nurses Association's (2015) position statement on nursing and human rights, affirms that, "(N)urses establish relationships of trust and provide nursing services according to need, setting aside any bias or prejudice" (ANA, 2015, p. 1). This statement on ethics and human rights provides the foundation and context for all other position statements related to the practice of nursing.

Nevertheless nurses are human beings and susceptible to the problem of dehumanizing those for whom they are ethically responsible. This can happen for a variety of reasons such as personal troubles, moral distress about not being able to practice well over a period of time, pressures to go along with others expectations, encountering people who are difficult, among other causes as discussed shortly. Being mindful that we can be guilty of dehumanization and that this is problematic for individuals and society is one way of mitigating the problem. Additionally, imagining oneself, or someone one cares deeply about, being in a dehumanizing situation can serve as a reminder that any of us could end up in the category of persons who are deemed less than fully human and can then be treated as such.

10.2.5 Human Rights Infractions: Insights from Cognitive Psychology

Before discussing the actual history of human rights abuses and the subsequent need for independent oversight of research studies, some insights from cognitive psychology about how human minds work and why abuses occur, are helpful. In fact, one of the early studies in cognitive psychology, *The Stanford Prison Experiment* of 1971 sought to understand whether punitive behavior on the part of prison guards stemmed from their nature or was situational. The study used college students, some assigned as guards and some as prisoners, and observed their behavior over a period of several weeks. The experiment had to be prematurely stopped as it became obvious the students started to assume their assigned roles and the potential emotional damage to them became obvious. As Zimbardo (2005) noted, "the power of social situations to distort personal identities and long cherished values and morality as students internalized situated identities in their roles as prisoners and guards" was remarkable. This study was conducted prior to the institution of national research regulations in the United States and would not meet current research ethics standards for a variety of reasons, it nevertheless provided important insights since validated in later studies. Moreover, we have learned that when people feel powerless to change their situation, they can either blind themselves to the seriousness of the situation, what Chambliss (1996) calls the "routinization of disaster" (Chapter 1 Heading) or actively continue to participate in unethical practices. Importantly, knowing these sorts of predispositions allows us to be vigilant and mindful about what is happening and resist following those whose motivation has become distorted.

10.2.6 A Very Brief History of Human Rights Abuses in Research

Most healthcare professionals are broadly aware that there have been serious human rights violations related to research. These abuses are not anomalies. Although we would like to think that the most egregious would not be possible now, history shows us that without critical mindfulness and objective analyses new abuses are possible and do occur. The most well-known and wide-spread abuses occurred during World War II. During the Nazi era, researchers exposed those imprisoned in concentration camps to "extreme cold, pressure, diseases, and unproven therapies" (Murphy, 2004, p. 2), without their consent. The concentration camp prisoners were predominantly Jewish, although also included others deemed undesirable and a drain on society. Post-war trials of these mostly medical researchers, as part of the International War Crimes Tribunal, held in Nuremberg, Germany in 1947 resulted in the Nuremberg Code which detailed the conditions of permissible research. Around the same time there were also reported research abuses sponsored by the Japanese government. These involved "vivisection, battlefield injuries, hypothermia, and exposure to lethal infective diseases" (Murphy, 2004, p. 2).

10.2.6.1 The Nuremberg Code

The Nuremberg Code details several essential aspects necessary for a research study to be deemed ethical. Most importantly is the prescription of "voluntary consent". For consent to be voluntary, the person should be free from coercion or other restraint and have the information needed as well as the capacity to consent. Moreover, the study should be able to provide new knowledge that cannot be gained by other means.

It should be well designed, carried out by qualified persons and capable of meeting its goals; potential harms must be anticipated and reduced (Annas & Grodin, 1995).

Interestingly, while we tend to think of the Nuremberg Code as being the first to introduce formal guidelines for the conduct of research on human subjects, similar regulations for research did exist in pre-war Germany but apparently either were not taken seriously or were not seen as applying to those in concentration camps. The Nuremberg Code, important as it was, did not initially have a widespread impact, perhaps because researchers in many countries disassociated themselves from the Nazi doctors whose actions were seen as aberrations (Grace, 2018).

Further, one of the critical criteria of the Nuremberg Code was seen as problematic. This is the voluntary participation criterion. Some argued that it was too narrow and would leave out people who were not deemed capable of voluntary consent to participate yet whose cohort might benefit from the fruits of the research. For example, children and those with cognitive challenges would not be eligible. Yet most people would agree that research involving human subjects has provided great benefits, thus it is an issue of justice to leave out of consideration for participation those whose cohort might benefit from advances in knowledge (Munson, 2008). Consider for example people suffering from dementia for which there is currently not a cure. Those in the later stages would not qualify as they are unable to provide voluntary, informed consent and are considered vulnerable. Yet, without their participation, this population is also left unable to fully benefit from the fruits of research activity.

10.2.6.2 The Declaration of Helsinki—1964 and Later Revisions

In response to the Nazi actions, the World Medical Association (WMA), initially an alliance of 27 countries, formed in 1947. The purpose was "to ensure the independence of physicians (from political pressures), and to work for the highest standards of ethical behaviour and care by physicians at all times" (WMA, 2021a). In 1964 the WMA promulgated a set of criteria for research and term it the Declaration of Helsinki, the declaration has undergone several revisions the latest in 2013 (WMA, 2021b). The 1964 and later versions were intended to correct the problem of only allowing voluntary consent. The idea of proxy consent was introduced. Proxy consent makes it permissible for a representative of the potential research participant to determine whether it is appropriate for that person or child to participate in a trial.

A second problem addressed was that of therapeutic versus non-therapeutic research. Therapeutic research is the testing of potential new treatments and interventions "for their ability to provide benefit to those suffering from an ailment" (Grace, 2018, p. 179). An example would be a proposed regimen of cancer drugs to treat a particular form of cancer. The term 'therapeutic' is a little misleading because there should be uncertainty about whether the protocol will achieve its aims—the condition of equipoise which is explained later—and not all participants receive the new regimen (some would receive a placebo). However, therapeutic research is distinguished from non-therapeutic research which does not have the aim of potential treatment. Such research often involves participation by 'healthy' volunteers. For example, the testing of potential COVID-19 vaccines involved healthy volunteers.

10.2.6.3 The Belmont Report and World Health Organization

Although the Declaration of Helsinki provided some important clarifications and its guidelines remain influential, ethical problems associated with research involving human subjects persisted internationally. For example in the United States, anesthesiologist Henry K. Beecher (1966) published an article documenting 22 cases of unethical research—he had actually accumulated many more cases but met resistance from medical journals related to publishing these. Subsequent to the Declaration of Helsinki and in response to publication of ongoing abuses, including the Tuskegee study of syphilis in African American men (1932–1972) a Government Commission was formed. As a reminder, the Tuskegee study was initiated by the U.S. Public Health Service (USPHS). At the beginning there was a plan to treat infected men with what was available at the time, but the USPHS ran out of funds. It was decided to continue the study as observational following untreated syphilis in a cohort of several hundred African American men, some who had syphilis and some who did not (Munson, 2003). Macon county, Alabama, was a rural area of predominantly African American population where poverty was rife. Infected subjects were not treated even after treatment became easily available. They were deceived into thinking some interventions were therapeutic. Moreover, "the researchers actively conspired with physicians … to prevent the subjects from obtaining treatment" (Murphy, 2004, p. 4) even when Penicillin became available.

This and reports of other unethical studies led to the passing of a National Research Act (1974) in the United States and subsequently the formation of an advisory commission—*the National Commission for the Protection of Human Subjects of Biomedical and Biobehavioral Research*. This commission led to rules for the conduct of research that would cover studies funded by the government, exceptions were studies conducted by the military and privately funded research (Murphy, 2004). Studies would be approved by an Institutional Review Board (IRB)—prior to their commencement and reviewed at predetermined intervals. Additionally, in the Commission's report—the Belmont Report—governing ethical principles were defined. Many countries both adopted the principles from the Belmont report and developed their own Human Subjects Review Boards to protect participants of studies. These boards are independent in nature and thus outside of the influence of researchers. In the United States the minimum make-up of these committees is regulated and consists of "at least 5 members of varying backgrounds, both sexes, and (more than) 1 profession. At least 1 scientific member, 1 nonscientific member, and 1 unaffiliated member" (Grady, 2015) moreover members must be qualified to review the protocols. The most significant charge for the review board is to ensure that the study has been well designed, is capable of meeting its goals, protects human subjects from anticipatable harms and puts into place mechanisms to quickly address and minimize unanticipated harms. While individual nations do have their own stipulations for the nature and membership of Human Subjects Review Boards (AKA IRBs), the general guiding principles are equivalent.

10.2.7 Ethical Principles Guiding Human Subjects Research

Three principles critical for facilitating ethical research on human subjects, were identified and defined in the Belmont Report. These are: *Respect for Persons, Beneficence, and Justice*. These principles for the most part are closely aligned with ideas behind Beauchamp and Childress' (2019), four ethical principles governing healthcare, *Autonomy, Beneficence, Non-maleficence and Justice* but are specific to research. As Jonsen (2005), a member of the Commission notes, the Commission settled on two principles originally discussed in an article by Englehart, *Respect for persons* and *Beneficence* and one from the writings of James Childress, *Justice as Fairness*. We introduce the three principles briefly here and elaborate upon, and exemplify them, following these brief descriptions.

10.2.7.1 Respect for Persons

The philosophical roots of this principle lie in moral theory about what is important about human beings such that they should not be treated as a means to someone else's ends. It is aligned with ideas about autonomy and the rights of persons to make their own decisions. The Belmont Report (National Institutes of Health, Office of Human Subjects Research [NIHOHS], 1979) states, "respect for persons incorporates at least two ethical convictions: first that individuals should be treated as autonomous agents, and second, that persons with diminished autonomy are entitled to protection" (Principle 1). What this means, in terms of research participants that have decision-making capacity, is that a person is entitled to the information they need to decide whether or not to enroll in a study. The information should be both tailored to their ability to process information and sufficiently detailed for the person to judge whether participation would be in line with their goals and preferences. Secondly, when a person is deemed not to have decision-making capacity (and in the case of children), the surrogate or proxy decision-maker should be also given the information needed to make a decision that is in the best interests of their charge. Additionally, researchers have a responsibility to ensure that the proxy decision maker is in fact making a decision that is in their charge's best interests. This principle is exemplified shortly along with strategies for addressing contraventions.

10.2.7.2 Beneficence

For research purposes Beneficence is defined as being dual-faceted, "do not harm, and maximize benefits" (NIHOHS, 1979). This seems like a simple definition; however it can be very tricky to safeguard against all possible harms when they may not be known. Also balancing the likely good for society produced by the research against possible harms to subjects is a very complex and tricky undertaking as exemplified in Sect. 10.3.2.

10.2.7.3 Justice

There are many definitions of Justice available in the literature. The one relied upon for research purposes is justice as fairness. First the question is what constitutes an ethically sound study such that asking people to participate does not waste their time or subject them to unfair risks and (2) "who ought to receive the benefits of research and bear its burdens?" (NIHOHS, 1979). As exemplified in the Tuskegee study, an injustice was perpetuated on unsuspecting persons who would not benefit from the study and many were actually harmed.

10.3 Common Problem in Research Settings

While there are endless permutations of problems in research settings that threaten one or more of the research ethics principles, there are general themes that can be identified. We exemplify some of these and offer possible actions that nurses can take to advocate for research subjects directly or via a proxy decision maker in the case of persons who do not have decision making capacity. They are grouped under the pertinent research ethics principle. Perhaps an important place to start is to understand some important issues that apply to the design and conduct of trials.

A major reason for undertaking research generally is quite simply that we do not know something. This condition of uncertainty is known as **equipoise**. As a clinical study progresses and results are analyzed the condition of equipoise may tilt towards validation of the novel treatment or drug. However, there must be sound empirical support for findings before concluding that the intervention (drug or other) is safe and effective. This criterion might mean enrolling more participants. On occasion, the usual levels of certainty gained by completing all phases of the study may be overridden when a drug is showing promise and those with the target illness are at extreme risk of harm because there is no effective treatment available. This was the case in the 1980s with the drug AZT (azidothymidine). The organized advocacy of, and request by, persons with acquired immunodeficiency syndrome (AIDS) for access to treatment (Institute of Medicine, 1991) for non-study participants was effective. This is also known as an exception to usual research processes based on compassionate use or an "emergency use authorization". At the time of this writing, COVID-19 was also posing concerns about timely accessibility of emerging promising vaccines. The processes of evaluating potential vaccines were compressed (see Box 10.1 for phases of drug studies) but the vaccines underwent a careful review process before they became publicly available.

Earlier we discussed the problem of **therapeutic misconception**. As a reminder this "exists when individuals do not understand that the defining purpose of clinical research is to produce generalizable knowledge, regardless of whether the subjects enrolled in the trial may potentially benefit from the intervention under study or from other aspects of the clinical trial" (Henderson et al., 2007).

Both of these common problems are recognizable by nurses who are caring for patients on a clinical trial or advising patients or potential research subjects about whether it is in their interests to participate. Some more specific problems that nurses may encounter associated with research protocols are described next. Perhaps the most important issue is that of informed consent and its adequacy for persons in determining whether to participate in a study. Many clinical studies are extremely complex and require a process of time for the intricacies and likely meaning in a person's life to be grasped. Ensuring that the process of informing is adequate for potential participant decision making is required by the research ethics principle of *Respect for Persons*. The principle of *respect for persons* coupled with the *principle of beneficence* obligates all members of a protocol—including the principal investigator (PI)—involving human subjects to prioritize the wellbeing of the participant above everything else. Understanding this point gives nurses a perspective when encountering problems where research ethics principles seem to be disregarded in favor of study completion.

10.3.1 Respect for Persons

10.3.1.1 Inadequate Informed Consent

This is a problem of patients or subjects who do not seem to understand the goals of the research. They may hope for benefit when that is not the intent of the study, this problem is especially pressing in drug studies. Additionally in a randomized control trial (RCT), where the person might be assigned either to a placebo arm or to standard treatment rather than to the drug or intervention under study, there is no guarantee to which arm the person will be assigned. Inadequate informed consent fails to respect a person's right to make an autonomous decision. Nurses have an important role to play in helping people to ask the right questions—a strategy for this is provided later—and to re-evaluate in the process of a study whether the subject's desire to continue has changed.

> **Box 10.1: Phases of Drug Trials**
>
> Grace, P. J. (2018). *Nursing ethics and professional responsibility in advanced practice.* Jones & Bartlett Learning. www.jblearning.com. Reprinted with permission.
>
> Research that involves the development and testing of new drugs generally takes place in four phases. Each phase is distinct and involves different groups of subjects. -Following is my synthesis of the pertinent literature over time including the National Institutes of Health (NIH)
>
> **Phase 1**
>
> Occurs after testing in animals when feasible. Uses a small group of people. The aim is to see both what is a safe dose and what dose is effective for the purpose designed. May use healthy subjects or subjects with a disease process. Is not designed to benefit the subject, although it sometimes provides a placebo effect (Grace, 2006) and in some cases has an effect on a patient's disease process. Often called safety and efficacy trials. Escalating doses of a drug are given to successive patients or patient groups
>
> **Phase 2**
>
> Uses larger groups of people, usually those who have the condition targeted, to further test for safety, side effects, and effectiveness
>
> **Phase 3**
>
> Uses a large group of subjects who have the condition the drug is designed to treat. Further tests safety and effectiveness, generally over a longer time frame. The number needed for the study is based on statistical estimates of what is needed to validate findings. Subjects are usually monitored by their physicians and the study PI
>
> **Phase 4**
>
> After Food and Drug Administration (FDA) approval of the drug for general use, these studies monitor for adverse findings over a period of time

10.3.1.2 Vulnerable People Being Exploited

All sorts of adults and children are vulnerable to exploitation whether this is inadvertent or intended. For example, prisoners are vulnerable to coercion by virtue of their situation. They may be offered benefits if they participate. There are safeguards built into the oversight of research in most countries that are meant to protect the vulnerable. However, in the day-to-day work of a study subtle and not so subtle pressures can be applied for a participant to continue when they have indicated they would like to leave the study. Children are especially vulnerable because decisions to enroll them in a study are made by parents or guardians. They are dependent on adults for their everyday needs. For the most part the adult has their best interest in mind but there may be monetary or other inducements to enroll a child. While a child who is able to understand reasons for engaging in research is generally given the opportunity to assent, they too may be influenced by the desires of the parent. As Munson (2008) writes, "one of the most controversial areas of all medical research has been that involving children as subjects" (p. 14). Each of these situations warrants a longer discussion that is beyond the scope of the chapter. Nurses who encounter such problems, can help parents think about the goals of the study and the risks to their child including the risk of loss of trust in the family when a child is enrolled in a study to which they have not assented.

10.3.1.3 Pressures to Stay in the Study

There are many circumstances under which a subject may decide they want to withdraw from a study. Among the reasons are: the study is taking up too much of their time, they are having uncomfortable side effects, or their personal circumstances have changed. Regulations in most countries support the right of participants to withdraw at any time, and the informed consent process in most studies spells out this right. Nevertheless, PIs and/or other team members are interested in the integrity of the study and its timely completion so pressures may be applied to keep the person in the study. It is important for nurses who are encountering such a problem to ascertain why the subject wishes to withdraw, ensure that they have the information they need and support the person's informed wishes.

10.3.1.4 Privacy and Confidentiality

The principle of respect for persons also applies to a subject's personal and medical information. It includes the right of subjects to know how their information will be safeguarded, who will have access to it and under which circumstances it would be shared. In genetic-related research this can pose significant problems as the information may concern other family members. Usually all of this is detailed in the informed consent process, but participants or potential participants may need help processing the meaning of that part of the informed consent process. One advocacy role of nurses encountering subjects with these sorts of concerns is to help the potential subject ask the pertinent questions of the PI or research coordinator.

10.3.2 Beneficence

Beneficence is the obligation to provide a good, as noted above in the brief section defining the three principles of research ethics. In healthcare ethics using Beauchamp and Childress (2019) four principles, beneficence generally refers to actions on behalf of an individual. In the context of research, the principle covers both individuals and society. As stated in the Belmont Report: "The obligations of beneficence affect both individual investigators and society at large, because they extend both to particular research projects and to the entire enterprise of research" (National Commission, 1978). In research settings, unlike in healthcare settings, the principle of Beneficence also covers the idea of Nonmaleficence. The Belmont Report asserts that as a result of their deliberations the committee framed the idea of Beneficence as including both "(1) do not harm and (2) maximize possible benefits and minimize possible harms" (National Commission, 1978).

10.3.2.1 Subjects Who Are Suffering and Unaware of Alternatives

One example of a failure of beneficence might be Ms. Timewell 68-year-old who has advanced breast cancer for whom prior chemotherapy regimens have failed. Ms. Timewell initially agreed to enroll in a study using a novel drug combination after discussing with her oncologist. This regimen if successful is not expected to be curative so much as extend her life. She had hoped to attend her granddaughter's high school graduation. However, the side effects from this combination are increasing her suffering. She is constantly nauseated, has mouth ulcers and has trouble managing her pain. She has been hospitalized for the second time. Beneficent actions on the part of the research team, perhaps in concert with nurses who are witnesses to her suffering, would be to discuss alternatives such as palliative care or hospice. Nurses could discuss with her what her goals are and "under what conditions she might wish to continue" (Grace, 2018, p. 199) on the research protocol.

10.3.2.2 Subjects Who Do Not Have or Lose Decision Making Capacity

Besides children who are reliant on adults to make decisions about their best interests, some adults lose their decision-making capacity in the course of a study. The principle of beneficence requires reevaluation of whether continuing the study is still what they would likely want. Some subjects who enter a trial have decision making capacity at the beginning of the study, for example a person with early-stage dementia. However, as the study continues they lose their ability to continue to consent. At this point a surrogate or proxy maker is needed to guard the continuing interests of the person.

10.3.2.3 Researchers and Team Members Who Are Acting Unethically

As noted earlier there are all sorts of pressures on research PIs and other members of the research team to complete a given study with sufficient subjects to demonstrate the success of the study. Additionally, the integrity of a study requires adherence to aspects of the protocol design. These pressures can cause members of the research team to lose focus on what is best for the subject. This is another area where a nurse who is witnessing the problem should advocate for the subject's wellbeing. For example, Mr. Jim Diebold was visiting his daughter 50 miles distance from his house when he suffered an acute myocardial infarction (AMI) and was hospitalized in Grantham Academic Medical Center. He is now ready for discharge but is to continue with a cardiac rehabilitation program. His daughter investigated and discovered such a program in Mr. Diebold's town and 5 min from his house … he lives alone but has two dogs and a cat that neighbors are caring. He has told Ms. Nguyen his nurse that he is eager to get home to his pets. As she is preparing his discharge Ms. Nguyen overhears Dr. Dwyer, the coronary care unit physician trying to persuade Mr. Diebold to join a research study he is conducting related to cardiac rehabilitation. The study would require Mr. Diebold to attend twice a week. She hears Dr. Dwyer say, "you will get much better oversight and care than you could at your home center". Ms. Nguyen knows that Dr. Dwyer has had trouble getting enough subjects, but she also knows that entering the study would not serve Jim's interests.

10.3.2.4 Surrogate Decision Makers Acting Against a Subject's Interests

Not infrequently persons who are acting as a surrogate or proxy decision maker for an adult or a child, make decisions that are not in the interests of that person. It may be that the decision maker has not understood what is at risk, is making decisions based on their values and preferences rather than those indicated by their ward's history, or is in the case of a child, their rather than the child's needs. In an example taken from Grace (2018), 10-year-old Timmy's discharge from hospital is delayed in order that he completes a drug study. Timmy has some uncomfortable, although not life-threatening side effects and there are alternative treatments available—Timmy has had these prior—with fewer side-effects. Timmy tells his nurse Clara that he badly "wants to go home". Clara overheard a conversation between Timmy's mother and stepfather that made her suspicious that Timmy's stepfather is counting on the monetary compensation from the study and is trying to persuade his wife to agree to keep him in hospital to complete the study.

10.3.3 Justice

The third principle defined in The Belmont Report is that of justice. Related to research on human subjects the *Principle of Justice* is about the fair distribution of the benefits and burdens of research. Since research using human subjects is for the purpose of providing knowledge that can improve individual and social good in a fair way, care must be taken not to unfairly place the burdens of research participation either on the least well off or the otherwise most vulnerable. However, the second part of the idea of justice as fairness is that people are not left out of research the findings of which might benefit them or their cohort. Thus, in formulating and enacting a research study the two questions that must be addressed are: Is the proposed study the study ethically sound"? and "How should the benefits and burdens be distributed"?

10.3.3.1 An Ethically Designed Study

Ethical considerations in the design of a study include: that it has been the thoughtful and carefully constructed by knowledgeable and skilled researchers, aims to add—and is capable of adding—knowledge that can improve human lives, does not arbitrarily include persons based on convenience, and does not leave out people or groups of people who might benefit. Additionally, the researchers have identified potential risks or harms and have strategies in place to address or minimize these.

10.3.3.2 Fair Selection of Subjects

In the past some studies selected participants based on convenience. For example, prisoners have been solicited into studies because they were easy to access. Other studies used subjects who were easy to deceive. Some persons whose cohort might benefit from a study have been left out of consideration. Justice is relevant to the selection of subjects of research at two levels: the social and the individual.

Individual justice in the selection of subjects would require that researchers exhibit fairness: thus, they should not offer potentially beneficial research only to some patients who are in their favor or select only "undesirable" persons for risky research.

> Social justice requires that distinction be drawn between classes of subjects that ought, and ought not, to participate in any particular kind of research, based on the ability of members of that class to bear burdens and on the appropriateness of placing further burdens on already burdened persons. Thus, it can be considered a matter of social justice that there is an order of preference in the selection of classes of subjects (e.g., adults before children) and that some classes of potential subjects (e.g., the institutionalized mentally infirm or prisoners) may be involved as research subjects, if at all, only on certain conditions. (National Commission for the Protection of Human Subjects, 1978)

10.4 Nurses Roles and Advocacy Strategies

There are a variety of roles that nurses have related to human subjects of research. Below is a non-exhaustive list.

1. Nurses may encounter patients in the clinic or hospital ward who are enrolled in a study but are receiving unrelated care.
2. Patients who are on a drug or intervention protocol are hospitalized secondary to side effects.
3. Patients are placed on a study protocol while hospitalized
4. Nurses are part of a research team in an inpatient or outpatient setting
5. Nurses are hired as a study coordinator
6. Nurses may also be asked for their advice by a friend or colleague about whether to enroll in a trial or not.

The chapter's first author Grace for several years served as an ethics resource for nurses in the Research Unit of a Large Metropolitan Hospital and heard first-hand some of the problems faced. However, the nurses also shared some of the successful strategies they used to advocate for subjects who were struggling with whether to leave a study. DeBruin et al. (2011) in their study of problems encountered by research nurses, assert that "nurses do the majority of the work of clinical trials" (p. 122) and thus have insights into the problems that occur. However, their study was one of the very few to-date that actually asked nurses for their insights.

10.4.1 Questions to Ask Before Entering a Study

A friend of the first author (Grace) had been diagnosed with idiopathic pulmonary fibrosis. Her pulmonologist suggested a research study of a drug that it was hoped could slow the progression. She was given the protocol information and informed consent document to study. It was quite complex and detailed and entailed many trips to the research site. We worked through it together and as a result I was able to give her questions to ask at the next meeting with the study coordinator. Each study is different, thus some of the questions asked will also vary. The following questions are helpful in advising a potential research subject. A caution is that our role is not to advise whether or not a person should enroll but rather to elicit the person's goals, desires, expectations and understanding of what is being proposed. Additionally, in working through the consent form to remind them that they have the right to leave the study at any time (the exception might be a surgical intervention that is irreversible or has been completed).

- What are the subject's goals? hopes? Expectations of the study?
- How likely is it that this study will satisfy these? Is there an inactive arm (placebo or usual treatment)? How will they feel if they discover they were not receiving the study drug?
- In what ways might this study interfere with the person's life?
- Why is the investigator interested in studying this?
- What aspects will be investigated, and which will not? Why these?
- What is the rationale for subject selection and exclusion?
- Whose interests are served by this project? Are there monetary inducements? Who is sponsoring the study?
- Whose interests are ignored or discounted?
- Have there been safety issues so far? What are these? How well have safety issues been addressed?
- How honest, complete, and understandable is the consent form?
- Will I have my own doctor/nurse as well as the research doctor/nurse
- Who will have my interests foremost?

10.4.2 Examples of Problems and Strategies for Resolution

10.4.2.1 Case: Rushing an Impaired Patient

Ms. Lopez comes into the emergency room with chest pain. She is medicated for pain and anxiety and tests indicate angina and impending myocardial infarction. The cardiologist talks to her about a study he is doing using a new stent. He says it is relatively urgent that the stent be placed as soon as possible. The emergency room nurse is concerned that Ms. Lopez has no one accompanying her, is drowsy and is not able to process the information. What should the nurse do?

Actions. She should relate her concerns to the cardiologist using the language of research principles and focusing on respect for persons and informed consent. While this may be a new type of stent, there are nonexperimental alternatives. Thus she should not be rushed into a decision. There may be a conflict of interest if Ms. Lopez does not have another physician overseeing her care. That is, the cardiologist may be putting his stent study before the good of the patient (a failure of beneficence). While there are some emergency procedures for which informed consent can be waived, these are usually life or death situations, and the ER staff would have been briefed on these. The nurse can ask Ms. Lopez if she has someone who could help her make this decision. Finally, if problems remain the nurse can seek the help of his or her supervisor and or discuss with a member of the human subjects' research board.

10.4.2.2 Case of Mistaken Trust

Mr. Abdul is in a memory care nursing home with mid-stage dementia. His niece is his surrogate decision maker. It has been suggested that Mr. Abdul would be a good candidate for a research trial using a drug that is hoped to reduce anxiety. His niece Amma, says to you the supervising RN, "I think I will sign him up for it as Dr. Barlow is so kind and trustworthy" she would not suggest something that would be bad for him.

Actions. As the advocate for the patient who has knowledge of what should be considered in deciding whether to enroll one's ward in a study, one would explain the responsibilities of a surrogate. First, to thoroughly review the available protocol information and informed consent process. Perhaps using some of the questions suggested earlier. Provide her with the questions to ask of the researcher and help her to think about Mr. Abdul's prior preferences and life goals as a way to think about what he might want.

10.5 Thought Experiment

Imagine that you have been diagnosed with a type of lung cancer that has a low chance of survival. Three years is the best-case survival scenario. However, you have heard that there is a promising new drug combination that has been tested in animals and is now in Phase 2 (see Box 10.1). If successful, the drug combination is anticipated to add a couple of years of life. Make a list of questions that you would like to ask of the researcher before deciding whether you would like to participate.

10.6 Suggestions and Questions

- If you notice problems with a participant, consider the problem in ethical terms. Is it a justice (someone is being excluded, the protocol is not being followed diligently, the study can't meet its goals), respect for persons (the person is not being told the details they need to make an informed decision to continue or discontinue participation), or a beneficence problem (side effects are too severe)?
- Discuss what you are noticing with a supervisor, the project manager, principal investigator or a member of the human subjects' review board or equivalent. You may need to go up the chain of responsibility: project staff → project manager → principal investigator → chair or member of the human subject review board that approved the study.
- Empower the subject, subject's family or proxy to ask salient questions of the research team.
- Review research ethics mechanisms in your country—who is responsible for reviewing studies for human subject or participant protections.
- Obtain an informed consent document from your IRB or Human Subjects Review Board and review all of the aspects covered.

10.7 Summary

Nurses frequently encounter patients who are the subjects of, or participants in research studies. While the goals of research differ somewhat from the goals of healthcare, nevertheless the safety and wellbeing of the subject or participant is of supreme importance. Human beings must not be treated as a means to someone else's ends regardless of the possibility that a study is not of any likely benefit to them but is rather to increase knowledge for the society. Arguably, what is important about societies is the individuals who comprise them. When nurses are acting in a nursing role related to research, professional goals persist. When nurses are hired to manage a research project because of their nursing knowledge and skills, nursing goals take precedence. However, it is also important that nurses attend to the need for study integrity (the likelihood that the study can achieve its aims—a justice issue). So a balance is needed. Decision-making strategies of balancing risks (to persons) versus benefits to society can be used.

References

American Nurses Association. (2015). *Code of ethics for nurses with interpretive statements.*
Annas, G. J., & Grodin, M. (Eds.). (1995). *The Nazi doctors and the Nuremberg Code.* Oxford University Press.
Beauchamp, T. L., & Childress, J. F. (2019). *Principles of biomedical ethics* (8th ed.). Oxford University Press.
Beecher, H. K. (1966). Ethics and clinical research. *New England Journal of Medicine, 274,* 1354–1360.
Chambliss, D. (1996). *Beyond caring: Hospitals, nurses and the social organization of ethics.* University of Chicago Press.
DeBruin, D. A., Liaschenko, J., & Fisher, A. (2011). How clinical trials really work: Rethinking research ethics. *Kennedy Institute of Ethics Journal, 21*(2), 121–139.
Grace, P. J. (2006). The clinical use of placebos: Is it ethical? Not when it involves deceiving patients. *The American Journal of Nursing, 106*(2), 58–61.
Grace, P. J. (2018). *Nursing ethics and professional responsibility in advanced practice* (3rd ed.). Jones and Bartlett Learning.
Grady, C. (2015). Institutional review boards: Purpose and challenges. *Chest, 148*(5), 1148–1155. https://doi.org/10.1378/chest.15-0706
Henderson, G. E., Churchill, L. R., Davis, A. M., Easter, M. M., Grady, C., Joffe, S., Kass, N., King, N. M., Lidz, C. W., Miller, F. G., Nelson, D. K., Peppercorn, J., Rothschild, B. B., Sankar, P., Wilfond, B. S., & Zimmer, C. R. (2007). Clinical trials and medical care: Defining the therapeutic misconception. *PLoS Medicine, 4*(11), e324. https://doi.org/10.1371/journal.pmed.0040324
Hurley, E. A. (2019). Why we need to keep the term "Research Subject" in our research ethics vocabulary. *Journal of Clinical Research Best Practices, 15*(2). https://www.magiworld.org/Journal/2019/1902_Participants.pdf
Institute of Medicine. (1991). *Expanding access to investigational therapies for HIV infection and AIDS: Roundtable for the development of drugs and vaccines against AIDS.* Accessed January 20, 2021 from: https://www.ncbi.nlm.nih.gov/books/NBK234125/pdf/Bookshelf_NBK234125.pdf
International Council of Nursing. (2012). *Code of ethics for nurses.* Author. Accessed January 11, 2021 from: https://www.icn.ch/sites/default/files/inline-files/2012_ICN_Codeofethicsfornurses_%20eng.pdf
Jonsen, A. R. (2005). On the origins and future of the Belmont Report. In J. F. Childress, E. M. Meslin, & H. T. Shapiro (Eds.), *Belmont revisited: Ethical principles for research with human subjects.* Georgetown University Press.
Kant, I. (1965). Foundations of the metaphysics of morals. In A. I. Melden (Ed.), *Ethical theories a book of readings* (pp. 317–366). Prentice Hall.
Kong, W. M. (2005). Legitimate requests and indecent proposals: Matters of justice in the ethical assessment of phase I trials involving competent patients. *Journal of Medical Ethics, 31*(4), 205–208.
Lidz, C., & Appelbaum, P. (2002). The therapeutic misconception: Problems and solutions. *Medical Care, 40*(9) (Suppl. 9), V-55–V-63.
Munson, R. (2003). *Outcome uncertain: Cases and contexts in bioethics.* Thompson/Wadsworth.
Munson, R. (2008). *Intervention and reflection: Basic issues in medical ethics* (8th ed.). Wadsworth/Thompson Learning.
Murphy, T. F. (2004). *Case studies in biomedical research ethics.* MIT Press.

National Commission for the Protection of Human Subjects of Biomedical and Behavioral Research. (1978). *The Belmont Report: Ethical principles and guidance for the protection of human subjects of research*. Department of Health, Education and Welfare.

National Institutes of Health. (2018). *Types of human subjects research*. Accessed January 10, 2021 from: https://www.nidcr.nih.gov/research/human-subjects-research/types-of-human-subjects-research

National Institutes of Health, Office of Human Subjects Research. (1979). *The Belmont Report: Ethical principles and guidelines for the protections of human subjects of research*. Accessed January 16, 2021 from: https://www.hhs.gov/ohrp/regulations-and-policy/belmont-report/read-the-belmont-report/index.html

The Stanford Prison Experiment. (1971/2021). Accessed January 12, 2021 https://www.prisonexp.org/

United Nations. (1948). *The Universal Declaration of Human Rights*. Accessed January 21, 2021 from: https://www.un.org/en/universal-declaration-human-rights/

Vaes, J., Paladino, M. P., & Haslam, N. (2021). Seven clarifications on the psychology of dehumanization. *Perspectives on Psychological Science, 16*(1), 28–32. https://doi.org/10.1177/1745691620953767

van Gaal, S., De Lange, F. P., & Cohen, M. X. (2012). The role of consciousness in cognitive control and decision making. *Frontiers in Human Neuroscience, 6*, 121.

Varden, H. (2017). Kant and women. *Pacific Philosophical Quarterly, 98*(4), 653–694.

Weston, A. (2011). *A practical companion to ethics* (4th ed.). Oxford University Press.

World Health Organization. (2011). *Standards and operational guidance for ethics review of health-related research with human participants*. WHO Press. Accessed January 10, 2021 from: https://www.who.int/ethics/publications/9789241502948/en/

World Medical Association. (2021a). *About us. What is the WMA*. Accessed January 16, 2021 from: https://www.WMA.net/who-we-are/about-us/

World Medical Association. (2021b). *Declaration of Helsinki*. Accessed January 16, 2021 from: https://www.wma.net/policies-post/wma-declaration-of-helsinki-ethical-principles-for-medical-research-involving-human-subjects/

Zimbardo, P. (2005). *Professional profile*. http://Zimbardo.socialpsychology.org

Chapter 11
Organizational Influences on Ethical Action

Aimee Milliken and Pamela Grace

Abstract In this chapter we discuss some of the major factors affecting nurses' work within institutions of various sorts such as hospitals, clinics, schools, and prisons, among others. We discuss the conflicts and contradictions that can arise between the ostensible public mission of an institution and the need of the institution to be economically viable. Ways in which conflicts can influence nursing practice and ultimately patient care are explored and strategies for nurses to use are provided. The remedy of institutional barriers to good care tends to require knowledgeable, skillful and collaborative action and may be beyond the ability of a sole nurse to resolve without the support of colleagues and other experts.

11.1 Introduction

Nursing practice is inevitably situated within the context of an organization of some sort, formal or informal. Whether a hospital, clinic, school, or community organization, the mission, vision, and values of the organization can, and should, be facilitative of ethical action. In some institutions these ideals serve as the anchor for structures and innovative practices aimed at actualizing the service aims of the institution. However, in other cases they may not be taken seriously at best, or merely serve as a public façade at worst. Thus, nurses and other healthcare professionals may face barriers to their ethical practice and to the provision of good patient care. It is an important professional responsibility that nurses identify barriers to ethical action and, when possible, work to address them at an organizational level (American Nurses Association, 2015; International Council of Nurses, 2012) and perhaps in collaboration with others. In this chapter, we describe the role of an institution's mission, vision, and values statements and how these can be used to argue for needed change.

A. Milliken (✉)
William F. Connell School of Nursing, Boston College, Chestnut Hill, MA, USA
e-mail: aimee.milliken@bc.edu

P. Grace
William F. Connell School of Nursing, Boston College, Newton, MA, USA
e-mail: pamela.grace.2@bc.edu

© The Author(s), under exclusive license to Springer Nature B.V. 2022
P. Grace and A. Milliken (eds.), *Clinical Ethics Handbook for Nurses*, The International Library of Bioethics 93,
https://doi.org/10.1007/978-94-024-2155-2_11

We then describe both effective and ineffective organizational structures, specifically those that allow for open moral spaces and other practices supportive of interdisciplinary communication and decision-making. We explore the important collaborative role the nursing perspective plays in the development and implementation of organizational policy. Finally, we provide case examples for discussion.

11.2 Institutional Mission, Vision, and Values

The widespread development and use of mission statements for institutions of various sorts is a relatively recent phenomenon. As noted in the Encyclopedia of Local History (Wilson, 2017):

> The Ford and Carnegie foundations' scathing critiques of the lack of rigor in business schools in 1959 resulted in a growing emphasis on management, finances, and strategic planning informed by such diverse fields as economics, psychology, sociology, engineering, and mathematics. Mission statements became part of the toolkit for corporate success by codifying the company's ideals and providing a set of principles to guide its actions and decisions (Index—Mission Statements).

An organization's "mission" statement serves as a description of its purpose. It is a publicly available explanation of why the organization exists and is meant to be aspirational. The "vision" statement provides a picture of the organization's aims for the future and often includes measures for defining success. In other words, it is an aspirational description of the organization in its idealized state. Finally, the "values" statement involves a description of the core principles that guide the organization, and delineate the boundaries the organization will work within to achieve the vision (Richmond, 2020). The mission, vision, and values vary depending on the type of organization. Additionally, there are likely to be linguistic, cultural, and regional variations. For example, a public hospital may have a different mission than a private, for-profit hospital. For countries with a partly or fully nationalized healthcare system, institutions may share common mission, vision, and value statements. Mission, vision, and values may also differ significantly by geographic location and population served. Nevertheless, because institutions that in some sense are involved in providing healthcare or promoting health and wellbeing in theory exist to provide a service aimed at providing a public "good," essential themes in their aspirational propositions are often discernible.

It is evident, then, that an organization's mission, vision, and values serve as an important ethical framework and represent critical considerations that can impact nursing practice. They can sometimes be used by nurses to hold their institutions accountable for implicit or explicit policies that do not serve patients well. However, influencing policies requires nurses to be knowledgeable about the structure of their institution, and be willing to serve on institutional committees where decisions are made, or to collaborate with others who have similar concerns. Nurses should be aware of their organizations' goals and values, as external pressures, such as financial constraint or political influence, may cause these values to be challenged. When searching for a place of employment, it can also be helpful to understand the mission, vision, and values of the prospective employer, in order to assess the degree of fit between the organization and the nurse's personal and professional values and the degree to which they can uphold the code of ethics governing nurses in that country.

11.3 Supportive Unit Structures

An organization's values can directly impact the degree of support nurses experience within the organization. Leadership style is another important factor to consider. Healthcare leaders who create supportive environments and demonstrate behavioral integrity have been found to decrease employee silence about critical issues, including feedback that could benefit the organization (Erkutlu & Chafra, 2019). Behavioral integrity involves alignment between the leader's words and their actions; in other words, it is the extent to which employees believe their leaders are keeping promises (Erkutlu & Chafra, 2019; Simons et al., 2007). Nurses, in particular, may, in certain situations, believe that speaking up is unsafe or will not make a difference, especially in environments entrenched in hierarchy (Morrow, Gustavson, & Jones, 2016). Thus, unit structures that are facilitative of ethical practice are critical in ensuring nurses can speak up and feel heard and are able to provide the safest and best possible care to patients.

Safe care is a critical component of ethical care. The ethical principle of non-maleficence, as discussed in earlier chapters, is relevant to the idea that institutions are responsible for anticipating and keeping persons safe from incidental and preventable harms such as medical errors, failure to rescue from an acute decline in condition, and nosocomial infections. For example, inadequate staffing may mean that a patient's decline is not noticed before it becomes a life or death emergency. Supportive unit structures are those in which attention to quality and safety are paramount, and where nurses' concerns are noted and acted upon. It has been well documented in the literature, for example, that when nurses are responsible for more patients than can be adequately monitored and cared for higher rates of mortality, failure to rescue, and nurse burnout and job dissatisfaction follow (Aiken et al., 2002).

Interdisciplinary communication is another important element of a safe and supportive clinical environment. Communication challenges have been connected to medical error and other serious complications for patients (Rosenstein & O'Daniel, 2008; Sutcliffe et al., 2004). In the authors' own experiences as well as from the literature, when nurses feel hampered in their ability to voice concerns, emerging ethical problems go unaddressed and the risk of practice error increases.

"Physicians, nurses, and allied healthcare providers have different interactions with patients based on role responsibilities, personal characteristics, and time spent engaged with the patient" (Grace et al., 2007, p. 8). Thus, nurses and physicians may view their moral obligations in different ways (Pavlish et al., 2019), and these differing perspectives can naturally lead to disagreement about the plan of care and sense of what is "right" for the patient. Being able to respectfully communicate about these disagreements, in an environment conducive to doing so, is an important element of a supportive healthcare environment. This type of dialogue may be more routine in certain clinical environments and geographic areas; other areas may maintain a more hierarchical approach to communication, where nurses may fear they will face repercussions for speaking up or expressing disagreement about a plan of care. In any case, it is essential that nurses have a process for communicating about ethical concerns that arise in the course of patient care. As noted in earlier chapters, when nurses feel they are ineffective in articulating their concerns or taking what they feel is the best action in a given case they can experience transient or lasting moral distress which in turn affects both them and their future practice (Epstein et al, 2019).

11.3.1 Moral Spaces

First described by feminist philosopher Margaret Urban Walker, moral spaces have been defined as "those patterns, structures, routines, and channels of communication that clarify the moral responsibilities and mutual accountability of all parties" (Walker, 1993a, p. 45, 1993b). Though this could be an actual physical space, it can be helpful to think of a "moral space" simply as one where respectful communication about ethical issues can occur, regardless of location (Hamric & Wocial, 2016). These sorts of opportunities are important in facilitating a supportive environment where nurses feel safe and comfortable raising concerns about the ethical challenges they face in practice. In turn, this type of dialogue can generate ideas about interventions for addressing the issues at hand, and can mitigate moral distress (Reilly & Jurchak, 2017). They are also facilitative of preventive ethics. That is, they allow learning from the past and present that can mitigate future problems from exacerbating.

Hamric and Wocial (2016) identify four key factors necessary for an effective moral space: (1) available ethics resources must be knowledgeable and have the skills to reason ethically, (2) they must be known to healthcare professionals and available during all shifts, (3) they must be available and able to respond in a time-sensitive fashion, and (4) they must be sanctioned by hospital and clinical leadership in order to be effective. They also encourage ethics resources to work in a proactive fashion when possible, in order to address the "everyday" issues that arise rather than only functioning as a reactive resource when a crisis arises.

While the availability of these types of ethics resources varies widely, nurses can create opportunities for this type of discussion within their own units or organizations. For example, regularly scheduled unit-based ethics rounds, focusing on discussing a particularly challenging case, can be helpful in increasing nurses' sense of being valued, decreasing self-reported levels of moral distress, and increasing perceptions of an ethical practice environment (Reilly & Jurchak, 2017). These sorts of rounds, ideally, would be supported by nursing leadership in order to facilitate staff buy-in. If individuals with ethics expertise are not readily available, journal articles and other prompts, such as the case studies available in this book, can be used to facilitate discussion.

11.3.2 Interdisciplinary Collaboration

Moral spaces can also facilitate communication and collaboration, particularly when these discussions are conducted in an interdisciplinary way. Interdisciplinary discussion about complex issues can help with "perspective-taking." In other words, it may help nurses to understand the unique perspectives and challenges that their physician colleagues face, and in return it may help physicians to understand these aspects of the nursing perspective. Role play, where participants "play" a character with a different professional background from their own, can be particularly helpful in this regard (Grace et al., 2014; Robinson et al., 2014). In the Clinical Ethics Residency Program that took place in 2 major academic medical centers in the US each year for three years, participants were often surprised at how strongly they assumed the role they were given to play and how emotional it could be. They described how this influenced their interactions both with non-nurse colleagues and family members (Lee et al., 2019).

Open discussions in a morally safe environment can also facilitate a model of interprofessional shared decision-making (IP-SDM). IP-SDM is defined as: "a collaborative process among clinicians that allows for team involvement in important clinical decisions, such as those pertaining to the goals and extent of treatment or other complex medical decisions and taking into account the available evidence and combined expertise as well as the patient's values, goals, and preferences" (Michalsen et al., 2019, p. 4). IP-SDM holds promise in facilitating environments where the perspectives of multiple professions, including nursing, can be heard and incorporated into the plan of care. As such, it is possible that the IP-SDM model could mitigate troublesome experiences including moral distress. Additionally, if dis-empowerment among nurses is experienced as the genesis of moral distress then the IP-SDM model can provide a venue where their perspective is heard and accounted for in the same way as that of others involved in the decision-making process (Epstein et al., 2019).

11.4 Nursing Ethics and Institutional Policy

Institutional policies that influence nursing practice can create ethical challenges, particularly if the perspective of the bedside nurse is not sufficiently incorporated in the development of them. For example, austerity efforts can limit the availability of certain treatment options or alter staffing ratios in a way that makes it more challenging to provide high quality patient care (Morley et al., 2019). While these efforts are ostensibly about conserving organizational resources they often work in opposition to the mission, vision, and values of the institution and end up being more costly in terms of patient wellbeing and recidivism or longer periods in the institution. Some authors argue that these sorts of financial constraints can cause avoidable moral distress (Morley et al., 2019). Nurses have also identified unsupportive organizational cultures, including those with perceived inadequate staffing, as barriers to delivering compassionate care (Valizadeh et al., 2018). As such, the perspective of the bedside nurse is critical in the development of organizational policy that is facilitative of ethical action and for actualizing the expressed core tenets of the institutions.

Nurse participation on organization-wide committees, unit-based practice councils, and other sorts of decision-making bodies within an organization are examples of shared-governance models that support the integration of the nursing perspective in organizational policy. Shared governance structures, opportunities for professional development, collegial relationships and supportive leadership have all been associated with increased nurse retention (Twigg & McCullough, 2014). Increased levels of nurse engagement are also associated with increased ratings of patient satisfaction, and nurse-rated levels of quality and safety (Kutney-Lee et al., 2016).

Despite the promise of such structures, implementing a shared practice model may prove challenging in organizations that are highly physician-centric, or in areas of the world where nurses have not historically been encouraged to speak up or play an active role in decision-making. In such cases, starting at the local, unit-based level may be feasible. For example, a unit-specific nurse-practice council, where nurses can discuss unit norms, expectations, and practices could be a first step.

11.5 Strategies for Change: Cases for Discussion

Case 1: The nurses in a cardiac intensive care unit in a large, academic teaching hospital notice that they often feel left out of the decision-making processes for their patients. Despite participating in daily bedside rounds with the medical team, they often find themselves questioning the plan of care and worried about "where things are headed" for their critically ill patients. Without a forum for discussion about these issues, they begin experiencing moral distress.

1. What action might this group of nurses take to develop a solution to this problem?
2. Who should they speak to, and why?
3. What institutional resources might they consider engaging as they problem solve?
4. How might they approach the situation if they are not comfortable discussing their concerns with the medical leadership of the unit?

Case resolution: The nurses in this case brought their concerns to their nurse manager. After a series of conversations between the unit's nursing and medical leadership, a plan was implemented for a once-weekly "support" rounds, where any clinician could bring up a case that they were concerned about for an interdisciplinary conversation. Rounds are attended each week by bedside staff, nursing leadership, the unit medical director, the attending of the week, and an ethics consultant, and provide a forum for discussing challenging and distressing cases.

Case 2: Critical care nurses who commonly cared for patients receiving extracorporeal membrane oxygenation therapy (ECMO) noticed that families of their patients seemed surprised by how sick their loved ones were while on the ECMO circuit and did not seem prepared for certain interventions that were commonly implemented. ECMO is a machine, similar to a heart–lung-bypass machine, that pumps blood outside the body in order to oxygenate it and allow the heart and/or lungs to rest. This knowledge deficit caused significant stress for families, and at times seemed to interfere with the quality of care the nurses felt they were able to provide, and they noticed increasing conflicts over the goals of care at the end of life for these patients.

1. What action might this group of nurses take to develop a solution to this problem?
2. Who should they speak to, and why?
3. What institutional resources might they consider engaging as they problem solve?
4. How might they approach the situation if they are not comfortable discussing their concerns with the medical leadership of the unit?

Case resolution: The nursing staff worked closely with their respiratory therapy colleagues to develop an informational brochure for patients and families, with important information about questions that frequently came up. They presented the brochure to their unit leadership, and it was well-received. After additional input from the medical team, the brochure was approved and is now distributed to patients and their families prior to ECMO initiation.

Case 3: An experimental surgery to spare the affected limb of adolescent patients with advanced sarcoma troubled the nurses and residents charged with caring for them after surgery. Among the side effects were bladder and bowel incontinence, intractable pain and severe body image disturbances. Nurses in the pediatric intensive care unit were becoming increasingly concerned as they encountered patients for whom it seemed loss of a limb might be preferable to the suffering they experienced. They noticed that in some cases the resident physicians avoided talking with the parents, and were reluctant to evaluate those children whose experience of side-effects was severe and intractable. They seemed to feel helpless to intervene. Additionally, the nurses encountered parents who said if they had known the severity of the sequelae they would never have agreed to the surgery.

1. What action might this group of nurses take to develop a solution to this problem?
2. Who should they speak to, and why?
3. What institutional resources might they consider engaging as they problem solve?
4. How might they approach the situation if they are not comfortable discussing their concerns with the medical leadership of the unit?

Case resolution: Several of the nurses spoke with the nurse manager about the problem. The nurse manager had recently completed an extensive ethics course. Together the nurses and nurse manager were able to clearly delineate their concerns during the conversation, listed them and decided that they needed to discuss the problem with the surgeon. It turned out that the surgeon was also worried about the populations of patients who did not seem to benefit but found it hard to deny the surgery when parents plead with him to do something to help their child. A subsequent multidisciplinary team meeting with physicians, surgeons, nurses, social workers, child life specialists, physical therapists and family members resulted in a more stringent pre-surgery evaluation and informed consent process. This process led to a more accurate determination of who could benefit, reduced the incidence of severe sequelae, and better prepared the family and child. The process with its clear criteria also lifted some of the pressure from the surgeon as it was a team determined process.

11.6 Summary

Organizations and the policies implemented by them have the potential to support or obstruct ethical nursing action. Nurses should be attuned to these issues, and, where possible, work to address the barriers they face in practice. There are a variety of organizational structures and practices that are supportive to nurses, and therefore supportive of ethical care. Nurses ought to have the opportunity to participate in decision-making at the institutional-level, however even in environments where this may not be the norm, there are actions nurses can take to promote ethical practice.

References

Aiken, L. H., Clarke, S. P., Sloane, D. M., Sochalski, J., & Silber, J. H. (2002). Hospital nurse staffing and patient mortality, nurse burnout, and job dissatisfaction. *JAMA, 288*(16), 1987.https://doi.org/10.1001/jama.288.16.1987

American Nurses Association. (2015). *Code of Ethics for Nurses.* http://www.nursingworld.org/DocumentVault/Ethics_1/Code-of-Ethics-for-Nurses.html

Epstein, E. G., Whitehead, P. B., Prompahakul, C., Thacker, L. R., & Hamric, A. B. (2019). Enhancing understanding of moral distress: The measure of moral distress for health care professionals. *AJOB Empirical Bioethics, 10*(2), 113–124. https://doi.org/10.1080/23294515.2019.1586008

Erkutlu, H., & Chafra, J. (2019). Leader's integrity and employee silence in healthcare organizations. *Leadership in Health Services, 32*(3), 419–434. https://doi.org/10.1108/LHS-03-2018-0021

Grace, P. J. Willis, D. G., & Jurchak, M. (2007). Good patient care: Egalitarian inter-professional collaboration as a moral imperative. *American Society of Bioethics and Humanities. Exchange, 10*(1), 8–9.

Grace, P. J., Robinson, E. M., Jurchak, M., Zollfrank, A. A., & Lee, S. M. (2014). Clinical ethics residency for nurses. *JONA: The Journal of Nursing Administration, 44*(12), 640–646. https://doi.org/10.1097/NNA.0000000000000141

Hamric, A. B., & Wocial, L. D. (2016). Institutional ethics resources: *Creating moral spaces. Hastings Center Report, 46*(October), S22–S27. https://doi.org/10.1002/hast.627

International Council of Nurses. (2012). *The ICN Code of Ethics for Nurses.* http://www.icn.ch/images/stories/documents/about/icncode_english.pdf

Kutney-Lee, A., Germack, H., Hatfield, L., Kelly, S., Maguire, P., Dierkes, A., & Aiken, L. H. (2016). Nurse engagement in shared governance and patient and nurse outcomes. *Jounal of Nursing Administration, 46*(11), 605–612. https://doi.org/10.1097/NNA.0000000000000412.Nurs

Lee, S., Robinson, E., Grace, P.J., Jurchak, M. & Zollfrank, A. (Published Online ahead of print April, 28, 2019). Developing a moral compass: Themes from the clinical ethics residency for nurses (CERN) final essays. Nursing Ethics. https://doi.org/10.1177/0969733019833125

Michalsen, A., Long, A. C., DeKeyser Ganz, F., White, D. B., Jensen, H. I., Metaxa, V., & Curtis, J. R. (2019). Interprofessional shared decision-making in the ICU. *Critical Care Medicine, 1,.* https://doi.org/10.1097/ccm.0000000000003870

Morley, G., Ives, J., & Bradbury-Jones, C. (2019). Moral distress and austerity: An avoidable ethical challenge in healthcare. *Health Care Analysis, 27*(3), 185–201. https://doi.org/10.1007/s10728-019-00376-8

Morrow, K., Gustavson, A., & Jones, J. (2016). Speaking up behaviours (safety voices) of healthcare workers: A metasynthesis of qualitative research studies. *International Journal of Nursing Studies, 64*, 42–51. https://doi.org/10.1016/j.ijnurstu.2016.09.014

Pavlish, B. C. L., Brown-Saltzman, K., Raho, J. A., & Chen, B. (2019). A national survey on moral obligations in critical care. *American Journal of Critical Care, 28*(3), 183–192. https://doi.org/10.4037/ajcc2019512

Reilly, K. M., & Jurchak, M. (2017). Developing professional practice and ethics engagement: A leadership model. *Nursing Administration Quarterly, 41*(4), 376–383. https://doi.org/10.1097/NAQ.0000000000000251

Richmond, S. (2020). Mission, vision, and values facilitation. Retrieved July 20, 2020, from Stanford Graduate School of Business website: https://www.gsb.stanford.edu/alumni/volunteering/act/service-areas/mission-vision-values-facilitation

Robinson, E. M., Lee, S. M., Zollfrank, A., Jurchak, M., Frost, D., & Grace, P. (2014). Enhancing moral agency: Clinical ethics residency for nurses. *The Hastings Center Report, 44*(5), 12–20. https://doi.org/10.1002/hast.353

Rosenstein, A. H., & O'Daniel, M. (2008). A survey of the impact of disruptive behaviors and communication defects on patient safety. *Joint Commission Journal on Quality and Patient Safety, 34*(8), 464–471. https://doi.org/10.1016/S1553-7250(08)34058-6

Simons, T., Friedman, R., Liu, L. A., & McLean Parks, J. (2007). Racial differences in sensitivity to behavioral integrity: Attitudinal consequences, in-group effects, and "trickle down" among Black and non-Black employees. *Journal of Applied Psychology, 92*(3), 650–665. https://doi.org/10.1037/0021-9010.92.3.650

Sutcliffe, K. M., Lewton, E., & Rosenthal, M. M. (2004). Communication failures: An insidious contributor to medical mishaps. *Academic Medicine, 79*(2), 186–194. https://doi.org/10.1097/00001888-200402000-00019

Twigg, D., & McCullough, K. (2014). Nurse retention: A review of strategies to create and enhance positive practice environments in clinical settings. *International Journal of Nursing Studies, 51*(1), 85–92. https://doi.org/10.1016/j.ijnurstu.2013.05.015

Valizadeh, L., Zamanzadeh, V., Dewar, B., Rahmani, A., & Ghafourifard, M. (2018). Nurse's perceptions of organisational barriers to delivering compassionate care: A qualitative study. *Nursing Ethics, 25*(5), 580–590. https://doi.org/10.1177/0969733016660881

Walker, M. U. (1993a). Reply to scofield. *Hastings Center Report, 23*(5), 45.

Walker, M. U. (1993b). Keeping moral space open: New images of ethics consulting. *The Hastings Center Report, 23*(2), 33–40. https://doi.org/10.2307/3562818

Wilson, A. H. (2017). *Mission statements. Encyclopedia of local history* (3rd ed.). Rowman & Littlefield.

Chapter 12
Social Justice, Structural Disparities and Nursing Responsibilities

Pamela Grace, Aimee Milliken, and John Welch

Abstract In this chapter we present an overview of the ways in which unjust social structures and institutions contribute to long and short term poor health outcomes in individuals and groups of individuals. Different theories of justice are briefly explored and highlighted for their potential to remediate those injustices that matter most to health and to the ability to live a minimally decent life. The implications of these theories for nurse moral agency are outlined. We make the case that identifying injustices contributing to poor health for our populations of immediate concern is a professional responsibility of all nurses, although the level at which they are addressed will depend on the level of nurse capacity and perhaps level of nurse education achieved. Finally, we discuss the issue of structural disadvantage as a global issue and propose a range of strategies for nurses to use from the local to the global.

12.1 Introduction

Current events have reminded us how important it is for all nurses to be aware that longstanding socioeconomic and racial disparities affect the health of many of those for whom we provide care. As the largest cohort of healthcare providers in almost all countries we could have power to identify and work towards the remedy of injustices, especially those that affect health which is, perhaps arguably, most of them. We see the results of injustices firsthand or hear the stories of our structurally/systematically disadvantaged patients and their families when we take time

---

P. Grace (✉)
William F. Connell School of Nursing, Boston College, Newton, MA, USA
e-mail: Gracepa@bc.edu

A. Milliken
William F. Connell School of Nursing, Boston College, Chestnut Hill, MA, USA
e-mail: aimee.milliken@bc.edu

J. Welch
Boston Children's Hospital, Health, Boston, MA, USA

Partners in Health, Boston, MA, USA

© The Author(s), under exclusive license to Springer Nature B.V. 2022
P. Grace and A. Milliken (Eds.), *Clinical Ethics Handbook for Nurses*, The International Library of Bioethics 93,
https://doi.org/10.1007/978-94-024-2155-2_12

to listen carefully. However as members of a profession we have been inconsistent in amalgamating and using our power to influence change. There are many reasons for paucity of action related to injustice. Structural injustices are notoriously difficult to address by individuals working alone. Anecdotally, from years of practice and teaching, busy nurses argue they do not have time to address issues outside of their immediate practice area. There are questions about how broadly any activism should go. Are we responsible for addressing injustices generally? One of us has argued elsewhere (Grace, 2001) that while some are prepared to address social injustices at a policy level, we are at least responsible for adding our voices and advocating in what ways we are capable for those whose problems are visible in our practice. If we do not do this then we are failing to work towards providing good care for our patients because the root causes of their problems are not addressed and we are essentially only—metaphorically speaking—'binding their wounds so they can go out into battle again'. Understanding our professional responsibilities related to identifying and addressing injustices and developing our moral agency to overcome obstacles to action, facilitates effective collaborations. Such collaborations are necessary for the conception and institution of good healthcare and just social policies; those that benefit all in society and that can especially address the health of those with disparities of various sorts. For bedside nurses this may mean taking small steps such as bringing stories to the attention of those who can use them to influence policies. A US example of this would be that a nurse in a unit that cares for patients with vascular problems, recognizes that many of his diabetic patients end up with limb amputations as a result of poor to no primary preventive care and raises this issue with unit leadership and with the policy leaders in his professional organization or association.

Disparities in health and in healthcare are indisputably injustices. Caught at the frontlines of the COVID-19 pandemic, nurses' own history as subjects of various injustices has been highlighted by the current situation. They have been asked to care for burgeoning numbers of those suffering from the highly infectious coronavirus, often with inadequate personal protective equipment. Some have been exposed to unnecessary risk by lack of administrative foresight at institutional and societal levels. They have worried about putting their own families at risk. Some of these problems were exacerbated in the US at least by chronic defunding of public health nationally and locally.

Additionally, the current prevalent practice in the US and elsewhere of outsourcing the manufacture of healthcare supplies to other countries has been revealed as resulting in complex and intricate problems that in spite of warnings from public health experts were not anticipated (Choi, Rogers & Vakil, 2020; Francis, 2020). All of this is to say that nurses cannot distance themselves from socio-political problems. Political processes affect every part of nursing practice as well as affecting our own wellbeing. We need to learn how to involve ourselves. The type of involvement we engage in will of course differ based on type and location of practice and educational preparation. At their most basic, nurses' actions can bring attention to the stories of the people they see in practice and how policies and social environment have worked against them having a 'minimally decent life' (Powers & Faden, 2006) as discussed in more detail later. Collectively, they can bring pressure to bear on policy makers and others to initiate change. They can also educate the public and stimulate their engagement in change. Health policies at all levels affect those for whom nurses care, thus among our responsibilities is that of educating ourselves about the health policymaking environment (Loversidge & Zurmehly, 2019).

In this chapter we briefly outline different perspectives and definitions of social justice. We take health and healthcare as human rights' issues, thus issues of social justice, and exemplify what we mean by this. Many injustices that accrue or develop in groups and populations are structural in nature. Structural injustices are those that occur because of the way a society constructs and maintains its social and economic institutions (e.g., government, schools, healthcare, banks and so on). Structural injustices are those that enable some individuals or groups to have access to many more resources than others and hinder some from engaging in the process of determining the nature of, and rules for communal living. Structural injustices can also be imposed by one society upon another in which the dominant society has the means of influence (Alfredson, 2018). Finally we offer some strategies for nurses to use in identifying and addressing injustices as they occur at different levels.

12.2 Perspectives on Social Justice

Social justice is a relatively new concept that emerged around the same time as the industrial revolution (1750–1830) and the associated radical widening of the gap between the well off and the poor. While aspects of modern ideas of social justice are visible in the writings of ancient and medieval philosophers, the idea that every human being ought to have the same sorts of opportunities to benefit from living in a society as everyone else is relatively recent (Jackson, 2005). The moral foundation, or the 'why' we need theories of social justice varies among theorists. Some like John Rawls (1971) build their theories on Immanuel Kant's arguments that each person because they are human and have the (potential) ability to reason logically must be treated with respect and not used exclusively as a means to someone else's benefit. This idea is discussed in more detail in Chapter 3. Theological arguments derive their force from the idea that the nature of human beings derives from the character of a loving and wise God, thus we should treat others as we would want to be treated (Cherry, 2009). Secular arguments revolve around the idea that all human beings have interests in living a 'minimally decent' life and in not having their interests overridden by the interests of those holding more power.

One of the problems with discussing issues of *social justice* is that there are different theories of what the concept means and how it could be actualized as discussed shortly. Roughly, social justice means that people would equally share the benefits and burdens of living in a society. This concept is of course inextricably related to the idea of justice. Justice is historically about treating people as they deserve to be treated, and offers explanations about why they deserve to be treated a certain way. For example in an education setting a student who works hard and knows the material deserves a good grade. A person whose property has been stolen deserves to have it restored. A just society sets out guidelines via a system of justice—a legal system for what is unfair, what can be claimed against others and how problems can be adjudicated. Social justice more particularly is about how the benefits and burdens of societal living are distributed, reinforced and redistributed fairly. Sometimes social justice is also called 'justice as fairness'. There are two major concerns associated with equating social justice with justice as fairness (distributive justice). Not all theories of social justice account for the aftermath of long term injustices—such as slavery, discrimination, or poverty. Thus, some people need much more assistance and empowerment before they can make use of opportunities, even so-called equal opportunities. This is the fundamental problem with equating equality (treating everyone as a placeholder for everyone else) and equity—the idea that some need extra help to get them to the place where they can be successful. A second problem is that we live in an increasingly Global world. Even if we could secure just systems and arrangements within a society this would be insufficient in dealings across societies (Jackson, 2005).

Social justice as a global or societal ideal is unattainable for many reasons, as noted by Powers and Faden (2006) among others. Reasons include: the complexity of human contexts and relationships, the varying characteristics and needs among human beings, difficulties determining what constitutes equality when types of needs, and individual capacities and talents vary greatly (Grace & Willis, 2012). Additionally, contemporary studies in cognitive and moral psychology have highlighted some of the unexpected ways the human mind works (Doris et al., 2010). There is evidence of predispositions in some human beings to seek advantage. Mussel and Hewig (2019) discuss one of these predispositions that they term a 'greed' trait. The greed trait evident in some people "predicts selfish economic decisions that come at the expense of others in a resource dilemma" (p. 1). So how is the problem of social justice to be solved? Power and Faden (2006) have provided a framework for looking at the problem of socially derived injustices that obstruct health and healthcare access that does not rely on the idea of striving to achieve social justice more generally, given the aforementioned challenges with this goal. Before discussing their ideas in more depth, a brief look at why theories of social justice do not provide clear guidance to nurses and other healthcare clinicians may be helpful.

12.2.1 Ancient to Contemporary Theories of Justice

The ancient Greeks such as Plato and Aristotle were concerned with Justice as a characteristic of people that could be cultivated. Aristotle made a "distinction between distributive and corrective justice" (Jackson, 2005, p. 360). *Distributive* justice was concerned with ensuring that the meritorious received what they deserved because of their efforts in the society and was more political than material in focus – about involvement and positions in political institutions. However, *commutative* justice was about resolving harms caused to a person by another person.

Not until around the mid-eighteenth century, for reasons given earlier related to movements of society towards large commercial enterprises did philosophers and social reformers become concerned with the plight of the poor (Stedman Jones, 2004). Attitudes began to reflect a shift in ideas from thinking the poor are an inevitable subset of society, in some ways not like everyone else—thus dehumanized, to ideas that no-one deserved to be poor. Indeed, there was growing recognition that the actions of some within society perpetuated the impoverishment of others. The problem of distribution was seen as bounded by the borders of a particular nation or state, to be resolved within that state. Each citizen was to be considered of equal consideration and a placeholder for every other person. How to go about determining what are fair distributions of the burdens and benefits of societal living, however, is very difficult.

12.2.1.1 John Rawls Theory of Justice as Fairness

Rawls (1971), a political philosopher, developed an in-depth philosophical theory of justice. "Philosophical theories of justice try to show what are or would be sound justifications for the rules of distribution" (Grace, 2018, p. 25). The idea is to conceptualize which social institutions would result in fair distributions of goods such as "education, food, shelter, and healthcare" (p. 25). What Rawls does is use a hypothetical strategy. His theory is complex and cannot be explained in depth here. Importantly though he starts from the assumption, following Kant as noted earlier, that the nature of persons is that they are primarily rational beings, capable of making moral rules for themselves. Thus persons who are placed in an ideal position—he calls this the *original position* (Rawls, 1971, p. 12) or the *veil of ignorance*—not knowing what their particular talents, assets and place in society will be, would construct the sorts of institutions that are most fair to all the least and the most well off (Rawls, 1971). He theorized that people in this imaginary situation would derive two principles for governing how the institutions function. "First: each person is to have an equal right to the most extensive liberty compatible with a similar liberty for others. Second: social and economic inequalities are to be arranged such that they are both (a) reasonably expected to be to everyone's advantage and (b) attached to positions and offices open to all" (Rawls, 1971, p. 60). An important point is that if there are differences in benefits to persons these would go to the least well off. In healthcare settings justice as fairness has been used as an important principle especially with regards to allocation of scarce resources but is not without its criticisms. Among the most compelling perhaps from both a cognitive science and feminist perspective is that even if just institutions could be constructed, there would be a continuous jostle by those seeking various sorts of advantages and power. Additionally, a problem is that many root causes of ill health lie in the social environment that worsens the long term health of the least well off. So far, the basis for healthcare professionals to adhere to principles of social justice may seem unattainable. On what can we depend to help us remedy those injustices that exist and interfere with the wellbeing of those disadvantaged by them? Powers and Faden's (2006) work on social justice offers us some ways of looking at these problems that can give rise to remedial strategies. They challenge us to change our focus from the Sisyphean task of trying to achieve social justice to those injustices that matter most in terms of health.

12.2.1.2 Powers and Faden

Powers and Faden (2006) in their book *Social justice: the moral foundations of public health and health policy,* explore the issue of social justice and the disadvantaged. They argue that the pursuit of the ideal of social justice is not necessary and probably not possible for good healthcare and social policies. "Our quest to identify the right public policy for women and children during the dark days of the AIDS epidemic left both of us with a deep conviction that the non-distributive aspects of well-being are essential to evaluating the justice of health policy" (p. viii). They were worried that resources directed to the most 'high risk' pregnant women, in the era before treatment or prevention of transmission were possible, while providing some benefit in terms of screening their infants, might further stigmatize the women who were disproportionately poor women of color. This provoked their exploration of what kind of theory would work to reduce or eliminate identified injustices that lead to poor health.

Their work led them to consider which 'inequalities matter most" (Powers & Faden, 2006, p. 3). They concluded that there are six identifiable essential dimensions of human living that are necessary for living a 'minimally decent life'. These essential dimensions are shared by human beings across cultures and societies. They propose that these essential dimensions are all necessary. Should any one of the dimensions be deficient in some way it will effect a change in the other dimensions (Grace, 2018; Grace & Willis, 2012) and lead to an inability to achieve even a minimally decent life. "Our list contains six core dimensions: health, personal security, reasoning, respect, attachment, and self-determination" (Powers & Faden, 2006, p. 16).

An example of how their theory would allow us as nurses to first identify and then work to remedy injustices leading to poor health is provided by Grace and Willis (2012). Mapping the themes from Willis' qualitative study of 50 men who reported themselves as healing from child abuse (including neglect) against Powers and Faden's assumptions, they found congruence. Interestingly one of the main findings was that healing from child abuse is a long and arduous road for those who do actually find resolution. Many of course do not heal. In brief, child abuse has long term effects on mental and physical health. It leads to hypervigilance as the ability to trust and sense of security is lost. Reasoning is distorted as the interpretation of the intentions of others becomes skewed by distrust. The ability to respect one's self and others is diminished as one has experienced chronic denigration this also leads to loss of ability to attach to others emotionally. "Finally, self-determination is compromised because the person strives to determine what the best choices are under seriously compromised perceptions of what is possible or desirable (a moral agency problem). Survivors are challenged to achieve a sense of self when in the past they have been treated as merely an object by the abuser" (Grace & Willis, 2012, p. 205).

Powers and Faden, then, provide a useful way for nurses to identify injustices that affect the wellbeing of their populations and work to remedy those. They provide a lens for the advocacy actions of nurses.

12.3 Health and Healthcare as Human Rights' Issues: Disparities and Nursing Advocacy

Fundamentally, health and healthcare are human rights issues, and as such are core concerns within nursing ethics. While access to care is often framed as a policy-level issue, it is also an issue concerning the capacity for healthcare professionals, and nurses in particular, to adhere to their codes of ethics. In much of the world, and especially in the United States where healthcare is privatized, nurses operate in a system where wealth and power are determinants of access to care. As such, it is often difficult for nurses to meet our professional aims of ensuring individual and social good. Moreover, nurses in the United States are often faced with patients who are suffering needless severe effects from poor access to primary care. We also know that a (Global) history steeped in slavery, colonialism, systematic oppression, and extraction of natural resources has driven deep health inequities in the world's poorest countries (Mukherjee, 2018). Lack of access to healthcare is not just about economics and how well the system is integrated to ensure a focus is on promoting and protecting health as well as treating disease. It is also about lack of health literacy, distrust of healthcare providers, untrustworthiness of healthcare providers, scarcity of resources and especially problems of structural injustices. Colonial systems were not only not interested in the health of indigenous people, they were systematically dehumanized (Mukherjee, 2018) and suffered horrendous conditions. One example of this is the forced separation of children of indigenous people in a variety of countries for the ostensible purpose of 'civilizing' them (Williams, 2018). Societal structures which perpetuate suffering have interests in keeping their actions and the results of their actions hidden. Thus one basic role for nurses related to social justice is to work towards raising consciousness and bearing witness (Djkovich et al., 2019).

Nursing's professional aims commit us to considering healthcare a human right; this is the fundamental social "good" we aim towards. The American Nurses Association's Code of Ethics (2015) serves as the normative, non-negotiable standard set forth by the nursing profession in the United States (US). This document establishes nurses as advocates (Provision 3) and endorses health as a human right (Provision 8). This perspective has been reiterated by the United Nations General Assembly (2015) which recently set a Sustainable Development Goal of Universal Health Coverage (UHC) (United Nations, 2015). Despite what we know about systematic injustices, and despite efforts to bring such injustices to light, we continue to fail to address the root causes of ill health as lying in such inequities.

12.3.1 Defining Health and Healthcare

Taking the position that healthcare is a fundamental human right leads to more questions than it perhaps answers, however it is a starting point. Nurses have a "persisting commitment both to the welfare of the sick, injured, and vulnerable in society and to social justice. Nurses act to change those aspects of social structures that detract from health and well-being" (American Nurses Association, 2015, p. vii). This is not an easy charge, but it is one we have promised to take on. In part, this requires a definition of what we mean by both health and healthcare.

12.3.1.1 Health

In chapter 1 we discussed the concept of health in some detail and provided a working definition of nursing's perspective on health. As a reminder, we use Willis et al (2008) definition whereby health is seen as a multifaceted-concept that is signified by sense of integrity or wholeness regardless of physical limitations or disease processes, or trajectory towards death. Thus health is in a large part a subjective concept for cognitively intact persons who can articulate their values, desires and preferences. What constitutes 'health' for persons who have lost or never had sufficient reasoning capacity may well be more of an objective evaluation that considers both evidence of suffering and of enjoyment in light of an understanding of the person's usual physical and emotional patterns.

What is also important, in any discussion about social justice and health equity, is to consider what this means at the family, community, and population levels. Effective person-level interventions to achieve health equity tend to have community- or population-level impacts. For example, it was found that effective treatment of individuals with multidrug resistant tuberculosis in poverty-stricken Haiti required more than just medication administration to the patients. Community-level interventions like improved access to safe drinking water, concrete (rather than dirt) floors, and tin (rather than leaking, thatched) roofs are also required (Farmer, 1999). Health, therefore, cannot be achieved on an individual level without an evaluation of and interventions aimed to support population health. The health of a population and an equitable approach to achieving it has inextricable links to economic justice and racial justice, such that effective health interventions are found at the intersection of all three of these things. Delivery of such interventions are considered healthcare.

12.3.1.2 Healthcare as a Human Right

Healthcare can best be defined as a system of goods and services aimed at preventing illness in, and protecting, promoting and restoring the health of, a population. The provision of healthcare varies among countries, some are organized as national entities with integrated services and some, like that of the US are series of unconnected services, what Elhauge (2010) has called 'fragmented' and which many have critiqued as unethical and unjust. Dernier (2005) persuasively notes that to assert healthcare as a human right entails meeting four criteria:

1. A "collective moral obligation, that is, an obligation on the part of society to ensure that everyone has access to some level of healthcare services" (p. 24) exists.
2. The obligation is morally binding and should take precedence in societal debates especially when considering scarce resources. Utilitarian arguments (the greatest good for the greatest number) do not supersede the need to provide healthcare to individuals.
3. "a basic right to healthcare implies that access to healthcare is owed to those who have the right" (p. 25)
4. All human beings within the scope of the society have the right simply because they are human beings.

The implications of these criteria include that everyone, regardless of their legal status in a country has access to the right to healthcare. This is a collective social responsibility (Dwyer, 2004). A conversation about health as a human right cannot stop with achieving universal health coverage. Building equitable health delivery systems will end the cycle of fragile health systems, mistrust of malfunctioning healthcare delivery, and poor health outcomes. Nurses have an important role to play in identifying and addressing injustices from the level of the individual to the global level as discussed shortly. In our codes of ethics and historical writings nurses have been powerful advocates for the marginalized and we are needed more than ever to advocate for just health policies and practices (Fowler, 2017). It might be argued that some injustices are too widespread and entrenched for us to effect change. Nevertheless, we live in a globalized world as has become starkly evidenced by recent events, not only do we have a professional responsibility to inform ourselves, we have a personal responsibility to understand the fragility of life and life circumstances. As Emily Friedman (1997) noted, any of us at any time could find ourselves looking over the 'abyss'.

12.4 Structural Injustice and Health Disparities

12.4.1 Structural Injustices Local and Global

As established in discussing the historical perspectives of social justice above, interest in the subject piqued as the gap between rich and poor became a chasm that could no longer be ignored. This divide, however, and the suffering of the world's poor are not the inescapable fates of societal evolution. Social suffering can find its origins in society, the decisions of the powerful, and attempts to maintain power and influence. That is, injustice is a direct result of the actions or inactions of humans. Since it is the responsibility of nurses to ease suffering, it should be of particular interest to nurses to understand these injustices and their root causes.

The injustices of the world, which perpetuate health inequity and poor health outcomes, are not casual, intermittent occurrences. Rather, they are the direct effects of historical systems like colonialism and slavery, the legacies of which maintain marginalization of entire populations—they are structural in nature, deeply embedded in the political, societal, and economic processes. The *outcome* of these structural injustices may include ongoing suffering, misery, or death and is therefore violent. The term structural violence is sometimes used to describe systemic marginalizations that results in devastating outcomes.

This structural violence is nearly always perpetrated against minorities and is based on race, ethnicity, religion, gender identity, sexual orientation, economic status, or social class and occurs across many sectors from healthcare, education, governmental representation, and economic mobility. Intersectionality refers to the compounding of structural violence against individuals who identify with multiple marginalized groups. For example, in the United States, trans women of color suffer from structural violence in far greater proportions than any one group individually (Forestiere, 2020). A report by the Harvard Civil Rights-Civil Liberties Law Review notes these individuals have unemployment rates four times the general population, experience homelessness at a rate of 41%, and are disproportionately at risk for violent attacks. In the US, there are few federal or state laws that protect this population and, in fact, some state laws allow perpetuation of violence with little to no protection of the victim (Forestiere, 2020) and efforts are underway to further strip legal protections from this group. It is via the combination of being pushed to the margins and a failure to create appropriate protections and support, that intersectionality deepens the injustices many patients experience. The intersections of marginalization are not just a US problem, however. Around the world, colonial tendencies and the legacy of slavery have amplified punishing neoliberal economics—policies rooted in laws of supply and demand that seek to privatize social support provision like healthcare—such that impoverished countries are forced to allow "invisible" market forces to drive access to and financing of healthcare (Mukherjee, 2018). These policies collide with centuries of untamed infectious diseases, disproportionate maternal and child mortality, extraction and export of natural resources, external interventionism, and global indifference. The intersectionality of geography, history, and impoverishment can be exponentially devastating in terms of life expectancy.

It is essential for good practice that nurses understand the complex and deeply ingrained structural injustices that impact the lives of the patients and communities they serve. Knowledge of the roots of injustice and the implications of intersectionality on patient outcomes are necessary if we are to serve patients well both in the moment and in envisioning social and policy changes. Mitigation of the effects of injustice on a patient's health should be a priority for nursing practice. Understanding the role of environment and circumstance in a patient's suffering, provides the bases for advocating for systematic and structural change that will prevent inequitable health outcomes.

12.4.2 COVID-19 and Injustices

The COVID-19 pandemic of 2020 has starkly highlighted the impact that historic and structural injustices continue to have on communities of color, persons with disabilities, and other vulnerable populations. As a result of structural racism and economic inequity, these groups are more vulnerable to the virus and less able to practice prevention measures, such as remote work and social distancing (Berlinger et al., 2020; Manchada et al., 2020). Additionally, many essential workers belong to communities of color, and due to the nature of their work face an increase in exposure to the virus. In addition, those with comorbidities and chronic conditions like hypertension, pulmonary disease, and diabetes are more severely impacted by the virus. These chronic conditions disproportionately impact communities of color in the US (Betancourt, 2020). As such, the devastating impacts of COVID-19 have overwhelmed these communities (Center for Disease Control & Prevention, 2021). As of February 2021, in the United States, Black people have died at 1.5 times the rate of white people (The Atlantic Monthly Group, 2021).

12.4.2.1 Crisis Standards of Care

These inequities were perpetuated in early attempts at developing Crisis Standards of Care guidelines (Manchada et al., 2020; Milliken et al., 2020). Crisis Standards of Care guidelines aim to provide guidance for allocating resources in the event that the demand outstrips supply (Gostin & Hanfling, 2009). In the Spring of 2020, after the initial pandemic surges in China and Italy, there was growing anxiety that available critical care resources, including beds and ventilators, would be insufficient to meet the demand created by the spread of the virus in the US. States across the country attempted to develop triage mechanisms to aid clinicians in deciding how to allocate these scarce resources. However, many of the mechanisms developed relied on assessments of long-term prognosis which is both difficult to objectively assess (and therefore subject to bias) and may be impacted by the presence of comorbidities that disproportionately impact communities of color and/or the presence of disabilities. As such, there was concern that these algorithms may serve to perpetuate racial injustices and ableism, further disadvantaging these already vulnerable populations. As of this writing, many states have adjusted their Crisis Standards of Care algorithms to attempt to mitigate these issues, however ethical challenges remain (Milliken et al., 2020).

12.4.2.2 Vaccination

The rapid development, testing, and emergency use authorization of multiple novel COVID-19 vaccines was a major scientific feat. However, as vaccine distribution began, additional concerns about injustice and structural inequity came to the fore. Long standing and well-founded mistrust in the healthcare system, brought on by exploitation and injustices such as but not exclusive to, the Tuskegee experiment (referenced elsewhere in this book) resulted in vaccine hesitancy, particularly in the Black community (Berlinger et al., 2021). This hesitancy has thus far created disparities in the proportion of the Black population that has been vaccinated as compared to the white population (KHN et al., 2021).

In addition to vaccine hesitancy, access to vaccines has been challenging. While different areas of the world have used different approaches, there remains much confusion about which segments of the population fall into which "priority groups." There have been concerning examples of "cutting the line," where the rich and privileged have gained access to vaccination ahead of frontline workers and the medically vulnerable. Additionally, people with disabilities have not consistently been considered in the first wave of priority groups, raising concerns about discrimination on the basis of disability (Contrera, 2021).

12.4.3 Common Injustices Recognizable By Nurses

Among the injustices that fall within the everyday practice arena of nurses but that require mindfulness, vigilance and trust-building to uncover and address are such things: as human trafficking, the plight of undocumented immigrants and their children, poor care related to implicit and unreflected upon biases, inadequate staffing in eldercare or nursing home facilities, elder neglect and abuse, and the dehumanizing attitudes of clinicians from all disciplines towards those they see as 'other'. It is beyond the ability of this chapter to discuss each in detail however next we offer some strategies for nurses to use in addressing local issues and in collaboration with others to address systematic and structural injustices and at the end of the chapter we provide some examples for thought and group discussion.

12.5 Strategies for Nursing: Identifying and Addressing Injustices

We have described how nurses have an important role in identifying and addressing injustices. As with other issues of injustice, nurses have professional responsibilities to attune themselves to these emerging issues and work to address them. While the nurse at the bedside may not be involved in developing Crisis Standards of Care or vaccine allocation schemes, they will be impacted by them. Nurses can take an active role by writing to their local governments, responding when requests for public comment are raised, and by helping to educate their patients and the public about issues like vaccination. This does mean keeping up-to-date both with evidence and emerging evidence as well as understanding, for example sources of mistrust related to vaccine hesitancy. Building trust is essential to changing minds when this is essential to the health of the other or the patient (Gaylord, 2018).

12.5.1 Nurses' Contributions to Just Environments and Policies

12.5.1.1 Professional Advocacy

There are many definitions of advocacy in the nursing literature, on one definition nurses are responsible for addressing patient rights infringements, on another advocacy is about speaking up when a patient is not getting what he or she needs whether or not that person knows that they are not getting optimal care. As Lisa Newton (1988) argues, a moral expectation of a professional is that they "respond…if practices in his field are inadequate … if the client is unhappy; if he is happy but … the state of the art is not adequate to his real needs" (p. 49). Another definition is related to the nurse-patient relationship, which is limited in its application to remedying injustices for populations.

Additionally, nursing scholars have undertaken concept analyses of advocacy to try to become clearer about its meaning in nursing practice. These analyses include research on nurses perspectives. Such concept analyses reveal the many ways which nurses think of advocacy but cannot tell us how nurses ought to think of advocacy. To derive a moral obligation from the ways nurses think is to commit the philosophical fallacy of deriving fact from value. That is, the fact that nurses think advocacy means a certain thing does entail that they ought to act in accord with this perspective. To provide a moral foundation for action requires a philosophical argument about why nursing exists, what services the profession provides, the nature of its implicit contract with the society and ways in which the service 'good' is furthered as discussed earlier.

A broader perspective on advocacy that includes obligations to address the root causes of certain problems, especially for the most disadvantaged is that of professional advocacy. Grace (1998, 2001) undertook to clarify the notion of 'Advocacy', as it relates to nurses and nursing, both because of varying definitions, some of which seem to require nurses to take risks for their jobs and/or relationships with colleagues and because definitions that existed did not adequately account for obligations to work towards rectifying broader social injustices. She traced the idea of advocacy back to its origins in the law and highlights why this adversarial view of arguing for the rights of one person against the claims of another cannot work for nurses as we do not have only one person for whom we are responsible. Instead, the notion of Professional Advocacy is more apt. Professional advocacy (Grace, 2001).

> consists in those actions taken to further the goals of the profession with regard to 'health'. It is an equivalent notion to professional role in that the actions of nurses while assuming a nursing role are directed at fulfilling the goals of the profession. These role actions have a moral component in that they are directed towards provision of a 'good'. Thus, they can be criticized to the extent that they are, or are not, honestly focused on achieving that good. So advocacy is an obligation of professional role but not solely in the narrow sense of speaking up for, or acting on behalf of, individuals or groups in specific situations.This is because necessarily included in the nurse's moral decision-making is consideration of which actions will be most supportive of the profession's goals. (p. 160)

Thus advocacy includes actions taken to address root causes of problems and our ethical obligations include advocating for a system that will provide the best care to the most people, including preventive care as well as clearly articulating what are the needs of individuals in our immediate care environment when these are not being heard or anticipated.

The origins of policies from local to national need to be examined and critiqued, along with who has vested interests, and who stands to benefit the most. This is important as Laperriere (2008) explains, because we tend not to look to expose "the powerful sources behind a social problem" (p. 393).

12.6 Chapter Summary

Nurses have an obligation, founded in the goals of our profession, to work towards addressing sources of injustice that impact the populations we serve. Frameworks, such as those offered by Powers and Faden (2006), can aid in identifying key areas where intervention can be most impactful. Though individual nurses may not be situated to ameliorate sources of structural inequity on their own, they are optimally positioned to identify these issues at the point of care and raise attention to them.

12.7 Book Summary

We developed the book to serve as a resource for point-of-care nurses practicing in a variety of clinical settings. We wanted the book to be both deeply informative and practical. Its contents, it is hoped, will also be helpful for others working in the necessarily interdisciplinary settings of contemporary healthcare. Understanding the reason-for-being of modern healthcare as that of providing a human good, rather than economic gain is foundational to grasping one's responsibility to individuals and the society. For nurses, ethical care is equivalent to good care.

However the complexity of contemporary healthcare environments can work against the provision of good care in many ways, regardless of country of practice, as discussed throughout this book. Thus developing the knowledge, characteristics, skills, and tools facilitative of moral agency especially in the face of practice barriers fortifies good practice and facilitates engaging in preventive ethics. Emerging evidence reveals moral agency can serve as an antidote, or mitigating factor, for moral distress (Lee et al., 2020; Traudt et al, 2016). Thus, we emphasized the importance of context, communication and collaboration in providing optimal care to patients and/or human subjects and in advocating for local, regional and even national initiatives that permit improved access to appropriate care, especially for the least advantaged.

References

Alfredson, G. (2018). Structural injustice. *World Encyclopedia of Law.* Accessed February 9, 2021 from: https://lawin.org/structural-injustice/

American Nurses Association. (2015). *Code of Ethics for Nurses.* http://www.nursingworld.org/DocumentVault/Ethics_1/Code-of-Ethics-for-Nurses.html

Berlinger, N., Wynia, M., Powell, T., Hester, D. M., Milliken, A., Fabi, R., & Jenks, N. P. (2020). *Ethical Framework for Health Care Institutions Responding to Novel Coronavirus SARS-CoV-2 (COVID-19) Guidelines for Institutional Ethics Services Responding to Managing Uncertainty, Safeguarding Communities, Guiding Practice* (Vol. 2). https://www.thehastingscenter.org/ethicalframeworkcovid19/

Berlinger, N., Wynia, M., Powell, T., Milliken, A., Khatri, P., Marouf, F., & Crane, J. (2021). *Ethical challenges in the middle tier of COVID-19 vaccine allocation: Guidance for organizational decision-making.* https://www.thehastingscenter.org/ethicalframeworkcovid19/

Betancourt, J. (2020). Communities of color devastated by COVID-19: Shifting the narrative. Retrieved February 13, 2021, from Harvard Health Blog website: https://www.health.harvard.edu/blog/communities-of-color-devastated-by-covid-19-shifting-the-narrative-2020102221201

Center for Disease Control and Prevention. (2021). Health Equity Considerations and Racial and Ethnic Minority Groups. Retrieved from COVID-19 website: https://www.cdc.gov/coronavirus/2019-ncov/community/health-equity/race-ethnicity.html

Cherry, M. J. (2009). Religion without God, Social justice without Christian charity, and other dimensions of the culture wars. *Christian bioethics: Non-Ecumenical Studies in Medical Morality, 15*(3), 277–299. https://doi.org/10.1093/cb/cbp020

Choi, T. Y., Rogers, D., & Vakil, B. (2020). Coronavirus is a wake-up call for supply chain management. *Harvard Business Review.* Accessed February 8th, 2021 from: https://hbr.org/2020/03/coronavirus-is-a-wake-up-call-for-supply-chain-management

Contrera, J. (2021). People with disabilities desperately need the vaccine. But states disagree on when they'll get it. The Washington Post. Retrieved from https://www.washingtonpost.com/dc-md-va/2021/01/13/disabled-coronavirus-vaccine-states/

Dernier, Y. (2005). On personal responsibility and the human right to healthcare. *Cambridge Quarterly of Healthcare Ethics, 14*(2), 224–234.

Djkowich, M., Ceci, C., & Petrovskaya, O. (2019). Bearing witness in nursing practice: More than a moral obligation?. *Nursing Philosophy, 20*(1), e12232.

Doris, J. M. & The Moral Psychology Research Group. (2010). The moral psychology handbook. Oxford University Press.

Dwyer, J. (2004). Illegal immigrants, health care, and social responsibility. *Hastings Center Report, 34*(5), 34–41.

Elhauge, E. (2010). *The fragmentation of the U.S. healthcare system: Causes and solutions*. Oxford University Press.

Farmer, P. (1999). Pathologies of power: rethinking health and human rights. *American Journal of Public Health, 89*(10), 1486–1496.

Francis, J. R. (2020). COVID-19: Implications for supply chain management. *Frontiers of Health Services Management, 37*(1), 33–38. https://doi.org/10.1097/HAP.0000000000000092

Forestiere, A. (2020). America's War on Black Trans Women. Harvard Civil Rights – Civil Liberties Law Review, Sept 23. Retrieved March 2021 from: https://harvardcrcl.org/americas-war-on-black-trans-women/

Fowler, M. D. (2017). Why the history of nursing ethics matters. *Nursing Ethics, 24*(3), 292–304.

Friedman, E. (1997). Managed care, rationing, and quality: A tangled relationship. *Health Affairs, 16*(3), 174–182.

Gaylord, N. (2018). Nursing ethics and advanced practice: Children and adolescents. In P. J. Grace (Ed.), Nursing ethics and professional responsibility in advanced practice (3rd ed.) (pp. 237–257). Jones & Bartlett.

Grace, P. J. (1998). A philosophical analysis of the concept 'advocacy': Implications for professional-patient relationships (Unpublished Dissertation). University of Tennessee-Knoxville, TN. http://proquest.umi.com. Publication No. AAT9923287, Proquest Document ID No. 734421751.

Grace, P. J. (2001). Professional advocacy : widening the scope of accountability. Nursing Philosophy, 2, 151–162. https://doi.org/10.1046/j.1466-769X.2001.00048.x

Grace, P. J. (2018). Nursing ethics and professional responsibility in advanced practice (3rd ed.). Jones & Bartlett Learning.

Grace, P. J., & Willis, D. G. (2012). Nursing Responsibilities and Social Justice: An Analysis in Support of Disciplinary Goals. *Nursing Outlook, 60*(4), 198–207.

Gostin, L. O., & Hanfling, D. (2009). National preparedness for a catastrophic emergency: Crisis standards of care. *JAMA—Journal of the American Medical Association, 302*(21), 2365–2366. https://doi.org/10.1001/jama.2009.1780

Jackson, B. (2005). The conceptual history of social justice. *Political Studies Review, 3*(3), 356–373.

Kaiser Health News (2021). Black Americans are getting vaccinated at lower rates than white Americans (Reported by Hannah Recht and Lauren Weber, January 17th). Retrieved from https://khn.org/news/article/black-americans-are-getting-vaccinated-at-lower-rates-than-white-americans/

Laperriere, H. N. (2008). Developing professional autonomy in advanced nursing practice: The critical analysis of sociopolitical variables. *International Journal of Nursing Practice, 14*(5), 391–397. https://doi.org/10.1111/j.1440-172X.2008.00700.x

Lee, S., Robinson, E. M., Grace, P. J., Zollfrank, A., & Jurchak, M. (2020). Developing a moral compass: Themes from the clinical ethics residency for nurses' final essays. *Nursing Ethics, 27*(1), 28–39. https://doi.org/10.1177/0969733019833125

Loversidge, J. & Zurmehly, J. (2019). Evidence-informed health policy. Sigma Theta Tau International. Supplemental materials for Evidence-Informed Health Policy. https://sigma.nursingrepository.org/handle/10755/17098

Manchada, E., Couillard, C., & Sivashanker, K. (2020). Inequity in crisis standards of care. *New England Journal of Medicine, 1–3*,. https://doi.org/10.1056/NEJMp2011359

Milliken, A., Courtwright, A., Grace, P., Eagan-Bengston, E., Visser, M., & Jurchak, M. (2020). Ethics consultations at a major academic medical center: A retrospective. *Longitudinal Analysis. AJOB Empirical Bioethics, 11*(4), 275–286.

Mukherjee, J. (2018). *An introduction to global health delivery: Practice, equity, human rights.* Oxford University Press.

Mussel, P., & Hewig, J. (2019). A neural perspective on when and why trait greed comes at the expense of others. *Scientific Reports, 9*(1), 1–7.

Newton, L. H. (1988). Lawgiving for professional life: Reflections on the place of the professional code. In A. Flores (Ed.), *Professional ideals* (47–56). Wadsworth.
Powers, M., Faden, R. R., & Faden, R. R. (2006). Social justice: the moral foundations of public health and health policy. Oxford University Press.
Rawls, J. (1971). *A theory of justice*. Belknap/Harvard University Press.
Recht, H., & Weber, L. (2021, January 17). Black Americans are getting vaccinated at lower rates than white Americans. Kaiser Health News.
Stedman Jones, G. (2004). *An end to poverty? A historical debate*. Profile Books.
The Atlantic Monthly Group. (2021). The COVID Racial Data Tracker. Retrieved February 13, 2021, from The COVID Tracking Project website: https://covidtracking.com/race
Traudt, T., Liaschenko, J., & Peden-McAlpine, C. (2016). Moral agency, moral Imagination, and moral community: Antidotes to moral distress. *The Journal of clinical ethics, 27*(3), 201–213.
United Nations. (2015). Transforming our world: The 2030 agenda for sustainable development. Retrieved from http://www.un.org/ga/search/view_doc.asp?symbol=A/RES/70/1&Lang=E
Williams, J. H. (2018). Child separations and families divided: America's history of separating children from their parents. *Social Work Research, 42*(3), 141–146. https://doi.org/10.1093/swr/svy021
Willis, D. G., Grace, P. J., & Roy, C. (2008). A central unifying focus for the discipline: Facilitating humanization, meaning, choice, quality of life, and healing in living and dying. *Advances in Nursing Science, 31*(1), E28–E40.

Index

A
Access to care, 178, 181, 193, 243
Advanced care planning, 103–107
Advance directives/Advanced directives, 95, 103–108
Advocacy, 5, 26, 27, 169, 191, 215, 218, 221, 243, 249, 250
Applied ethics, 7, 9, 45, 53
Autonomy, 12, 24, 38, 45–47, 49, 88, 95, 103, 106, 107, 116, 121, 143, 144, 156, 182, 186–188, 190, 214

B
Baby Doe rules, 138
Belmont Report, 47, 213, 214, 218–220
Beneficence, 24, 45–48, 95, 190, 207, 215, 218, 219, 223, 224
Bentham, Jeremy, 44, 48
Best interest, 23, 42, 48, 50, 87, 95, 126, 138, 140–147, 161, 186, 188, 214, 217, 219
Biases, 14, 15, 22, 28, 29, 45, 50, 94, 116, 120, 122, 123, 129, 130, 137, 148, 176–178, 180, 196, 206, 210, 247, 248
Biobanks, 168, 169
Bioethics, 4, 6, 7, 9, 10, 23, 38–41
Biomedical ethics, 39, 40, 129
Biotechnology, 7, 10, 39–41, 53, 207

C
Care ethics, 40, 51
Care redirection, 138, 139
Central unifying focus (CUF), 22, 121
Child abuse, 138, 147, 183, 208, 242

Clinical ethics, 6, 9, 39, 52, 86, 88–91, 93, 97, 106, 118
Clinical ethics consultation. *See* Ethics consultation
Clinical Ethics Residency for Nurses (CERN), 4, 10, 14, 148
Clinical judgment, 4, 26, 50, 51, 148, 186, 191
Codes of ethics, 7, 8, 21, 38, 44, 48, 116, 127, 129, 167, 178, 190, 197, 229, 243, 245
Communication, 5, 10, 12, 16, 26–28, 46, 53, 60–62, 64, 65, 67, 71, 73, 75–78, 80, 81, 83, 93, 94, 97, 101, 103, 116, 126, 145, 176, 191, 193, 228–231, 251
Communication skills, 16, 94
Confidentiality, 47, 91, 164, 165, 170, 183–185, 218
Confucian, 45
Conscience, 8, 121, 124, 126
Conscientious objection, 124, 126
Consequentialism, 42, 44, 207
Countertransference, 187, 197
COVID-19 impact
 emotional, 122, 195
 physical, 36, 195
 psychological, 36, 194, 195
Crisis Standards of Care, 247, 248
Cultural competence, 118–120
Cultural differences, 116, 123, 129
Cultural Engagement model, 118
Cultural factors, 115
Culturally embedded, 116, 117
CURES Act, 182

D

Data sharing, 184
Decision-making frameworks, 41, 50, 52, 96, 98
Declaration of Helsinki, 212, 213
De-escalation, 166, 189–191
Deontology, 42, 44
Dilemma, 7, 23, 38–41, 52, 94, 95, 97, 117, 163, 181, 240
Direct to consumer testing (DTC), 162, 163
Discipline, 5–10, 14, 38–41, 53, 86, 93, 121, 167, 248
Discrimination, 7, 138, 157, 165–167, 170, 180, 240, 248
Disparities, 119, 168, 179, 181, 185, 237, 238, 243, 245, 248

E

Elder abuse, 183
Equipoise, 212, 215
Ethical awareness, 15, 22–24, 29, 154
Ethical conflict, 97, 100, 101, 106
Ethical decision-making, 15, 42, 50–53, 106, 124, 148, 186
Ethical principles, 8, 16, 24, 42, 45, 46, 53, 86, 88, 95, 96, 106, 213, 214, 229
Ethical sensitivity, 24, 25
Ethics, 4, 6, 9, 12, 14, 16, 22, 24, 26, 28, 38, 39, 44, 52, 53, 86, 88–94, 96–99, 101, 103, 106, 116, 117, 127, 141, 147, 148, 161, 164, 165, 207, 210, 211, 215, 216, 218, 222, 224, 230, 233, 234
Ethics consultation, 4, 39, 86, 89–94, 99–101, 106, 118
  ethics consultation approaches, 52
Ethics education, 4, 23, 24, 53, 91, 92, 148
Ethics policies, 92
Eugenics, 159, 166, 170

F

Feminist ethics, 51
FESOR framework, 95
Fidelity, 46, 50

G

Genetic counseling, 159, 162, 164, 167, 168
Genetics, 10, 41, 120, 136, 153–170, 178, 218
Genetic screening, 154, 156, 170

Genetic testing, 142, 147, 154–156, 159–163, 168, 170
  genetic testing types, 159
Genomics, 153, 154, 158, 159, 167, 168, 170
Goals of, 60, 82, 91, 93, 101, 103, 105, 127, 160, 170, 180, 187, 189, 192, 207, 216, 218, 224, 233
  healthcare professions, 8, 12, 21, 45, 48, 60, 159, 250
  nursing, 21, 120

H

Health, 5–7, 9, 11, 12, 16, 21, 37, 39, 42, 48, 49, 51, 53, 60, 86, 91, 98–100, 115–118, 120, 122, 124–126, 131, 144, 154, 160, 162, 163, 165–168, 178–182, 188, 192–194, 196, 198, 208, 228, 237–246, 249, 250
Healthcare, 3–6, 8–12, 14, 16, 24, 27, 28, 36–51, 53, 61, 86, 87, 89–91, 93, 97–99, 101–107, 116, 119, 121–123, 127, 129, 130, 137, 138, 140–146, 149, 153, 155, 158, 162, 166–168, 170, 176–178, 180–185, 187, 193, 195, 196, 207, 211, 214, 218, 219, 224, 227–230, 237–246, 248, 250, 251
Healthcare as a human right, 245
Healthcare ethics committees (HECs), 86–94, 97, 100, 106
Healthcare professions, 5, 6, 8, 9, 21, 22
Health definitions, 5, 6, 244
Health literacy, 243
Historical trauma, 121, 122
History of Medicine, 35
Human Genome Project, 153
Human rights, 46, 47, 103, 130, 140, 166, 209–211, 239, 243–245
Human subjects research. *See* Research
Human Subjects Review Board, 213
Hume, D., 44, 48

I

Implicit bias, 123, 168, 176–178, 196
Informed consent, 47, 127, 156, 158, 159, 161, 162, 164, 169, 170, 184, 188, 209, 212, 216, 218, 222–224, 234
Institutional Review Board (AKA Human Subjects Review Board), 158, 161, 165, 208, 213, 214, 224

Interdisciplinary, 5, 7, 16, 22, 26–29, 53, 60, 71, 92, 96, 102, 142, 228, 229, 231, 232, 250
Interpretation, 128, 158, 163, 242
Involuntary admission, 188
Involuntary treatment, 187

J
Justice, 41, 45, 49–51, 86, 179, 181, 212, 215, 220, 221, 224, 239, 240, 242, 244
Justice as fairness, 46, 49, 215, 220, 240, 241

K
Kant, I., 42, 43, 46, 47, 49, 51, 143, 209, 239, 241

L
Language difficulties, 129. *See also* Communication
Life sustaining treatment (LST), 87, 92, 106, 140
Living will, 103, 104, 107, 108. *See also* Advance directives

M
Managerialism, 12
Mandated reporting, 183
Medical ethics, 6–9, 23, 38, 40
Medical futility, 139, 142
Medically Ineffective Treatments, 139
Mental health, 5, 71, 120, 121, 175–181, 184, 193–198
Microaggression, 121, 129
Mill, J.S., 44, 48
Mindfulness, 177, 178, 196, 211, 248
Miracles (believe in), 125
Moral, 7–9, 14, 23, 24, 27–29, 36, 40–44, 46, 49, 52, 94, 95, 97, 102, 117, 118, 123, 124, 126, 129, 130, 137, 139, 143, 180, 192, 194, 206, 208–210, 214, 228–232, 238–242, 245, 249–251
Moral Absolutism, 116, 117
Moral agency, 4, 13–16, 22, 23, 26, 27, 29, 102, 238, 242, 251
Moral character, 26, 29, 129
Moral communities, 28, 29

Moral distress, 5, 9, 23, 27–29, 61, 136, 137, 146, 180, 192, 194, 208, 210, 230–232, 251
Moral judgment, 25, 26
Moral motivation, 25
Moral philosophy, 7, 9, 22, 39, 41, 87
Moral Relativism, 116
Moral spaces, 228, 230, 231
Moral status, 139, 140
Moral Subjectivism, 116
Moral theory, 41, 42, 44, 45, 47, 51, 206, 214

N
Narrative ethics, 51, 52
Neonatal intensive care, 136
Neonatal intensive care units (NICU), 136–139, 141, 149
Non-maleficence, 24, 45, 47, 140, 161, 229
Nuremberg Code, 211, 212
Nursing advocacy, 243
Nursing education, 23, 183
Nursing ethics, 6, 8, 9, 22, 23, 148, 184, 231, 243
Nursing goals, 24, 41, 102, 120, 131, 224

O
Open Notes, 182
Organizational ethics, 92, 97, 99, 100, 106

P
Parental decision-making, 141, 146
Paternalism, 49
Patient preferences, 104, 105, 125
Patient Self Determination Act (PSDA), 103
Personal behaviors, 67
Philosophers, 7, 27, 39, 41, 42, 44, 46, 86, 239, 241
Philosophical inquiry, 41
Philosophy of medicine, 40
Post-traumatic stress disorder (PTSD), 105, 179, 180
Power structures, 51
Prejudices, 14, 15, 29, 50, 116, 123, 129, 180, 210
Prenatal diagnostic tests, 156, 157
Preventive ethics (PE), 5, 24, 99–101, 106, 147, 230, 251
Primum Non Nocere, 36, 47
Principal investigator in research, 207, 216

Principles, 7, 12, 16, 24, 36, 42, 45–49, 51, 53, 60, 86, 88, 98, 117, 125, 129, 130, 137, 143, 144, 161, 186, 191, 192, 207, 213–216, 218–220, 223, 228, 241
Privacy, 11, 47, 91, 158, 163–165, 170, 183–185, 187, 197, 218
Professional advocacy, 249, 250
Professional ethics, 6, 7, 9, 37, 46
Professional responsibility or Obligation, 14, 15, 22, 25, 40, 53, 88, 106, 121, 154, 163, 164, 227, 238, 245, 248, 250
Professions, 4, 6–9, 14, 22, 37–39, 44, 60, 101, 231
Proxy consent, 212
Public health, 4, 6, 41, 44, 157, 158, 238

Q
Quality of life, 10, 22, 25, 94, 102, 104, 108, 121, 137, 139, 141
Quinlan, Karen Ann, 87

R
Racism, 45, 120, 178, 180, 185, 196, 247
Rawls, J., 49, 239, 241
Reflection on practice, 96, 148
Reflective practice, 28, 29
Religious influences, 11, 124
Research, 4, 9, 22, 24, 37, 39, 40, 47, 51, 67, 88, 90, 91, 93, 97, 102, 103, 136, 141, 142, 145, 153, 158, 161, 164–166, 168–170, 178, 182, 185, 206–209, 211–224, 249
Research definition, 208
Research ethics
   Ethical Principles Guiding Research, 214
   human rights abuses, 210, 211
   therapeutic versus non-therapeutic, 212
Resource allocation, 91, 92, 97
Respect for persons, 143, 207, 214, 216, 218, 223, 224
Rest's Four Components, 24
Restraints, 189, 190, 211
   chemical, 189, 190
   physical, 189, 190

S
SAVI®, 26, 60–62, 64, 67, 71, 78, 80, 81, 83
Scarce resources, 7, 40–42, 86, 97, 241, 245, 247
Secondary trauma (vicarious trauma), 176, 194, 195
Self-reflection, 22, 28, 29, 53, 96, 123, 129, 148, 178, 197
Shared decision-making, 98, 138, 231
Shared trauma, 121, 122
Social determinants, 178, 179, 196
Social justice, 40, 44, 49, 92, 122, 177, 221, 239–245
Spiritual influences, 124
Stereotype, 120, 176, 178, 196
Stigma, 176–178, 184, 193, 194, 196
Structural injustice, 238, 239, 243, 245–248
Structural violence, 246
Summum bonum, 41
SUPPORT study, 103
Surrogate, 47, 48, 87, 90–92, 95, 103–105, 125, 130, 209, 214, 219, 220, 223

T
Team decision-making, 137, 138
Telehealth, 185, 186
Telepsychiatry, 185, 186, 196
Therapeutic use of self, 176, 186, 197
Transference, 187
Trauma-informed care, 191, 192
Tuskegee experiment, 248

U
Utilitarianism, 44, 48
Utility principle, 44

V
Vaccination hesitancy, 248, 249
Values, 4, 5, 10, 11, 13, 14, 22, 24, 25, 28, 30, 42, 44, 45, 47, 48, 52, 53, 86, 91, 94–96, 99, 102, 104, 106, 109, 115–121, 123–125, 130, 131, 137–140, 147, 148, 155, 156, 158–160, 164, 167, 169, 185, 192, 193, 206, 208, 211, 220, 227–229, 231, 244, 249
Veracity, 46, 50, 129, 146
Virtue ethics, 52
Virtues, 40, 43, 45, 129, 130, 148, 185, 217

GPSR Compliance
The European Union's (EU) General Product Safety Regulation (GPSR) is a set of rules that requires consumer products to be safe and our obligations to ensure this.

If you have any concerns about our products, you can contact us on

ProductSafety@springernature.com

In case Publisher is established outside the EU, the EU authorized representative is:

Springer Nature Customer Service Center GmbH
Europaplatz 3
69115 Heidelberg, Germany

www.ingramcontent.com/pod-product-compliance
Ingram Content Group UK Ltd.
Pitfield, Milton Keynes, MK11 3LW, UK
UKHW022152230426
12049UKWH00003BA/51